Growing Older in World Cities

New York, London, Paris, and Tokyo

Victor G. Rodwin and Michael K. Gusmano,

Editors

Vanderbilt University Press

NASHVILLE

© 2006 Vanderbilt University Press
All rights reserved
First Edition 2006

10 09 08 07 06   1 2 3 4 5

Printed on acid-free paper.
Manufactured in the United States of America

Library of Congress Cataloging-in-Publication Data

Growing older in world cities : New York, London, Paris, and Tokyo /
Victor G. Rodwin, and Michael K. Gusmano, editors.— 1st ed.
     p. ; cm.
ISBN 0-8265-1489-8 (cloth : alk. paper)
ISBN 0-8265-1490-1 (pbk. : alk. paper)
     1. Older people—Long-term care. 2. Urban health.
[DNLM: 1. Long-Term Care—London. 2. Long-Term Care—New
York. 3. Long-Term Care—Paris. 4. Long-Term Care—Tokyo.
5. Geriatric Assessment—London. 6. Geriatric Assessment—New
York. 7. Geriatric Assessment—Paris. 8. Geriatric Assessment—
Tokyo. 9. Health Services for the Aged—London. 10. Health Ser-
vices for the Aged—New York. 11. Health Services for the Aged—
Paris. 12. Health Services for the Aged—Tokyo. 13. Socioeconomic
Factors—London. 14. Socioeconomic Factors—New York. 15.
Socioeconomic Factors—Paris. 16. Socioeconomic Factors—Tokyo.
17. Urban Health—London. 18. Urban Health—New York. 19.
Urban Health—Paris. 20. Urban Health—Tokyo.
WT 31 G884 2005]
I. Rodwin, Victor. II. Gusmano, Michael K.
RA564.8.G765 2005
362.198'97—dc22
                              2005005460

To the memory of Manny Tobier
Whose wit and wisdom encouraged this endeavor,
And to our children when they grow older:
May they live in interesting places!

Contents

Figures and Tables

Figures

Tables

Acronyms and Special Terminology

General

IADL	Instrumental activities of daily life
ADL	Activities of daily life
LTC	Long-term care
OECD	Organization for Economic Cooperation and Development
WHO	World Health Organization

France

ACTP	Caretaker allowance (allocation compensatrice pour tierce personne)
AGGIR	An indicator used in France to measure levels of disability among older persons. (Autonomie Gérontologique Groupe Iso-Ressources)
APA	Personal autonomy allowance (allocation personnalisée d'autonomie)
AP-HP	Public Hospital Corporation of Paris (Assistance Publique–Hôpitaux de Paris)
Canicule	Heat wave
CASVP	Center for Social Action for Paris (Centre d'Action Sociale de la Ville de Paris)
CNAMTS	French National Health Insurance Fund for Salaried Workers (Caisse Nationale d'Assurance Maladie des Travailleurs Salariés)
CRAMIF	Regional Health Insurance Fund (Caisse régionale d'assurance maladie d'Ile de France)
CREDES	Centre de Recherche et de Documentation en Economie de la Santé
DASES	Division of Health and Social Affairs for Paris (Direction des Affaires Sociales, de l'Enfance et de la Santé)
DRASS	Regional Office of Health and Social Affairs (Direction Régionale des Affaires Sanitaires et Sociales)
DREES	Division of Research, Studies, Evaluation and Statistics of the Ministry of Health (Direction de la Recherche, des Etudes, de l'Evaluation et des Statistiques)

EHPAD   Institutional long-term care beds
            (établissement d'hébergement pour personnes âgées dépendantes)
HBM   Low cost housing
            (habitation bon marché)
HID   Handicap, Disability, and Dependency Survey
            (Handicaps-Incapacités-Dépendance)
HLM   Public or social housing
            (habitation à loyer modéré)
IAURF   Urban and Regional Planning Agency for Ile-de-France
            (Institut d'Aménagement Urbain de la Région Francilienne)
INSEE   National Institute of Statistics and Economic Studies
            (Institut National de Statistiques et des Etudes Economiques)
OPAH   Program to Renovate Housing
            (Opération Programmée d'Amélioration de l'Habitat)
ORSIF   Regional Health Observatory of Ile-de-France
            (Observatoire Régional de Santé d'Ile de France)
PPIB   Permanent Panel of Insurance Beneficiaries of the CNAMTS
SESI   Division of Statistics, Studies and Information Systems, Ministry
            of Labor and Social Affairs
            (Service des Statistiques, des Etudes, et des Systèmes d'Information,
            Ministère du Travail et des Affaires Sociales)
SSIAD   Home nursing service
            (Services des soins infirmiers à domicile)
ONAC   National Office for Veterans
            (Office National des Anciens Combattants)
PSD   Disability allowance
            (prestation spécifique dépendance)

Tokyo

AGH   Alzheimer Group Home
HFE   Health Facilities for the Elderly
Kaigo
  Hoken   The public, mandatory long-term care insurance system
LTCH   Long-term care hospitals
LTCI   Long-term care health insurance
LTCIP   Long-term care insurance program
MHW   Ministry of Health and Welfare
MHLW   Ministry of Health, Labor and Welfare
SNHA   Special nursing homes for the aged
TMG   Tokyo Metropolitan Government

New York City

ALP	Assisted-Living Program
DFTA	New York City's Department for the Aging
DHMH	New York City's Department of Health and Mental Hygiene
DHHS	Department of Health and Human Services
EISEP	In-Home Services for the Elderly Program
HVS	Housing and Vacancy Survey
LTHHCP	The New York Medicaid Long-Term Home Health Care Program
NORC	Naturally occurring retirement community
NYC	New York City
SPARCS	Statewide Planning and Research Cooperative System

London

DOH	Department of Health
DWP	Department for Work and Pensions
GHS	General Household Survey
GLA	Greater London Authority
GP	General practitioner
HMSO	Her Majesty's Stationary Office
LHO	London Health Observatory
LLTI	Limiting long-term illness
LRC	London Research Centre
NHS	National Health Service
ONS	Office of National Statistics

PART I: INTRODUCTION

1. Growing Older in World Cities: Implications for Health and Long-Term Care Policy

Victor G. Rodwin, Michael K. Gusmano, and Robert N. Butler

Declining birth rates, increasing longevity, and urbanization have created a new challenge for cities: how to respond to an aging population. Although population aging and urbanization are not new concerns for national governments around the world, the consequences of these trends for quality of life in cities have received scant attention. No comparative studies of world cities have examined their health or long-term care systems; nor have comparisons of national systems for the provision of long-term care focused on cities, let alone world cities.

In this book, we investigate how the four largest cities among the wealthiest nations of the world—New York, London, Paris, and Tokyo—are coping with this challenge. Whether these world cities offer a model of what other cities will someday resemble as their populations grow older, or whether they will always be regarded as special cases in their respective nations, they share a host of important characteristics. Within them live the largest numbers of older persons in their nations, and in some neighborhoods the percentage of persons over sixty-five years far exceeds what the census demographers project for their respective nations in 2030. Thus, New York, London, Paris, and Tokyo may serve as laboratories to inquire about the implications of demographic change for health and quality of life, living arrangements and housing, and the provision of long-term care to older persons when they become frail.

New York, London, Paris, and Tokyo exercise a powerful influence in the world beyond their national borders. These "global city-regions" are centers of finance, information, media, arts, education, specialized legal services, and advanced business services, and contribute disproportionate shares to their national economies' gross domestic products.[1] As centers of medical excellence, they set a world standard for care through their medical-training programs, biomedical research institutions, and university hospitals. But are these influential centers prepared to meet the challenge posed by the "revolution of longevity?"[2] How will these world cities accommodate this revolutionary demographic change? Are they prepared to implement the health and social policy innovations that may be required to serve their residents, both old and young? Will they be able to identify the new opportunities that increased longevity may offer? Can they learn from one another as they seek to develop creative solutions to the myriad issues that arise? Finally, can other cities learn from the experience of these four giants as they confront this challenge?

The Convergence of Two Trends

Population aging. Population aging is the result of two demographic changes since World War II—declining birth rates and increasing human longevity. The decline in birth rates is well recognized by the general public. The increase in longevity has only recently penetrated public consciousness. Over the course of the twentieth century, life expectancy in the United States increased by approximately thirty years.[3] Part of this increase was due to continuing declines in infant mortality. An important part, however, reflects the extension of human longevity by three months a year over the later third of the century.[4]

Between 1970 and 2000, the population sixty-five and over in the United States increased from 9.9 to 12.4 percent of the population. Generally, older people are not only living longer; they are healthier and have fewer disabilities than did older people of previous generations. Nonetheless, there is a growing population of vulnerable persons eighty-five years and over. Between 1970 and 2000, this population grew from 1.5 to 4.2 percent of the population sixty-five years and over. As a share of the total population, this group doubled (from 0.7 to 1.5 percent). While these increases are remarkable, the United States remains relatively young compared with other developed countries.

Along with these trends, because of women's higher life expectancy compared to men's, from 1920 to 1980, women's share of the population increased steadily. As of 2000, women comprised nearly 60 percent of the older population; among the population eighty-five and over they outnumbered men by a factor of two to one.[5]

By 2020, one-third of the population in many nations will be over sixty years of age, and 20 percent will be over sixty-five years of age in nations belonging to the Organization for Economic Cooperation and Development (OECD). By the year 2050, every third person on the planet will be over sixty. The aging of older persons themselves magnifies these trends. As of 2000, 10 percent of the population older than sixty was over eighty years of age. The census projects that this figure will rise to 25 percent by 2050.

Among developed countries, Japan is aging at the fastest rate. In France, it took 115 years for the percentage of the population sixty-five years of age and over to rise from 7 to 14 percent (1865–1980), but Japan experienced the same increase in only twenty-six years (1970–1996).[6] By 2030, Italy and Bulgaria will be the only developed countries projected to have a higher percentage of older people than Japan's.[7]

Urbanization. Cities have been growing more rapidly than at any time in history, and the world's population is increasingly concentrated in urban areas. UN estimates indicate that 60 percent of the population will live in cities in 2030.[8] Although older people are less likely than younger people to live in urban areas, the majority of older people in the developed world live in cities, and UN demographers project that the number of older city dwellers will grow throughout the world.

Not only have the number and percentage of people living in urban areas grown; the populations and scale of cities have also grown. There are now at least twenty so-called megacities, defined by the United Nations as cities of over ten million people; by 2015, there will be twenty-three.[9] The fastest-growing megacities are in developing nations, and by 2015 all megacities—with the exception of Tokyo and New York—will be in developing nations.

Urbanization and the growth of larger cities have led to demands for more and better data at the urban level. For example, the National Academy of the Sciences' Panel on Cities recently called for the development of urban-level data sets. Despite the surge of interest in these cities, comparative studies of health and social policy, health systems, and health across cities are notably absent from the literature. The World Health Organization (WHO) launched a movement in the 1980s known as Healthy Cities, which continues to promote social and economic factors affecting health through demonstration projects and innovative programs in cities throughout the world.[10] The Healthy Cities network has sensitized local authorities to the health implications of various urban policies and developed a list of indicators in thirty-two health-related areas.[11] With the exception of preliminary comparisons, this movement has yet to make significant contributions to research.[12]

Most existing studies of health and long-term care systems fail to distinguish rural from urban and "dense inner urban" from suburban. This is problematic, not only because most older persons live in cities, but also because the institutions serving them in inner urban and suburban areas are different from those serving older persons in rural areas. In European capital cities, for example, recent evidence indicates that the old urban infrastructure does not accommodate well its rapidly aging population.[13] The magnitude of and diversity within world cities suggest that there are multiple communities of older persons with widely disparate incomes and needs.

The Consequences of Population Aging and Urbanization for Cities

The likely causes and consequences of human longevity and population aging have been the subject of sustained study worldwide and the topic for important expert meetings of the United Nations (Vienna, 1982; Malta, 1986; and Madrid, 2002). But there has been almost no attention paid to the impact of these trends on health and quality of life in cities where most of the world's population will reside in the future.

Growth of urban poverty. New solutions to the challenge of population aging must also operate within the context of growing urban poverty. Poverty among older persons is a serious problem in both urban and rural areas. As a result of urbanization, however, poverty is becoming concentrated in urban areas around the world and reaching unprecedented levels. Between 1970 and 1990, this trend was evident in the Western Hemisphere: the share of the poor living in cities almost doubled in Latin America (from 36 to 60 percent) and increased from 56 to 72 percent in the United States.[14] Since the majority of new urban dwellers in developing countries are poor, it follows that the rest of the developing world will also see a huge increase in its share of urban poverty as urbanization increases.[15]

The vulnerability of older people. The attacks of September 11, 2001, and the European heat wave of August 2003 highlight the vulnerability of older people in cities and the importance of understanding the health, social, and long-term care systems in urban areas. In New York City, the volume of services for older New Yorkers was cut, in some cases severely, in the days immediately following the attacks. Services supported by philanthropic funds, such as the city's Meals-on-Wheels program, which delivers food to older New Yorkers, were among the hardest hit because donations were redirected toward various World Trade Center relief efforts.[16] Four senior centers below Manhattan's Fourteenth Street closed for a week, although three were able to reopen after that.[17] At least six thousand older persons live in the immediate vicinity of the World Trade Center, twenty-four thousand if one includes the entire area below Canal Street affected by the attacks. Many frail older persons in this area who depend on home help and nursing care found themselves cut off for days from such assistance. For some, these services were the only link to the outside world, leaving them with an overwhelming sense of vulnerability

The attacks of September 11, as well as the large number of deaths among older persons in Paris during the August heat wave of 2003, highlight the importance of long-term care systems for social support of frail older persons in major population centers concerned with emergency-preparedness initiatives. As population aging and urbanization increase, we will need models of how to accommodate this growing at-risk population who live in cities. Many of the chapters in this book address these needs. Developing programs that identify vulnerable older people without violating their civil liberties is a crucial challenge for each of these four world cities.

Changing family structures and expectations. The increase in life expectancy has augmented the burden of family caregivers. Known as the "sandwich generation," a growing number of middle-aged people are providing care to older parents while caring for their own children. This development affects women disproportionately because they tend to adopt most of the responsibility for the care of older parents, and research indicates that women who are in the labor force are just as likely to act as caregivers as women who are not.[18]

The past thirty years have also seen a rise in the number of grandparents caring for grandchildren, a trend driven by the growth in single-parent families, women in the workplace, and the number of children orphaned by AIDS. In 1997, 4 million children under the age of eighteen lived in their grandparents' homes; 1.3 million of these children "had neither a father or mother present, and another 2.0 million had only one parent, usually the mother, present."[19] In the United States, grandparent caregiving is more prevalent among African Americans and among older people living in cities.

Custodial grandparents tend to be poorer and less well educated than grandparents who are not providing live-in care for their grandchildren. They are also more likely than other grandparents to have physical limitations and to be suffering from depression. This finding is consistent with other studies of caregivers, which show that caregiving can have a negative impact on physical and mental health.[20] Studies of caregiving have found that it is associated with physical and psychological stress, possibly because the demands of caring for children may force older persons to confront their limitations and make them more likely to report them.

Declining disability rates. The "compression of morbidity," a concept introduced by James Fries, refers to a reduction in the amount of disability among older persons and its compression into fewer years at the end of life.[21] Swedish geriatrician Alvar Svanborg was the first to observe and report on a decline in disability rates among older persons. In a study of three cohorts of seventy-year-olds in Gothenburg, Sweden, born in 1900, 1905, and 1910, Svanborg found improved functional status and health in each successive cohort. More recently, Kenneth Manton reported reductions in the instrumental activities of daily life (IADLs) and, to a lesser extent, activities of daily life (ADLs) among older persons in the United States.[22]

According to the 2000 National Long Term Care Survey, the prevalence of physical disability and cognitive impairment significantly decreased during the last two decades of the twentieth century. Between 1982 and 1999, the percentage of older persons with a physical disability dropped from just over 26 percent to less than 20 percent. Likewise, the percentage of older persons with cognitive impairment fell during this period (from 5.2 to 2.7 percent).[23] Consequently, not all older people will need long-term care. About 40 percent of people over eighty-five are fully functional. Nevertheless, the growth in the "older old" population suggests that there will be an increasing need for long-term care services. Persons age eighty-five years and over tend to be less healthy, more socially isolated, and therefore more vulnerable than people between sixty-five and seventy-four. For example, in the United States, Medicare beneficiaries eighty-five years and over are more likely than younger Medicare beneficiaries to have two or more chronic conditions, at least one functional limitation, and mobility and social activity limitations. They are also less likely to be engaged in paid employment and more likely to live below the poverty line.[24]

Why Examine Aging and Long-Term Care in World Cities?

The terms "world cities" and "global cities" have been used interchangeably to mean cities at the center of the global economy and hubs in the international world of transnational corporations, financial services, and information exchange.[25] A comparison of world cities can improve understanding of the unique challenges and opportunities these cities offer to older persons. For thousands of years, cities have been regarded, simultaneously, as "the natural center of everything that mattered" and "the source of corruption and evil."[26] When examining the characteristics of world cities and their implications for older persons, it is easy to understand this apparent paradox. High levels of congestion, pollution, and crime in world cities, as well as social polarization and the high cost of housing, may undermine quality of life for older people. Yet these cities offer greater access to public transportation, pharmacies and stores, world-class medical centers, museums, parks, concert halls, colleges and universities, libraries, and theaters and other venues for entertainment. They are important cases to study because they are unique within their national borders and because they share these characteristics.

A second reason for focusing on world cities among wealthy OECD nations is that, because of their relative wealth and dominance, their ties to the global economy, and their concentration of business, cultural, and scientific activities, they exercise a strong influence—for better or for worse—on the exploding megacities of developing nations. As urbanization and population aging increase, policy makers in megacities need models for how to organize the health and long-term care systems to accommodate this population shift. Policy makers around the world view these four cities as frontiers for health and social policy innovations that meet the challenge of population aging in an urban context. The experience of these world cities may provide useful lessons.

Third, our focus on world cities among OECD nations is due, simply, to the availability of data in comparison to data available on megacities of the developing world. A careful study of growing older in cities requires substantial demographic, socioeconomic, and policy information, but it is extraordinarily difficult to find comparable data across cities and their neighborhoods. Studying large cities in the developed world provides an advantage because more data is available about them. Even so, identifying comparable data among world cities remains a challenge.[27]

Fourth, as command-and-control centers in the global economy, world cities are marked by a growing number of wealthy and poor residents, a shrinking middle class, and increasing socioeconomic inequalities.[28] According to the world city hypothesis, a concentration in a few cities of financial, information, and other specialized service industries, as well as headquarters of transnational corporations, has accompanied the dispersion of production and distribution around the world.[29] As a result, these cities attract large numbers of highly affluent people to work in their financial, legal, and information-technology sectors. At the same time, globalization has created a great number of jobs in what Tobier (see Chapter 3) calls the "under the stairs" economy (in the hospitality industry—hotels, restaurants, tourism, convention centers; in health and home care; and in small businesses of all sorts). These relatively low-skill, low-wage jobs have attracted a large and growing number of immigrants to these cities. This dichotomy has helped produce stark inequalities, particularly in New York and London.[30]

It is important to understand better how older people are faring in this environment; there are reasons to believe that it may pose serious challenges to many. World cities offer tremendous cultural and entertainment opportunities, but they are expensive places to live. Only a small percentage of older persons have the financial resources to take advantage of the opportunities they provide. Tobier estimates, for example, that only one out of twenty older households has "enough" money to take full advantage of New York's unique opportunities for a higher quality of life (see Chapter 3). With the growth of a large population working in service industries, the next generation of older persons in these cities may have even greater need for assistance. The substantial costs associated with long-term care, particularly assisted living, home care, and other alternatives to institutionalization, put some options out of reach for many of the oldest old. New solutions to long-term care must be responsive to the economic constraints of older people living in these world cities.

Why Focus on New York, London, Paris, and Tokyo?

Some have argued that New York, London, Paris, and Tokyo are the only cities that meet the definition of a world city.[31] Indeed, some even question whether Paris and Tokyo are "global" cities to the same degree as are New York and London.[32] Even without adopting a strict definition of the term, there are at least three reasons why these cities are useful laboratories for exploring the issues raised by growing older in cities. To begin with, they share a similar scale and concentration of older residents. In addition, New York, London, and Paris share strikingly similar rates of older women living alone. While Tokyo provides a contrasting case, there is evidence that it too has a growing number of older women living alone. Finally, all four cities share a knowledge base and scholarly literature, which is fruitful to extend by examining some hypotheses in the supporting literature.

Scale and concentration. Among cities in the United States, New York has the highest concentration of persons over sixty-five years of age—close to a million (Table 1.1). London, Paris, and Tokyo have the highest concentration of older persons in their respective nations. These cities have all been affected by declining birth rates and a rising share of older persons. They already include neighborhoods in which persons sixty-five years and over exceed 20 percent, the level the U.S. Census Bureau projects for the entire United States in the year 2030. As a result, they can serve as social laboratories in which to test alternative interventions that address health and social needs of cities with aging populations.

Table 1.1. Number of Persons 65+: Four World Cities, 1999–2001

	Urban Core[a]	First Ring[a]	Total
New York City, 2000	186,776	751,081	937,857
Greater London, 2001	288,305	619,870	908,175
Paris and First Ring, 1999	327,335	521,388	848,723
Tokyo, 2000	372,060	964,229	1,336,289

Sources: New York City: U.S. Census 2000; Greater London: U.K. Census 2001; Paris region: INSEE 1999; Tokyo: Japan Census 2001.

[a] Paris was the prototypical "urban core" against which we selected a comparable urban core for New York, London, and Tokyo. Paris and First Ring includes the surrounding three departments (Figure 2.1). For New York City, this is Manhattan; for London, the fourteen boroughs known as Inner London; for Tokyo, the urban core of 11 inner wards. For a more detailed discussion, see Chapter 2.

Similarities and differences—older people living alone. In each of the four cities, large and growing segments of older persons live alone. Among the population sixty-five and over in the United States, 9.7 million (28 percent) live alone. Census demographers expect this number to rise to over 25 million in 2020, and the most vulnerable population of those eighty-five and older living alone is likely to more than double.[33]

Of the four cities, Inner Tokyo has the lowest percentage of persons eighty-five years and older living alone (23 percent in 2000), followed by Inner London and Manhattan (both 55 percent in 2000) and Paris (60 percent in 1999). Yet when the percentage of older persons living alone in the urban core of each city is compared to that of its first ring, there is a striking convergence. In all four cities, rates of living alone among older persons are higher in the urban cores. This is true for the population over eighty-five and more generally for those over sixty-five years (Table 1.2).

Perhaps the most striking aspect of those living alone in world cities is the high percentage of women eighty-five years and over in Manhattan, Paris, and Inner London (Table 1.3). Data on New York and London indicate that gender, ethnicity, and race are important factors in distinguishing among older persons who live alone. In New York City and Greater Paris, women are almost twice as likely to live alone (57.5 and 60 percent) as men (29 and 30 percent). In New York City, percentages of living alone are significantly lower among older Hispanics and Asians and slightly lower among African Americans than among their white counterparts. Likewise, in Greater London, percentages of living alone are higher among the white population than among the black Caribbean, Indian, and Bangladeshi populations.

The high incidence of living alone, among older women in the urban cores

Table 1.2. Persons 65+ and 85+ Living Alone: Four World Cities, 1999–2001 (as a percentage of age cohort)

	65+		85+	
	Urban Core	**First Ring**	**Urban Core**	**First Ring**
New York City, 2000	44.1	29.7	55.3	40.1
Greater London, 2001	50.4	39.3	57.4	52.3
Paris and First Ring, 1999	44.0	33.6	59.8	48.5
Central Tokyo, 2000	24.7	20.4	23.0	19.2

Sources: New York: U.S. Census 2000; London: UK Census 2001; Paris region: INSEE 1999; Tokyo: Japan Census 2000.

of world cities, raises intriguing questions. Living alone is a source of independence—but it may also be a sign of isolation. Given the great disparities in each of these cities, it is likely that some older persons living alone are doing quite well, while others are isolated and vulnerable.

Policy convergence? Hypotheses from the literature. The study of aging and long-term care in each city can build on the existence of significant data on each city as well as scholarship on their economic functions, architecture, urban design, and transportation infrastructure.[34] There is even a recent study of London's competitive advantage with New York, Paris, and Tokyo in the global economy.[35] And as noted earlier, there is a rich literature on the roles of world cities in the global economy

Table 1.3. Persons 85+ Living Alone, by Gender: Four World Cities, 1999–2001 (as a percentage of all persons 85+)

	Men	**Women**
Manhattan, 1999	41.3	67.9
Inner London, 2001	45.2	62.3
Paris, 1999	39.6	67.6
Inner Tokyo, 2000	15.9	26.4

Sources: Manhattan: New York City Housing and Vacancy Survey 1999; Inner London: UK Census 2001; Paris region: INSEE 1999; Inner Tokyo: Tokyo Metropolitan Government 2000.

and the ways the cities are affected by these economic functions. A number of prominent scholars suggest that the social and economic characteristics of world cities are converging. According to this literature, the mobility of capital on a global scale makes it difficult for these cities, or the nations in which they exist, to address this polarization and other social challenges for fear of driving business out of the city. The forces of globalization exacerbate the "privileged position of business" in capitalist democracies.[36] Because domestic capital has more "exit options" as the result of globalized production, there is at least the perceived risk or credibility of risk of domestic capital flight if domestic tax and expenditure policies do not favor short-term profitability.[37] If this model is correct, we should see a common pattern of retrenchment of social welfare programs in these cities. Critics assert that the convergence hypothesis advanced by much of the global-cities literature underestimates the power of the state and fails to account for important differences in social welfare programs.[38]

A complete examination of the convergence hypothesis associated with the global-cities literature is beyond the scope of this book. Nevertheless, in examining long-term care, we look for evidence of convergence in this important domain. To what extent do the pressures of globalization make it difficult for these cities, and the nations in which they exist, to respond to the needs of their aging populations? To what extent are the policy responses to population aging and the scope of available services for older people similar across these cities?

Cross-National Policy Learning

The Netherlands, Germany, and, most recently, Japan have adopted public long-term care insurance programs for their older citizens that may serve as models for the rest of the world. Indeed, one of the goals of this book is to learn more about the implementation of the Japanese long-term care insurance system in Tokyo, and to think about the lessons of this experience for other world cities.

One of the challenges of cross-national learning is to explore good practices, as well as interesting failures. In comparison to the typical study tour, the combination of our data on health and long-term care in world cities with case material on innovative programs allows knowledgeable practitioners to interpret what they see. Since local authorities can sometimes implement innovative initiatives faster than can their national governments, such information about world cities can be useful to their governments and program managers.[39]

Although these cities face a similar challenge, they do so within quite different national health, social, and long-term care policy contexts. With regard to heath care, Parisians and Tokyoites are covered by systems of national health insurance. The National Health Service (NHS) covers Londoners. Medicare (Parts A and B) covers most older New Yorkers, but there are significant gaps in Medicare coverage, such as that for prescription drugs.[40]

There are also differences in coverage of long-term care. Japan is the only country of the four with long-term care insurance. Home-help and home-nursing services for older persons are covered primarily by the national Long-Term Care Insurance (LTCI) scheme, and everyone forty years old and over contributes to this program. There are two broad categories of beneficiaries for LTCI. Those aged forty to sixty-four must pay insurance premiums but are eligible for services only if their long-term care needs are the result of one of fifteen aging-related diseases. Those sixty-five and over pay higher premiums, which are deducted from their pensions, and are eligible for home-care services regardless of the level of their needs. Users are expected to pay 10 percent of the cost of services, the other 90 percent being covered by a mix of municipal, prefectural, and national funds. Premiums in 2000 were around twenty-four dollars per person per month, but they vary across municipalities (including across Tokyo's wards).

Great Britain covers nursing and home-care services under the NHS, but these programs are means tested and availability is limited. The Home Care Services unit of each local authority provides home-attendant services directly or contracts with independent organizations for its provision.[41] Although increasingly rare, housekeeping services are provided as well. It is up to local authorities to decide whether to charge for these services, and some have instituted a weekly rate. Older home-care users who must pay generally do so with their Attendance Allowance, a weekly income supplement for personal care.

France covers medical services under its national health insurance (NHI) program, as well as nursing services provided in long-stay hospital beds, nursing homes, and residential/retirement homes, but individuals must pay the cost of room and board. France also provides limited access to social services. A variety of funding streams exists to pay for home help. In addition, the Old Age Insurance Fund's local social welfare services provide home help for those with lower levels of dependency. Beginning in April 2002, the central government established a cash-allowance program to finance home help for frail older persons based on assessment of levels of dependency.

Public financing for long-term care in the United States is more limited than in the other countries we examine. Medicare pays for only the first one hundred days of nursing-home care. Most older persons in the United States "spend down" their assets until they are eligible for Medicaid, which is means tested and limited to older persons with very limited incomes.[42] Both these publicly funded programs have limited home-care health programs, though New York State's is the most generous in the nation and accounts for more than half of Medicaid spending on home health care in the United States.

Beyond these national policy frameworks within which world cities operate, an area of discretionary local policy exists even in the most centralized unitary states such as France, Japan, and Great Britain. This discretion is particularly important with respect to the process of determining eligibility and subsequently arranging for home-nursing services and a host of social and home-help services. For example, local authorities in London have a critical role in the allocation of residential care for frail older persons; social services for older persons may vary greatly by *ku,* or ward, within Tokyo; and social welfare in Paris is reputedly more generous than in most other French departments, though there appears to be considerable variation within Paris.

The attempt to derive lessons from the experiences of other nations has a long history,[43] and there is an immense literature on cross-national comparisons of health and long-term care systems and policies in OECD nations.[44] The focus on national aggregates, however, masks important variations within nations, for example, between urban and rural areas, large and small cities, cities and suburbs, and—as we demonstrate in this book—urban cores and their surrounding first rings.

This book adopts a new approach to the comparative analysis of health-system performance. Since world cities have more characteristics and problems in common than do nation-states, they provide notable advantages for more refined comparisons and cross-national learning. As Marmor and Klein contend in their discussion of cross-national comparative policy analysis: "If the focus of concern is the transplantability of ideas or models, then it is clearly essential that the two environments not be too different."[45]

Since New York, London, Paris, and Tokyo share many sociodemographic characteristics than do their respective nation-states—including greater income inequalities and more ethnic diversity—but have different health and long-term care system characteristics, the comparative analyses we conduct can provide insights into the possible effects of these systems on disparities in the use of long-term care.

Plan of the Book

This book sums up what is known about older persons in New York, London, Paris, and Tokyo, as well as what is known on the organization, financing, and use of health, social, and long-term care services for them, based on existing city-specific information, documents, and existing research studies. Our studies on aging and long-term care highlight significant areas of convergence and difference among these world cities. For example, we see convergence in the percentage of older people receiving home care in the urban core of each city, but a great disparity in the density of nursing-home beds. The percentage of those aged eighty-five years and over living in long-term care institutions is higher in Manhattan than in Paris, and more than three times as high as in London and Tokyo. These data raise an abundance of intriguing questions for policy makers concerned with the future of long-term care.

The book is organized in six sections. In the next chapter, we present our approach for comparing these cities based on existing spatial units of analysis. The next four sections present a set of chapters about each city. They address two broad themes: the socioeconomic and health status of older persons and how these have evolved over time; and older persons' living arrangements and use of long-term care. In the final section of the book, we summarize and interpret the findings from these chapters, identify similarities and differences, explore the lessons for policy makers and service organizations that care for older people in cities, and present a research agenda for addressing the questions that remain.

Acknowledgments

No research project of this scope is the product only of its editors and authors. We are grateful to Robert N. Butler for his early embrace of the World Cities Project, a collaborative venture of the International Longevity Center (ILC-USA), New York University's Wagner School of Public Service, and Columbia University's Mailman School of Public Health. We acknowledge financial support from the Japan Foundation, Center for Global Partnership (CGP); a health policy investigator award to Victor Rodwin for his project on Megacities and Health from the R. W. Johnson Foundation; a grant from the Florence Gould Foundation to support the Paris and New York components of the project; a grant from the New York Community Trust to support the New York component of the project; and support from ILC-USA's sister organizations in Paris (ILC-France), London (ILC-UK), and Tokyo (ILC-Japan).

Many of the papers contributed to this book were first presented at a series of meetings held in Tokyo, London, and Paris. The Tokyo meeting (June 2000) was sponsored by ILC-Japan and the CGP; the London meeting (November 2001) was sponsored by ILC-UK and the National Health Service's London Regional Office. The Paris meeting (June 2003) was sponsored by ILC-France and the Research Division (Direction de la Recherche, des Etudes, de l'Evaluation, et des Statistiques (DRESS) of the Ministry of Health. ILC Directors Dr. Robert N. Butler, Baronness Sally Greengross, Dr. Françoise Forette, and Shigeo Morioka provided critical support at every stage of our research.

In addition to what we learned in these meetings, we are grateful to local government organizations in each of the cities: In New York, the Department for the Aging–DFTA (Commissioners Herb Stupp and Ed Mendez and Director of Research Jackie Berman); in London, the London Health Observatory–LHO (Bobbie Jacobson); in Paris, the city's Direction des Affaires Sociales, de l'Enfance, et de la Santé (DASES) and the Observatoire Régional de Santé for Ile-de-France; and in Tokyo, the Tokyo Metropolitan Government's Bureau of Social Welfare.

We wish to thank the following colleagues for assistance ranging from data acquisition to critical comments on our chapters. In New York, Birgit Bogler, Marilyn DeLuca, Irena Dushi, Susan Ghanbarpour, Margaret Hodgson, Keiko Honda, Jin Liu, Gabriel Montero, Charlotte Muller, Bridgit Simone; in London, Justine Fitzpatrick, Elizabeth Lowe, Olivia Nuamah, Wendy Sykes; in Paris, Marc Duriez, Marc Esponda, Jeanne Fagnani, Ruth Ferry, Christine Grouas, Loic Josseran, Roland

Moreau, Philippe Pépin, Robert Poinsard, Diane Slama-Lequet, Jeremie Sautter, Marc Simon, Marie-Sophie Schwalm, Alfred Spira, Florence Veber; in Tokyo, Tetsuo Fukuda, Junichi Kajiyama, Yukiko Kudo, Emiko Kobayashi Mikami, Yoko Shiro, Yoshiko Yamada, Shiro Yamasaki, Nobu Yasuda. We acknowledge Michael Curran and Kenny Green (ILC-USA) for supporting our Web site (ilcusa.org/projects/research) and producing camera-ready maps and figures. Finally we thank our families for continued support and for allowing us to travel to world cities.

Notes

1. Scott, A. 2001. *Global City Regions: Trends, Theory, and Policy.* New York: Oxford University Press.

2. Butler, Robert N. 1987. The Longevity Revolution. *Mount Sinai Journal of Medicine* 54(1): 5–8.

3. U.S. Census Bureau. 2001. *Demographic Trends in the 20th Century.* Washington DC: Government Printing Office.

4. Horiuchi, S. 2000. Greater Lifetime Expectations. *Nature* 405(6788): 744–745.

5. U.S. Census Bureau, *Demographic Trends.*

6. Ibid.

7. U.S. Census Bureau. 2000. International Data Base. www.census.gov/ipc/www/idbnew.html.

8. UN Population Division. 2001. *World Urbanization Prospects: The 1999 Revision* (New York: United Nations, 1999), 5 (www.un.org/esa/population/publications/wup1999/WUP99CH1.pdf); "Cities" here refers to "urban agglomerations," defined by the United Nations as the "population contained within the contours of a contiguous territory inhabited at urban levels of residential density irrespective of whether that population lives within or without the administrative boundaries of the city" (ibid.).

9. Ibid.

10. See, e.g., Aicher, J. 1998. *Designing Healthy Cities: Prescriptions, Principles, and Practice.* Malabar, FL: Krieger; Ashton, J. 1992. *Healthy Cities.* Bristol, PA: Open University Press; Duhl, L., and T. Hancock. 1998. *A Guide to Assessing Healthy Cities.* Copenhagen: WHO Healthy Cities Project Office.

11. Garcia, P., and M. McCarthy. *Measuring Health: A Step in the Development of City Health Profiles.* Copenhagen: WHO Regional Office for Europe.

12. WHO's Collaborating Center for Research on Healthy Cities, in the Netherlands, is conducting an evaluation of what has been accomplished in selected Healthy Cities (see www.rulimburg.nl-who-city/aswww.html). Also see Doyle, Y., D. Brunning, C. Cryer, S. Hedley, and C. Russell Hodgson. 1997. *Healthy Cities Indicators: Analysis of Data from Cities across Europe.* Copenhagen: WHO Regional Office for Europe.

13. Project Mégapoles. 1999. *Growing Old in Metropolitan Areas.* 2d rev. ed., Final Report, 1998–1999. See www.lho.org.uk/Publications/Attachments/PDF_Files/projmega.pdf; accessed May 2005.

14. Massey, Douglas. 1996. The Age of Extremes: Concentrated Affluence and Poverty in the Twenty-First Century. *Demography* (33)4: 395–412.

15. Ibid.

16. Doss, Lori. 2001. Starved for Donations, Citymeals-on-Wheels Fears Service Cuts. *Nation's Restaurant News,* October 15.

17. *MMR (Mayor's Management Report).* 2002. New York: Mayor's Office, 331.

18. Pavalko, Eliza K., and Julie E. Artis. 1997. Women's Caregiving and Paid Work: Causal Relationships in Late Midlife. *Journal of Gerontology: Social Sciences* 52B(4): 170–179.

19. Muller, Charlotte, and Marjorie Honig. 2000. *Charting the Productivity and Independence of Older Persons.* New York: ILC-USA, April.

20. Cantor, Marge H. 1983. Strain among Caregivers: A Study of Experience in the United States. *Gerontologist* 23:597–604.

21. Fries, J. F. 1980. Aging, Natural Death, and the Compression of Morbidity. *New England Journal of Medicine* 303:130–135.

22. Fries, J. F., Anthony J. Vita, Richard B. Terry, and Helen B. Hubert. 1998. Aging, Health Risks, and Cumulative Disability. *New England Journal of Medicine* 338:1035–1041; Svanborg, A., G. Bergstrom, and D. Mellstrom. 1982. Epidemiological Studies on Social and Medical Conditions of the Elderly. Report on a Survey. (Euro Reports and Studies 12). Copenhagen: World Health Organization.

23. Hodes, Richard J. 2002. Department of Health and Human Service, National Institutes of Health 2003 Budget Request. Testimony before the House Subcommittee on Labor-HHS-Education Appropriations. March 13.

24. Muller, Charlotte, James Nyberg, and Judith Estrine. 2001. Old and Poor in America. *Issue Brief,* ILC-USA. October. (See www.ilcusa.org/_lib/pdf/b20021121a.pdf.)

25. Hall, P. 1984. *The World Cities.* 3d ed. London: Weidenfeld and Nicholson; Sassen, S. 1981. *The Global City: New York, London, Tokyo.* Princeton: Princeton University Press; Focas, Carlampo. 1998. *The Four World Cities Transport Study.* London: London Research Center.

26. Zwingle, E. 2002. Feature: More to Explore. *National Geographic Magazine* On-Line, www.nationalgeographic.com/ngm/0211/feature3/index.html.

27. Short J., M. Kim, and H. Wells. 1996. The Dirty Little Secret of World Cities Research: Data Problems in Comparative Analysis. *International Journal of Urban and Regional Research* 20:697–717.

28. Hall, *The World Cities;* Sassen, S. 2001. *The Global City: New York, London, Tokyo.* 2d ed. Princeton: Princeton University Press; Sassen, S. 1994. *Cities in the World Economy.* Thousand Oaks, CA: Pine Forge Press; White, J. 1998. Old Wine, Cracked Bottle? Tokyo, Paris, and the Global City Hypothesis. *Urban Affairs Review* 33(4): 451–477.

29. Friedmann, J. 1986. The World City Hypothesis. *Development and Change* 17(1): 69–83; Sassen, *Cities in the World Economy.*

30. Fainstein, S., I. Gordon, and M. Harloe, eds. 1992. *Divided Cities: London and New York in the Contemporary World.* Oxford University Press.

31. Hall, *The World Cities.*

32. White, "Old Wine."

33. U.S. Census Bureau, 2000.

34. Hall, *The World Cities*; Sassen, 1981, *The Global City*; Sassen, *Cities in the World Economy.*

35. Department of Environment and Government Office for London, United Kingdom. 1996. *Four World Cities: A Comparative Study of London, Paris, New York, and Tokyo, 1996.* London, UK: Llewelyn-Davies, UCL Bartlett School of Planning and Comedia (see ld@easynet.co.uk).

36. Dahl, R. A. 1985. *A Preface to Economic Democracy.* Berkeley: University of California Press; Elkin, S. 1987. *City and Regime in the American Republic.* Chicago: University of Chicago Press; Lindblom, C. E. 1977. *Politics and Markets: The World's Political-Economic Systems.* New York: Basic Books.

37. Stryker, R. 1998. Globalization and the Welfare State. *International Journal of Sociology and Social Policy* 18(2/3/4): 1–49.

38. Gurr, T., and D. King. 1987. *The State and the City.* London: Macmillan; White, Old Wine.

39. For example, cities in the United States and Canada passed ordinances banning ozone-depleting chlorofluorocarbons in the 1980s, well before the 1996 deadline for eliminating them was set by an international treaty. O'Meara, M. 1999. *Reinventing Cities for People and the Planet.* Washington, D.C.: Worldwatch Institute, June.

40. The Medicare reform law adopted in 2003 provides a limited prescription-drug benefit that is scheduled to go into effect in 2006.

41. As of January 2004, primary care trusts are responsible for commissioning, providing, and monitoring health and social services. The primary care trusts include general practitioners and social workers from each local authority.

42. The eligibility for Medicaid is determined by each state within parameters set by the federal government.

43. Klein, R. 1983. Strategies for Comparative Social Policy Research. In A. Williamson and G. Room, eds. *Health and Welfare States of Britain.* London: Heineman Educational Books; Marmor, T. R., and R. Klein. 1994. Rationing: Painful Prescription, Inadequate Diagnosis. In T. R. Marmor, ed. 1994. *Understanding Health Care Reform.* New Haven: Yale University Press.

44. Organization for Economic Cooperation and Development (OECD) health data come from a CD-ROM available from the Paris or Washington office of the OECD. The most recent version (2004) uses a broad definition of "health" and includes a wide range of social and economic indicators.

45. Marmor and Klein, Rationing, 113.

2. How Can We Compare New York, London, Paris, and Tokyo? Defining Spatial Units of Analysis

Victor G. Rodwin and Michael K. Gusmano

Among the four world cities examined in this book, Tokyo surely stands out as most different from the other three. Beyond being the largest city in terms of population size and surface area, it is also the most culturally distinctive. While sharing the attributes of a modern metropolis with New York, Paris, and London, Tokyo preserves its Asian roots with regard to such social patterns as community organization, living arrangements, and family relationships.[1] Since older persons tend to embody tradition, it is intriguing to ask how they fare in a world city that stands at the forefront of westernization and modernity. In this sense, the chapters on Tokyo offer insights on the importance of culture in relation to more global economic forces and their impact on the lives of older persons.

Before one can address these issues in relation to our broader theme—the impact of human longevity and population aging on Tokyo—it is important to begin with one of the first problems that emerges in any comparative inquiry: how to define the relevant units of analysis. Tokyo Prefecture spreads well beyond the confines of the modern metropolis, which we refer to as Central Tokyo (twenty-three wards). It includes the western Tama district (twenty-seven cities) and a number of rural islands. The entire Tokyo Prefecture with its twelve million population, all under the administration of the Tokyo Metropolitan Government, might be compared to the New York Metropolitan region, the Greater London region, or Ile de France, which includes Paris and its two surrounding rings. But these vast agglomerations are not typically regarded as relevant units for defining world cities. Rather, the image of world cities is usually rooted in their historical and spatial development around an urban core. Moreover, their urban cores are most directly connected to their functions as centers of command and control in the global economy and to their centrality in the worlds of culture, education, and the media.

The Urban Core as a Unit of Analysis

In defining the urban cores of Tokyo, New York City, London, and Paris, our initial studies were guided by six criteria: historic and spatial development; population size; population density; social inequalities; spatial distribution of employment and commuter patterns; and density of health-system resources (hospital beds and physicians).

First, with respect to spatial development, Paris, Manhattan, and Inner London represent the historic centers from which these metropolitan regions grew. Although there is no generally accepted definition of Tokyo's urban core, the same can be said of the city's eleven wards inside the Yamanote subway line (see Figure 2.1). Second, in terms of population size, Manhattan, Paris, and Inner London range from 1.5 to 2.6 million.

Third, in terms of population density, Manhattan and Paris are similar: sixty-six versus fifty-three thousand inhabitants per square mile. Both have almost twice the population density of Inner London. Inner Tokyo's density, however, is much closer to Inner London's than to that of Manhattan or Paris.

Fourth, with regard to the presence of social inequalities, the urban cores of these cities reflect a mix of high- and low-income populations. Finally, a number of criteria derived from central place theory suggest three striking parallels between Manhattan, Paris, Inner Tokyo, and Inner London:[2]

Concentrated employment centers. The urban cores function as employment centers that attract large numbers of commuters. Approximately one-third of the first ring's employed labor force commutes to Manhattan, Paris, Inner Tokyo, and Inner London every day.

Physician density. All four urban cores are characterized by a high density of physicians, much higher than that of their first rings (Table 2.1). The core/first-ring ratio of physician density is higher for Inner Tokyo (3.9) and London (3.6) than for Manhattan (2.1) and Paris (2.3).

Acute care hospital beds. Manhattan, London, and Inner Tokyo have 2.5, 2.6, and 2.8 times as many acute care hospital beds as their respective first rings; Paris has 1.8 times as many. These ratios include acute care hospital beds in large university teaching hospitals in all the central cores (Table 2.1).

Summary. Paris—with 2.1 million inhabitants within its nineteenth-century walls and the peripheral freeway that surrounds its twenty *arrondissements*—was the prototypical "urban core" against which we selected comparable urban cores for New York, London, and Tokyo. The Paris population and area (105 square kilometers) are miniscule in comparison to Greater London's 7.3 million people and 1,590 square kilometers; New York City's 8 million people and 826 square kilometers; and Central Tokyo's 8.1 million people and 616 square kilometers. Rather, Paris is comparable to the urban core of these cities: for New York City, Manhattan with its 1.5 million population; for London, the fourteen boroughs known as Inner London with a population of 2.6 million.

For Tokyo, with no conventional definition of an urban core, we relied on the criteria noted earlier and arrived at an urban core comprised of eleven inner wards (*kus*) that cover an area of sixty-seven square miles and had a 1995 population of

Figure 2.1. Urban Core and First Ring Population Estimates: Four World Cities, 1999–2000

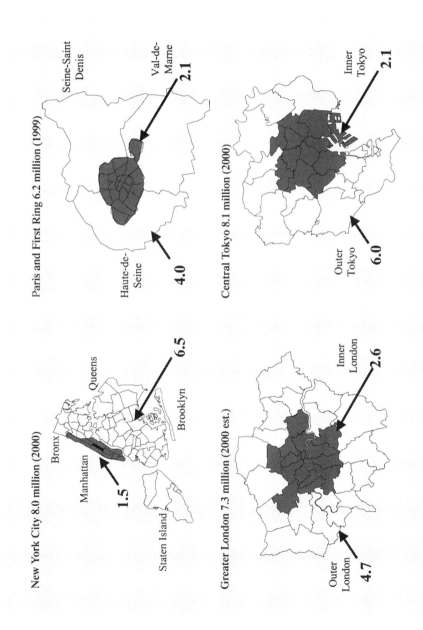

New York City 8.0 million (2000)

Bronx

Queens

Manhattan

Brooklyn

Staten Island

1.5

6.5

Paris and First Ring 6.2 million (1999)

Seine-Saint Denis

Val-de-Marne

2.1

Haute-de-Seine

4.0

Greater London 7.3 million (2000 est.)

Inner London

2.6

Outer London

4.7

Central Tokyo 8.1 million (2000)

Inner Tokyo

2.1

Outer Tokyo

6.0

Sources: NYC: U.S. Census, 2000; Paris and First Ring: INSEE, 1999; Greater London: ONS, 2000; Tokyo, Population Census, 2000.

Table 2.1. Physician and Acute Hospital-Bed Density: Four World Cities, 1997–2002

		Physicians[a]	Acute Hospital Beds[b]
New York City 2004/2002	Urban Core	85.5	7.0
	First Ring	20.5	2.4
	Ratio[c]	4.2	2.9
Greater London 1999/2000	Urban Core	36.9	3.7
	First Ring	10.3	1.4
	Ratio	3.6	2.6
Paris and First Ring 2002/2001	Urban Core	84.6	7.0
	First Ring	37.0	3.9
	Ratio	2.3	1.8
Tokyo (23 wards) 1998/2000	Urban Core	70.0	12.8
	First Ring	18.0	4.6
	Ratio	3.9	2.8

Sources: For physician density, New York City: United Hospital Fund, 2004; London: LHO, 2000; Paris: Ministère de l'Emploi et de la Solidarité, SESI—répertoire ADELI au 1er janvier 98; Tokyo: *Tokyo Statistical Yearbook*, 1996, and Tokyo Statistical Association, 1998. For hospital beds, New York City: *Health Care*, United Hospital Fund, 2002; London: LHO, 2000; Paris: DRASS SAE 1995 (rates based on 1995 population), and INSEE projection OMPHALE; Tokyo: *List of Medical Facilities,* 2000, Bureau of Public Health, Tokyo Metropolitan Government.
[a] Per 10,000 persons
[b] Per 1,000 persons
[c] Ratio = urban core/first ring

two million. This area is roughly comparable to Paris, Manhattan, and Inner London in terms of population size and area. Except for Shitamachi, these inner wards are within the Yamanote loop line and include such important hub stations as Shinjuku, Shibuya, Ikebukuro (Toshima Ward), Shinagawa (Minato Ward), and Tokyo (Chiyoda Ward); Inner Tokyo, as defined here, is thus the area to which most commuters to Tokyo come to work. Since these eleven inner wards are all within about a five-mile radius of the Imperial Palace, they may clearly be said to be "central locations" within Central Tokyo.[3]

So defined, Inner Tokyo includes the major loci of political, economic, and social activities. Japan's legislative, executive, and judicial bodies are located in the three central wards, along with offices of the major political parties. Headquarters of

Japan's major corporations are situated either in the three central business districts or in the new subcenters of Tokyo. Major parks, museums, and cultural facilities are also concentrated in the inner eleven wards. Finally, this definition of Inner Tokyo includes the city's past and present, as well as wards dominated by higher and lower occupational groups.

In addition to the problem of choosing appropriate units of analysis, another important issue in any comparative inquiry involves structuring the comparisons around similarities as well as differences among the units being compared.

Similarities and Differences as a Starting Point for Comparative Analysis

Similarities. All four urban cores have economies based on services and informa-tion, which are closely tied to national and international transactions. They are also centers of culture, media, government, and international organizations. And their resident populations include some of the wealthiest and poorest members of their respective nations.

The poverty rate, defined as the percentage of households with incomes below one-half the median, is almost twice as high in Manhattan (28.5 percent) as in Paris (12.8 percent).[4] Although household-income data are not available in the United Kingdom, occupational/class categories defined by the census may be used as a proxy. Although this is not comparable to the Manhattan and Paris figures, it allows us to observe a similar pattern in all three cities—poverty levels for the population of the urban core are slightly higher than those in their first rings. In the Paris agglomeration, the poverty rate is 10.2 percent; in New York, 25.6 percent.[5] In Greater London the share of lower "classes" is 14.9 percent as opposed to 17 percent in Inner London.

For Tokyo, since we have no data on poverty rates, we examine a proxy indicator of deprivation: the percentage of households receiving public assistance. In 1996, this was slightly higher in the urban core (2.08 percent) than in the periphery (1.56 percent).[6]

With the exception of New York, a similar pattern holds for the percentage of foreign-born populations. Roughly one-quarter of the population in Inner London and Manhattan, and about 20 percent of the population in Paris, was born abroad. In Paris and Inner London, this foreign-born population is higher than in the first ring, but in Manhattan the percentage of foreign-born population is lower than in the surrounding boroughs.

Tokyo collects data on "foreigners" rather than on the foreign born and has a far more homogeneous population than has either Manhattan or Paris. In Inner Tokyo, 3 percent of the population are foreigners; in the twelve outer wards, only 1.6 percent are foreigners. These data, however, understate the inter-Asian diversity within Tokyo, as they do not account for Japanese of Korean descent or illegal im-migrants from Asia.

Differences. Despite their common characteristics, these cities have many significant differences. Among the four, Manhattan is characterized by the highest level of inequality in the distribution of income. For example, intracity variation in average household income varies from a ratio of 2.1 in Inner Tokyo to 3.0 in Paris and 5.0 in Manhattan.[7] One of the characteristics of global cities is the polarization between the well-to-do and the poor. Opinions differ on the extent to which this is a common characteristic and also on whether there are important variations among cities. Paris has been called a "soft" global city in contrast to New York because it provides more family services, income support, and health services to the poor.[8] Tokyo is more like Paris, and London more like New York in this regard.

The percentage of single-parent families is also much higher in Manhattan (22.8 percent) than in Paris (14.7 percent), Inner London (9.8 percent), or Inner Tokyo (9.0 percent). Birth rates are highest in Inner London (64.6), roughly the same in Manhattan and Paris (around forty-eight per thousand females aged fifteen to forty-five), and lowest in Inner Tokyo (30.2).

Population projections for 2015 indicate that Inner Tokyo will have the highest percentage of persons sixty years old and over (35 percent) in comparison to Paris (20 percent), Manhattan (18 percent), and Inner London (14.3 percent). At present, however, Paris has nearly twice the percentage of persons eight-five years and over (2.8 percent) of Manhattan, Inner London, and Inner Tokyo (Table 2.2).

Most of these differences—poverty rates, birth rates, and family structure—reflect national patterns and policies with regard to income maintenance and immigration. Other differences—population density and percentage of the older old—are distinctive urban characteristics. Still other contrasts involve societal and institutional responses to the growing need for long-term care services.

Framing the Inquiry on Growing Old in Four World Cities

New York City, Greater London, Paris and its first ring, and Central Tokyo share some important characteristics. Older persons in their inner cores have higher rates of labor-force participation than have their counterparts in the surrounding city. In addition, there is a much higher percentage of older persons living alone and receiving home-care services and a lower percentage institutionalized in long-term care facilities (see Chapter 22). Despite these convergent characteristics, there are some striking differences among older persons living in the inner cores of these cities—differences in labor-force participation rates, percentage of persons living alone, systems for the provision of social care, and life expectancy at sixty-five and at eighty years.

What is the relationship among different patterns of labor participation, alternative living arrangements, greater use of home-care services, and the quality of life of older persons in Manhattan, Paris, Inner London, and Inner Tokyo? How are these cities adapting to a world in which baby boomers are aging? How do older city dwellers who have chosen to "age in place" and avoid retirement communities make use of

Table 2.2. Persons 65+ and 85+: Four World Cities and Their Nations, 1999–2001 (as percentage of total population)

	65+			
	Urban Core	**First Ring**	**Total**	**Nation**
New York City, 2000	12.2	11.6	11.7	12.3
Greater London, 2001	10.5	13.4	12.4	15.8
Paris and First Ring, 1999	15.4	12.9	13.7	16.0
Tokyo, 2000	17.7	15.9	16.3	17.2

	85+			
	Urban Core	**First Ring**	**Total**	**Nation**
New York City, 2000	1.7	1.5	1.48	1.5
Greater London, 2001	1.5	1.8	1.6	2.0
Paris and First Ring, 1999	2.8	1.9	2.2	2.0
Tokyo, 2000	1.8	1.5	1.6	1.3

Sources: New York: U.S. Census, 2000; London: U.K. Census, 2001; Paris: INSEE, 1999; Tokyo: Census 2000. National figures: OECD Health Data, 2002.

the present organization of health and social services? Finally, how is one to explain differences in life expectancy at birth, as well as in age-specific mortality rates, among the four cities? For example, death rates are higher in Manhattan than in the other urban cores for those between sixty-five and eighty-five but significantly lower for those eighty-five and over. This finding is consistent with Manton and Vaupel's analysis of cross-national data from the United States, Sweden, France, England, and Japan.[9] What, if anything, does it suggest about quality of life and its relation to social and health-care services for older persons in these world cities?

Starting from the concept of an urban core discussed earlier, we asked contributors to cover a broad range of topics across the following themes: population characteristics—demographic, socioeconomic, and migration patterns—of persons sixty-five years and over and eighty-five years over; health status of older persons; housing arrangements and institutional care; and health and social services.

Population Characteristics

Demographic perspective. How does the population of older persons in these cities compare to that in their surrounding region and nation? What is the spatial distribution of older persons within each city or urban core? How have their demographic characteristics evolved since 1980? What are the best demographic projections for 2010? 2020? Characterize trends over the past two decades and summarize information on current projections for the urban core and surrounding area.

Socioeconomic perspective. What is the economic, occupational, and educational status of older persons in each city (urban core) compared to those in its surrounding region and the nation? What is the ethnic and immigrant (foreign-born) mix among older persons? What are their labor-force participation rates?

Migration patterns. What is known about migration patterns of older persons in each city? What groups typically move out of the city and at what age? What groups are attracted by retirement or "productive aging" in each city?

Health Status of Older Persons

How does the health status of older persons in each of the cities compare to that of those in the surrounding regions and nation? Indicators range from life expectancy at sixty-five years to functional abilities, disabilities, mobility limitations, and age-specific mortality rates, including mortality rates by cause. For example, how do age-specific mortality rates, by cause of death, differ among geographic areas of the city? Can we find comparable data to make intercity comparisons?

Health and Social Services

What is known about hospitalization rates of older persons in these cities, where hospital services make up an important export sector? What is the mix of primary versus specialty medical services used by older persons? What are the hospitalization rates of older persons in the urban core? What are the principal causes of admission?

How are home-care nursing and/or medical services organized and financed in each city for older persons? How are day-care programs for older persons organized and financed? Are there significant programs to provide meals for frail older persons? What is the extent of variation in service level among local districts within each city? What is the range of indicators used to measure their scope and size?

Housing Arrangements and Institutional Care

For the urban core, city, and/or surrounding region and nation, what percentage of older persons (by age cohort) lives in long-term care institutions—nursing homes, long-stay hospitals, or retirement homes with medical support services? Among persons over eighty-five years, what proportion live alone? How are these persons distributed across a continuum of housing and household arrangements in the city?

A Cautionary Note

Although no single book could answer all these questions, our hope is that the mix of chapters in each section sheds light on many of these issues in the context of each world city. As far as we know, this study is the first of its kind.

Notes

We wish to thank Emiko Mikami for assistance in defining the inner core of Tokyo.

1. Bestor, T. 1989. *Neighborhood Tokyo*. Stanford, Calif.: Stanford University Press.
2. See, e.g., Berry, Brian. 1961. *Central Place Studies*. Philadelphia: Regional Science Research Institute; King, L. J. 1984. *Central Place Theory*. Beverly Hills, Calif.: Sage.
3. See, e.g., Cybriwsky, R. 1991. *Tokyo: The Changing Profile of an Urban Giant*. London: Bell Haven Press; Cybriwsky, R. 1998. *Tokyo: The Shogun's City at the Twenty-First Century*. New York: Wiley; Seidensticker, E. 1983. *Low City, High City: Tokyo from Edo to the Earthquake*. New York: Knopf; and Seidensticker, E. 1990. *Tokyo Rising*. New York: Knopf.
4. Household-income data for New York City are from *Current Population Survey*. 1994. U.S. Census. Washington D.C.: Government Printing Office. For Paris, figures are from Chambaz, C., F. Guillaumat-Tailliet, and J. M. Hourriez. 1999. Le revenu et le patrimoine des ménages. In *Données socials*. Paris: INSEE. For Manhattan, New York City, Paris, and the Parisian agglomeration, poverty level is the percentage of households with incomes below half the median income of that city or area. (The Paris agglomeration is slightly larger than Paris and its first ring.) Data refer to pretax income; for Manhattan, pretax income includes Social Security and welfare payments but not other transfer payments, such as food stamps.
5. Data for Paris for 1994 are from Chambaz, Guillaumat-Tailliet, and Hourriez, Le revenu. Data for New York are from *Current Population Survey*.
6. Tokyo Statistical Association.1998. *Tokyo Statistical Yearbook, 1996*.
7. These are ratios of average household income by neighborhood: twenty *arrondissements* in Paris, seven *ku*s in Inner Tokyo, fourteen boroughs in Inner London, and ten subborough areas in Manhattan. For Paris and Tokyo, the data are from the Ministry of Finance for all households that file income taxes; for Manhattan, from the New York City Housing and Vacancy Survey for subborough areas. This survey is sponsored by the NYC Department of Housing, Preservation, and Development and is conducted by the U.S. Census (census.ogv; hhes; www/housing/nychvs/html) (accessed April 25, 2005). All figures are for 1990 except Manhattan's (1989).
8. Body-Gendrot, Sophie. 1996. Paris: A "Soft" Global City? *New Community* 22(4 [October]): 595–605.
9. Manton, K., and J. Vaupel. 1995. Survival after the Age of 80 in the United States, Sweden, France, England, and Japan. *New England Journal of Medicine* (333)18:1232–1236.

3. Growing Old in the City That Never Sleeps: Aging in New York

Emanuel Tobier

Introduction

An apt variation on an ancient Chinese curse might be, "May you live in an interesting place." New York is just such a place. Barring Las Vegas, it comes as close as any city can to operating around the clock, seven days a week. Few of the city's longtime residents would disagree that it is growing more hectic and harried by the minute.

Many older (and mostly better-off) New Yorkers responding to these pressures have voted with their feet, and over the last half century there has been a steady stream moving out in substantial numbers (Tables 3.1 and 3.2). Few outsiders, though, choose the city as a place to grow old in. As best one can tell from what is almost wholly anecdotal evidence, the much vaunted "return to the city" among older persons still seems to be mainly confined to the very old and frail who go back to be near their families.

High rates of net out-migration notwithstanding, a great many older people (defined for our purposes as persons sixty-five years and over) reside in New York, 938,000 as of 2000.[1] Overwhelmingly, these have been long-term residents of the city. While sharing certain distinctive needs and limitations common to people at this stage of life, these individuals are diverse in their backgrounds, resources, and inclinations.

This chapter describes these differences and highlights the major changes that have taken place in the socioeconomic characteristics of New York City's older population over the last few decades. What can these trends tell us about the needs, existing and emerging, of the city's over-sixty-five population? The chapter sheds some light on the consequences for older persons of living in the midst of the unique environment formed by the New York City version of a world city.

Table 3.1. Components of Population Change: NYC, 1950–2000 (in thousands)

	1950	1960	1970	1980	1990	2000
Population <65	7,287	6,968	6,947	6,120	6,369	7,070
Population 65+	605	814	948	952	953	938
Total population	7,892	7,782	7,895	7,072	7,322	8,008
Births		1,640	1,579	1,162	1,190	1,311
Deaths		817	880	796	752	685
Total natural increase		823	699	366	438	626
Net migration 65+		-50	-134	-289	-139	-127
Net migration <65		-882	-452	-900	-48	208
Total net migration		-932	-586	-1189	-187	81
Net population change[a]		-109	113	-823	251	686

Sources: U.S. Census of Population 1950–2000; New York City Department of Health 1950–2000; estimates of net migration by author.

[a] Net population change = natural increase + net migration

Manhattan: New York's World City

The real-world workplace of the organizations and individuals that make New York a world city is wedged into a six-square-mile swathe of lower and midtown Manhattan in which more than 2.5 million people are employed by 110,000 or so establishments of various sorts (90 percent of them for-profit enterprises).[2] Adding in the adjacent residential areas, such as its Middle East and West Side districts, which are the neighborhoods of choice for a great many of the key people in these enterprises, brings the overall total to around twelve square miles with a live-in population of about four hundred thousand.

Within this jam-packed beehive is the latest version of what has proven to be one of the nation's most durable platforms for economic and cultural innovation. It is made up of enterprises that are part of industries such as the media, advanced professional and corporate services, finance, and headquarters operations. It is home as well to an incredible array of nongovernmental organizations and cultural institutions. Its participants, who are drawn from everywhere in the world and all walks of life, are engaged in transactions and activities that are complex in nature and extremely lucrative, on the whole require a considerable amount of creativity, and serve very large and geographically extensive markets, audiences, and constituencies.[3] There is no other place in the world like it.

Table 3.2. Components of Population Change: Manhattan, 1950–2000 (in thousands)

	1950	1960	1970	1980	1990	2000
Population <65	1,789	1,491	1,324	1,224	1,291	1,350
Population 65+	171	208	215	205	197	187
Total population	1,960	1,698	1,539	1,428	1,488	1,537
Births		328	268	190	197	226
Deaths		221	216	168	160	141
Total natural increase		107	52	22	37	85
Net migration 65+		-31	-56	-44	-28	-42
Net migration <65		-338	-155	-89	51	6
Total net migration		-369	-211	-133	23	-36
Net population change[a]		-262	-159	-111	60	49

Sources: U.S. Census of Population 1950–2000; New York City Department of Health 1950–2000; estimates of net migration by author.

[a] Net population change = natural increase + net migration

Manhattan and the Other City

But this part of Manhattan, as powerful an economic concentration as it represents, is—politically speaking—no more than a highly expensive piece of real estate that is part of the Greater City created by an act of the New York State Legislature in 1898. The rest of the city, or the other New York—comprising the outer boroughs—is home to four-fifths of the city's population and contains all but 5 percent of the city's physical land area. It is no exaggeration to say that the key people, businesses, and organizations involved in the life and times of the Manhattan-based world city regard the comings and goings of this other New York as peripheral to their most vital interests.

This is increasingly reflected in the rapidly growing social and economic divide between these two parts of contemporary New York, although, historically, Manhattan has always had a disproportionate number of the rich and well-to-do in its overall population mix, and it has always been where the highest-paying and most prestigious jobs have been located.[4]

However, in times past, these worlds were bridged by the existence of a substantial middle class into which those less well off or their offspring could rise, and whose members and their children in turn could aspire to even loftier heights. The post–World War II diminution of the city's middle class, both in Manhattan and in the other New York, has greatly reduced the extent to which this upward mobility takes place.[5]

Nevertheless, despite their increasing estrangement from the life of the other New York, the global economy's movers and shakers, a surprisingly large and diverse group, are hardly unaffected by its travails. For one thing, Manhattan's global economy is by far the city's principal source of taxable wealth and thus supports a wide array of public services (education, health care, mass transit, sanitation, police) that are consumed mainly by the other New Yorkers; it also generates, despite its increasingly elite character, a great many routine clerical jobs as well as an increasing number of what might be called under-the-stairs jobs—in health care, hotels, building maintenance, and the like—which are mainly held by other New Yorkers. These are indispensable to the daily functioning of the world city's global economy, as well providing the underpinnings of the other New York's livelihoods.[6]

A Century of Population Change

By the middle of the twentieth century, New York City's population, then at eight million, had reached what so far has proven to be its all-time peak (Table 3.3). Population growth had been particularly rapid in the earlier decades of the century. Between 1900 and 1930, it went from 3.4 to 6.8 million, the combined result of what were, by today's standards, a high rate of natural increase and soaring levels of immigration. Growth slowed sharply from 1930 to 1950 owing to the passage of severely restrictive immigration legislation in the mid-1920s and a sharp reduction in birth rates. Even so, the city added just over a million people to its population during these two decades—the Great Depression and World War II notwithstanding. Such rapid population growth in cities was a common feature of the U.S. demographic landscape in the first half of the last century, with New York simply leading the way as it consolidated its position as the nation's premier city.

The postwar era. While the city's overall population remained unchanged between 1950 and 1970, the social and economic characteristics of its residents altered a great deal. During this period, large numbers of the city's younger (and almost entirely middle-income) residents and their families moved to the suburbs. Overwhelmingly, they were of white European background and were responding in a prosperous time—an economic golden age, as it has been called—to the prospect of much better housing and more spacious (and auto-friendly) surroundings.

And, indeed, much the same story was being enacted throughout the United States during this period. But as a substantial fraction of the city's middle class moved upward and outward, large numbers of black Americans from the South, as well as natives of Puerto Rico, U.S. citizens by birth, were moving in. The movement of blacks from the South, where most still lived at the end of the 1930s, to the cities in the Northeast and Midwest was a major factor in the postwar demographic

Table 3.3. Selected Population Characteristics: NYC and Manhattan, 1950–2000 (in thousands)

	Total Population		Net Change		%65+ (n)		%65+ Female (n)		85+		85+ as % of 65+	
	NYC	Mhtn.	NYC	Mhtn.	NYC	Mhtn.	NYC	Mhtn.	NYC	Mhtn.	NYC	Mhtn.
1950	7,892	1,960			7.7 (605)	8.7 (171)	54.5 (330)	55.0 (94)	21	6	3.5	3.6
1960	7,782	1,698	-110	-262	10.5 (814)	12.2 (208)	55.0 (448)	55.7 (116)	32	9	4.0	4.5
1970	7,895	1,539	113	-159	12.0 (948)	14.0 (215)	58.7 (557)	59.5 (128)	57	14	6.0	6.4
1980	7,072	1,428	-823	-111	13.5 (952)	14.3 (205)	61.9 (589)	62.9 (129)	77	17	8.1	8.3
1990	7,322	1,488	250	60	13.0 (953)	13.3 (197)	62.6 (596)	63.0 (124)	103	23	10.8	11.8
2000	8,008	1,537	686	49	11.7 (938)	12.2 (187)	61.6 (578)	60.9 (114)	122	26	13.0	13.7

Sources: U.S. Census of Population 1950–2000: estimates by author.

transformation of urban America.[7] In the case of Puerto Ricans, though, the resettlement pattern was a more idiosyncratic one, as the destinations on the U.S. mainland to which they journeyed were concentrated to an unusual extent in New York City. There were soon to be more persons of Puerto Rican background in New York than in San Juan, the commonwealth's capital city.[8]

Between 1950 and 1970, the city's non-Hispanic white population fell by 28 percent, while its combined black and Latino population tripled (Table 3.4). These two flows—one involving whites and their growing families moving from the city; the other, blacks and Latinos and their even higher birth rates moving to it—turned out to be roughly comparable in scale. But the departing whites were much better educated and better off than the latest arrivals to the big city. And while the newcomers were able to improve their well-being in the 1950s and 1960s—a period in which New York still seemingly offered enough of the kinds of economic opportunities they were able to take advantage of—this did not make up for the significantly higher and more rapidly growing incomes of the suburban-bound white families.[9]

Thus, while inflation-adjusted median family incomes in New York City increased by 76 percent between 1950 and 1970, they lagged well behind income growth in the region and the nation. Median family income in New York City, only 7 percent below that of the New York metropolitan area in 1950, had fallen to 22 percent below by 1970. Considerably complicating matters, intergroup tensions and conflicts escalated as these changes unfolded.

New York's exceptionalism. In comparison with other big cities in the United States, the stability shown by New York's population during this period is nevertheless quite remarkable. As of 1950, nine of the ten largest cities in the United States, with New York the most populous, were located in either the Northeast or the Midwest regions of the country. Over the next twenty years, the other eight experienced an aggregate population decline of 25 percent, ranging from 10 percent for Chicago to St. Louis's 25 percent. New York's better showing was based on the resilience of its Manhattan-based economy, in which blue-collar weakness—though noticeable—was offset by white-collar strength. This was unlike the situation in other big U.S. cities of this time, in which blue-collar losses outweighed white-collar gains by substantial margins (Table 3.5).

The Terrible 1970s

With the 1970s, it seemed as if the city's luck had finally run out. In this tumultuous decade, New York's previously buoyant white-collar businesses, increasingly dominated by financial services, faltered at the same time that losses in its chronically weak blue-collar industries rose dramatically. America's principal headquarters city and its go-to place for financing big deals was looking shaky.[10]

Between 1969 and 1977, New York shed 700,000 jobs—10 percent of its total at

Table 3.4. Population by Age and Race: NYC, 1950–2000 (in thousands)

	White		Black		Hispanic		Other Races		All Races	
	65+	% Total	65+	% Total	65+	% Total	65+	% Total	65+	% Total
1950	94.4	87.3	4.6	9.2	0.8	3.1	0.2	0.3	100	100
(n)	(573)	(6,890)	(28)	(729)	(5)	(246)	(1)	(27)	(607)	(7,892)
1960	91.9	77.8	6.2	13.6	1.6	7.9	0.4	0.7	100	100
(n)	(760)	(6,053)	(51)	(1,060)	(13)	(613)	(3)	(56)	(827)	(7,782)
1970	85.5	62.9	9.1	19.6	4.3	15.2	1.1	2.3	100	100
(n)	(829)	(4,967)	(88)	(1,548)	(42)	(1,202)	(11)	(178)	(970)	(7,895)
1980	78.0	52.4	12.9	24.0	6.9	19.9	2.1	3.8	100	100
(n)	(743)	(3,703)	(123)	(1,695)	(66)	(1,406)	(20)	(268)	(952)	(7,072)
1990	67.3	43.2	18.1	25.1	11.3	24.4	3.4	7.4	100	100
(n)	(651)	(3,163)	(175)	(1,836)	(109)	(1,784)	(33)	(540)	(968)	(7,323)
2000	57.5	35.0	21.3	24.5	14.9	27.0	6.3	13.5	100	100
(n)	(539)	(2,801)	(200)	(1,962)	(140)	(2,161)	(59)	(1,084)	(938)	(8,008)

Sources: U.S. Census of Population 1950–2000; estimates by author.

Table 3.5. Median Family Income: Selected Cities and U.S., 1949–1999

	1950	**1960**	**1970**	**1980**	**1990**	**2000**
Baltimore	$3,275	$5,659	$8,814	$15,721	$28,217	$35,438
Boston	$3,249	$5,747	$9,133	$16,069	$34,377	$44,151
Chicago	$3,956	$6,738	$10,239	$18,776	$30,707	$42,724
Cleveland	$3,531	$5,935	$9,098	$15,991	$22,448	$30,286
Detroit	$3,955	$6,069	$10,038	$9,961	$22,566	$33,853
Los Angeles	$3,575	$6,896	$10,530	$19,467	$34,364	$39,942
St. Louis	$3,205	$5,355	$8,173	$15,265	$28,274	$28,274
NYC	$3,526	$6,091	$9,673	$16,818	$34,360	$41,887
Manhattan	$3,073	$5,338	$8,976	$16,326	$36,831	$50,229
Philadelphia	$3,322	$5,782	$9,361	$16,388	$30,140	$37,036
Pittsburgh	$3,314	$5,605	$8,787	$17,499	$27,484	$38,795
Washington DC	$3,800	$5,993	$9,576	$19,099	$36,256	$46,283
United States	$3,083	$5,660	$9,586	$19,917	$35,225	$50,046
As % of U.S.						
NYC	1.14	1.08	1.01	0.84	0.98	0.84
Manhattan	1.00	0.94	0.94	0.82	1.05	1.00

Sources: U.S. Census of Population for current dollars 1950–2000; Annual Average Consumer Price Index 1950–2000.

the beginning of the period. Its residents' inflation-adjusted median family income dropped by 7 percent during the 1970s after having rung up substantial gains in the two preceding decades. And in the mid-1970s, to avert municipal bankruptcy, severe cutbacks were imposed on the local public sector. Major development projects were shelved and office vacancy rates reached levels not seen since the Great Depression. Crime rates continued to rise, reaching new heights in the process.

This tide of misfortune triggered a massive exodus of people from New York City. Between 1970 and 1980, the city's population declined by over 800,000 persons, and the rate of net out-migration tripled. The city's white (and largely middle-class) population was now falling at an even faster rate than it had in the postwar period. The lure of the suburbs was now augmented by the push from a declining economy and growing concerns about personal safety. Moreover, incoming blacks or Puerto Ricans, who were also put off by the souring of what was now a declining local economy, were no longer filling the population gap thus created. Henceforth, the population of both these groups would continue to grow from natural increase factors but at a much more modest pace than previously.

New York Redux

Doomsayers freely predicted more of the same. But in the face of a good deal of pessimism about its prospects, the city's economy rebounded in the late 1970s. Within a decade or so, New York's private sector employment had regained virtually all its losses, with quickening white-collar growth now more than offsetting continuing blue-collar losses. In real terms, median family income in the city rose by 22 percent during the 1980s, a whopping increase and better than four times the national rate of growth.

Responding to this stimulus, New York's population began to climb again—increasing by 3 percent during the 1980s—while net out-migration plummeted to a mere 15 percent of its pace a decade earlier. At this time, though, other Frost Belt cities with very few exceptions continued their losing ways. Although the city's economy faltered once again at the end of the 1980s—several hundred thousand jobs were lost between 1989 and 1994—once the great bull market got its second wind and the new-economy firms thronged Manhattan's so-called Silicon Alley, New York's Manhattan-based economy went into orbit for the balance of the decade. The hard times at the beginning of the decade were quickly forgotten and euphoria reigned.

As tax revenues climbed, even as tax rates fell, public services were improved—with expenditures in such areas as police and fire protection enjoying particular favor. With crime rates dropping and welfare rolls declining, there was a widespread sense that the city had become a far better place for living as well as working. Population trends responded positively to resurgent economic growth, and New York's population rose by a remarkable 10 percent between 1990 and 2000 and ended the decade back at its all-time high of around eight million.

Only a handful of the other old cities in the United States saw their populations increase during this decade, and none came close to matching New York's rate of growth. And, for the first time in its post–World War II history, New York experienced a positive net in-migration of people as a result of the surge in its foreign-born population, echoing its experience at the century's beginning.

Every Silver Lining Has a Cloud

While population growth had resumed in the 1980s and 1990s, some trends did not change. The racial composition of the city, for example, continued to alter along earlier lines. By 2000, the city's white population had fallen to 36 percent of the total, from 90 percent a half century earlier. As of century's end, approximately 25 percent of the city's population was black, 25 percent Latino, and 10 percent

Asian. Compare this with fifty years earlier, when only one of one hundred New Yorkers was Asian.

But now within each group—whether white, black, brown, or Asian—the share that was either foreign born or of foreign-born parentage was rising. In the century's final decade, a disconcerting downside accompanied the city's irrepressible diversity. For while its economy, judging by such indicators as employment and payrolls, had been booming, the same could hardly be said of the economic fortunes of many of its residents. According to the U.S. Census Bureau, the median family income in New York City fell by 7 percent between 1989 and 1999, while the comparable national figure rose by 9 percent. This decisively reversed the pattern of the preceding decade, in which, as earlier noted, the median income of the city's families increased by 22 percent, approximately four times the national rate.

The reasons for this disconnect are still far from clear. It seems to be one of those awkward facts that are duly noted without any serious attempt at an explanation. In any event, this future now looks a good deal more problematic than it did a couple of years ago. To begin with, three years of a sharply falling stock market and the ensuing wave of corporate scandals have dealt a heavy blow to the city's financial services industry, its economic mainstay. What the long-term effects of this will be are still unclear, but unqualified optimism about the future of this critical New York industry would certainly seem unwarranted at this point. This blow was further compounded by a national recession in 2001, which, though brief and shallow, has been followed by a noticeably weak recovery. In any event, its localized impact on New York City is likely to be both more serious and longer lasting than was a similarly described national economic cycle in the early 1990s.

Finally, even when the national economy regains its stride—as it surely will—and even if we assume less assuredly that shell-shocked investors eventually will return in force to the equity markets, there is still the potentially more serious long-term impact of the events of September 11, 2001, on the city's economic future.

Implications for Older Persons

Having reviewed the long-term interactions between the city's economy and its overall population, we turn to how a particular subset of this population—those sixty-five years and over—has fared. This population is presumably less affected by current changes in economic conditions because most of its members are no longer part of the active labor force and their current incomes are derived largely from pensions based on their past earnings. However, their insulation from significant changes in their immediate surroundings is far from complete.

For example, many of today's over-sixty-five individuals came of age and then raised their own families in a time and place steeped in codes of behavior that stressed deference to authority and respect for one's elders. Today, such attitudes are widely viewed as comically dispensable, much to the discomfort of older persons. For they have seemingly grown old—"aged in place," as the sociologists put it—into a far different world from the one that they had imagined inhabiting at this stage of their lives.

Half a century ago, there were just over 600,000 persons over the age of sixty-five living in New York. Amounting to 8 percent of the city's overall population, their share had been rising sharply along with the growing life expectancy of older adults. Between 1950 and 1970, while the city's nonelderly population fell by 5 percent, the city's older population increased by 60 percent, from 607,000 to 970,000, with virtually all of this increase consisting of native and foreign-born whites born in the decades around the turn of the last century who had spent their adult lives in the city.

By 1970, the share of the city's population sixty-five years of age and over had risen to 12 percent of the total. It would have been greater still if it were not for the increasing number of older whites who were now relocating when they reached the customary age of retirement. Net out-migration of the over-sixty-five popula-tion from New York City more than doubled between the 1950s and 1960s (from 50,000 to 134,000). Economically, the ability of older persons to move had been significantly enhanced by the dramatic postwar improvements in benefits under the Social Security program and in private pensions. There was also a supply-side factor at work. This was the rapid development in this period of easy-to-reach retirement communities in Florida and other states catering to what was essentially a middle-class market (see Chapter 5).[11]

The city's older population declined for the first time ever in the 1970s in ab-solute terms, falling by 2 percent, from 970,000 to 952,000. But as there had been a much sharper drop in the size of its nonelderly population at the time—down by 12 percent—the share of the over-sixty-five population continued to increase. Out-migration among over-sixty-fives doubled between the 1960s and the 1970s, from 134,000 to 289,000. Virtually all out-migration during this period took place among whites, and the city's older white population declined by 20 percent.

As contrasted with younger whites, this stepped-up outflow was for older whites more a function of the difficulties they were experiencing or anticipating as a result of the stresses caused by the city's rapidly changing racial and ethnic makeup. It is the better-off residents who left, as was true among younger households as well. By 1980, the city's median family-income level had fallen to 20 percent below the comparable national figure.

In the 1980s and the 1990s (a period of renewed growth, as we have seen), while the city's population under sixty-five years increased by 16 percent, or just under a million persons, its over-sixty-five population more or less stabilized at the level it had reached in 1970. Thus, the city's population grew "younger" in the sense that its share over the age of sixty-five—unlike the nation's—declined slightly. The size of its older white population fell by another 24 percent from 1980 to 2000, while its minority over-sixty-five population, overwhelmingly blacks and Latinos, nearly doubled in absolute terms—thus just about canceling each other out. As of 2000, however, whites still accounted for 58 percent of the city's over-sixty-five population, quite a bit higher than their 32 percent share of its under-sixty-five population.

Incomes of older persons. Despite the increasing out-migration from the city of its higher-income older households, an apparent improvement took place in the economic fortunes of its nonmobile over-sixty-five population. Between 1970 and 1980, the poverty rate among the city's sixty-five-and-over population fell from 22 to 15 percent (in a period in which the poverty rate among its population under sixty-five years increased from 14 to 20.8 percent; see Table 3.6).

As in the postwar period, this improvement was primarily the result of further increases in Social Security payments. Nevertheless, during this period the relative economic standing of the city's older population, vis-à-vis the nation's, worsened. In 1970, the city's poverty rate for older persons (22 percent) was four percentage points below the national figure. But by 1980, it was on a par with the nation's. And worse was to follow. In the course of the following two decades, the poverty rate for the city's older population increased from 14 to 18 percent, while the poverty rate for the nation's sixty-five-and-over population declined to 10 percent.

Women have considerably higher rates of poverty than do men—from 36 percent more for those sixty-five to seventy-four to 55 percent more for those over seventy-five. Family arrangements as well bear on the well-being of older persons. Married older couples have poverty rates approximately 70 percent below those who live alone. Finally, race and ethnicity have a strong bearing on the distribution of poverty. The poverty rate among the city's older black, Latino, and Asian populations runs from two to three times that for whites.

Published local area data on the incomes of elderly persons (as opposed to pov-

Table 3.6. Poverty Rate among Persons 65+ and <65 Years: NYC and U.S., 1970–2000 (as percent of age cohort)

	Total below Poverty		Persons 65+ below Poverty		Persons <65 below Poverty	
	NYC	U.S.	NYC	U.S.	NYC	U.S.
1970	14.9	13.7	21.7	26.0	14.0	12.3
1980	20.0	12.4	14.4	14.8	20.8	12.1
1990	19.3	13.1	16.5	12.8	19.7	13.2
2000	21.2	12.4	17.8	9.9	22.2	12.3

Source: U.S. Census of Population, 1970–2000.

erty-rate data only) became available in the 1990 census. As of 2000, the median income of New York's households headed by persons sixty-five to seventy-four years of age was 13 percent below the comparable national figure, and 14 percent below in the case of households headed by persons seventy-five and over. Ten years earlier, the incomes of New York households in the age group from sixty-five to seventy-four had been 2 percent above the corresponding national figure, and 2 percent below for the seventy-five-and-over age group. Between 1990 and 2000, median household income for the age group sixty-five to seventy-four registered a 52 percent increase nationally, well above this period's inflation rate. For New York, however, its gain of 30 percent barely kept pace with inflation (Table 3.7).

Census data on poverty and income refer strictly to money income. This obviously falls short of providing a full picture of the trends in well-being among older people. For example, since the mid-1960s the Medicare and Medicaid programs have provided significant additions to the command over resources by the elderly in the form of heavily subsidized medical care and now, increasingly, of home care. The sums involved are quite substantial and obviously have made quite a difference in the amount and kind of personal and health care that older individuals receive. For example, as of 2000, expenditures on Medicare, which are overwhelmingly for health-care services to persons sixty-five years of age and over, were valued at 65 percent of the Social Security payments going to this age group.[12]

At the national level, a major source of wealth and potential income for older persons has been the appreciation that has taken place in the value of the homes they own. Nearly all the net worth of older-homeowner households takes the form of the value, net of mortgage debt, of their primary residence. By the time most homeowners reach the age of sixty-five, they are typically free and clear of all mortgage debt. And despite the need to pay the out-of-pocket costs of maintenance and property taxes—the latter often levied at reduced rates for older homeowners—that they are debt-free enables them to live at what amounts to reduced rents. Under a variety

Table 3.7. Median Income of Households Headed by Persons 65+: U.S., NYC, and Manhattan, 1990 and 2000

	1990		2000		% Increase	
	65–74	**75+**	**65–74**	**75+**	**65–74**	**75+**
U.S.	$20,653	$13,149	$31,368	$22,259	52	69
NYC	$21,050	$12,920	$27,271	$19,196	30	49
Manhattan	$21,440	$14,710	$29,925	$21,569	40	47

Source: U.S. Census of Population, 1990–2000.

40   Growing Older in World Cities   Part II: New York

of so-called reverse mortgage arrangements, they can, if they so desire, withdraw some of their accumulated wealth for current expenditure purposes.

By comparison, renters with equivalent current money income enjoy none of these advantages or options. Compared with most parts of the country, a much smaller proportion of older New Yorkers are homeowners. As of 2000, only 40 percent of the city's households headed by persons sixty-five and over owned homes, while the comparable national figure was 78 percent. The city's rate has been rising (it was only 35 percent in 1990), but even this figure is inflated, because a significant portion of housing classified as owner occupied by the census among the elderly in New York City takes the form of government-subsidized multifamily units, in which the owner's ability to cash in on rising property values is anywhere from highly constrained to nonexistent.[13]

Ominous signs ahead. New York's older population has become worse off by both national and regional standards over the last few decades and is falling further behind. It is likely that in the period ahead, the median older household in the city may even experience an absolute decline in its standard of living. One ominous sign of this possibility is that in the 1990s, the income of this typical older household in the city barely kept pace with inflation, even though the incomes of older households were then benefiting from much higher payments from private retirement programs, which were supplemental to their Social Security pensions.

While exact figures are not yet available from the 2000 census, it seems likely that at least 50 percent of the city's households headed by persons over the age of sixty-five receive some amount of retirement income in addition to their Social Security pensions (in which the extent of coverage is a good deal higher). Average retirement incomes for New York residents more than doubled in the 1990s—from $8,600 to $17,700 per household—while average Social Security payments increased by only 39 percent (from $7,700 to $10,800). The point is that in the foreseeable future it is highly unlikely that payouts from private pension schemes will come close to matching their performance of a decade earlier.

Among older persons, what groups are likely to be affected by this development? A good guess is that the beneficiaries of most private retirement pensions—including those operated by state and local governments for their retired employees—are in the upper quartile of the over-sixty-five household-income distribution. That means that three-quarters of older pensioners will not be affected all that much by these impending cutbacks. However, a substantial number of middle-class older households will still face the prospect of sliding real incomes over the next few years at least.

Even more troubling is that the percentage of older New Yorkers drawing Social Security pensions fell from 84 percent to 79 percent of the total sixty-five-and-over population between 1990 and 2000. The comparable national figure in 2000 was 94 percent, and this was unchanged from its 1990 level. There are a number of possible explanations for this significant (and alarming) discrepancy. One is that a great many older New Yorkers have never accumulated enough credits to qualify for Social Security. They could be either long-term undocumented immigrants or very recent but nevertheless legal immigrants brought in under family-reunification provisions of the immigration laws. Another dire possibility is that there is a sizable group of people who either habitually worked off the books at marginally paying jobs or were institutionalized for lengthy periods.

In response to this situation, there has been a substantial increase in the number of older New Yorkers receiving benefits under the federally funded Supplemental Security Income (SSI) program, which is restricted to and designed for persons whose income falls below the poverty level. Between 1990 and 2000, the number of New York's older SSI recipients increased by 27 percent, rising from 11 percent of the city's over-sixty-five population to 17 percent.[14]

The old get older. One of the inescapable consequences of the increasing life span of older adults is that the number of the much more problematic "old old" is increasing at a considerably faster pace than are the largely nonproblematic "young old" (or, as *The Economist* so politically incorrectly put it, the "hale wrinklies").[15] The number of New Yorkers between sixty-five and seventy-four years of age declined by 13 percent between 1970 and 2000, from 626,000 to 495,000, as the city's eighty-five-and-over population (the aforementioned "old old") more than doubled and now accounts for 13 percent (and still rising) of its over-sixty-five population. The in-between group, the seventy-five- to eight-four-year-olds, increased over this period by 21 percent, from 265,000 to 321,000. The aging of the aged is most pronounced among whites, who as of 2000 accounted for close to 70 percent of the city's eighty-five-and-over population and for more than three-fifths of its over-seventy-five group.

Because women outlive men by many years, the aging of the over-sixty-five population has meant its feminization as well. In 1950, there were 88 older men for every 100 women of the same age living in the city. By 1990, the comparable figure had fallen to 60 men to 100 women of a certain age. Among the old old, the ratio is 40 men for every 100 women. However, there seems to be light at the end of the tunnel for the male of the species, as the gulf between the mortality rates of the sexes has more recently begun to narrow. This statistic may account at least in part for the reversal in this very long-running trend in the 1990s, when the New York City sixty-five-and-over male/female ratio edged up to 62 per 100. But given the size of the existing longevity gap, among the elderly, men in New York and elsewhere will continue to be outnumbered by women for the foreseeable future.

As people age, their concern about being able to maintain some degree of autonomy mounts. Their overriding fear is having to go into a nursing home. One measure of the degree to which they actually succeed in maintaining their autonomy is reflected in census data on the household arrangements of older persons. On this score, it seems that 95 percent of older persons both locally and nationally are able to continue to live independently and only 5 percent are in group quarters of some sort.[16] Since midcentury, when it was at 7 percent, the share of New York's older population in group quarters fell by 1970 to just under 5 percent, where it has remained despite the sizeable increase in the proportion of the older old, with their much higher rates of institutionalization. Indeed, there was a very sharp drop between 1990 and 2000 in New York in the rate of institutionalization among the over-eighty-fives, from a bit over 18 percent to under 15 percent.

Among the young old, men have a somewhat higher rate of institutionalization than do women, but past that point their relative positions shift. Of women over the age of eighty-five, 17 percent live in group quarters, while only 11 percent of comparably aged males do. These rates, too, vary by race and ethnicity, with blacks having the highest rate, followed by whites, Latinos, and Asians, in that order. Elderly blacks are much more likely to live in group quarters than are elderly Latinos, and by far the lowest rate of group-quarters living exists among Asians, despite their incomes being lower than those of either blacks or Latinos, much less those of whites.

Within the past decade or so, the greater availability of Medicaid-financed home-care services have increasingly made it possible for older people, and particularly the very old, to remain in their own homes.[17] Obviously, the need for home care is extensive. As of 2000, 17 percent of older persons in New York reported having difficulties with personal care—bathing, food preparation, and the like—or with mobility outside the home; a third were disabled on both scores. As one might expect, disability increases with age: 13 percent among sixty-five- to seventy-four-year-olds and double that for those seventy-five years of age and over. Women report a considerably higher rate than men do—22 percent versus 16 percent—and the difference between the sexes widens with age.

As we have seen, relatively few of the elderly are shunted off to nursing homes, although with the progressive aging of the aged it becomes more and more difficult to keep their numbers from growing, even in cities like New York where the overall over-sixty-five population is not likely to change by much. That brings us to the question of what sorts of housing arrangements and household relationships the other 95 percent maintain. As of 2000, three-fifths of older New Yorkers lived in family households, that is, in separate living units occupied by two or more related people. Nationally, this figure is 64 percent, which suggests that older New Yorkers are more likely than are their national or suburban counterparts to be part of nonfamily households, that is, living arrangements in which two or more unrelated people share a home or, more typically, in which a woman lives alone. One further distinguishing feature of family living among older New Yorkers is that they are much less likely to be married. More of them live with other relatives or as parents in households headed by one of their children. This does not signify any great return to an earlier age in which much higher proportions of the elderly lived with their adult married children. While the rate at which older New Yorkers nest with their married or unmarried adult children is considerably higher than the national figure of 4 percent, it still represents only 8 percent of the total. Asians are the group in which this practice is most prevalent, accounting for an astounding 20 percent of older Asians, followed at some distance by Latinos, with whites showing the lowest rate of all.

However, given the differences in longevity between the sexes, living longer and independently also means that a significant part of the elderly population—women, to an overwhelming extent—will end up living alone as the surviving members of what were once married couples. Of older New Yorkers, excluding those who are institutionalized, 34 percent live in such circumstances, four percentage points above the national rate. Locally (as well as nationally), three-quarters are women. What is interesting, though, is that the percentage of older persons living alone has remained more or less unchanged both locally and nationally over the last couple of decades, despite the continued aging of the older population. One possible explanation is that because the rise in housing costs has outstripped the increase in the incomes of single older individuals, as opposed to the combined incomes of older households that typically contain more than one older person, more of the elderly who would have opted to live alone have been sharing residences.

It is widely believed that New York City has a disproportionately large gay and lesbian population, although it is impossible to say how large with any confidence, especially if one has to rely on census data. However, there are some clues that suggest the numbers are substantial. For example, 11 percent of older New Yorkers, better than one out of ten, have never married. This compares to 4 percent, fewer than one out of twenty, for the United States as a whole. This rate is strikingly higher in Manhattan, which has several longstanding gay and lesbian neighborhoods that have historically been magnets for young homosexuals throughout the United States and probably from everywhere in the world. It is of course true that younger people who are heterosexual are today marrying later in life and many apparently will, according to surveys of their intentions, never marry at all. But this trend reflects a change in lifestyle that was not widespread at the time the present cohort of elderly in New York was younger.

How Manhattan Became a World City

Manhattan is now viewed as one of the priciest residential real estate markets in the United States and, indeed, in the world. But that has not always been the case. During the long period in which its population was falling (most of the past century), while residential Manhattan contained disproportionate shares of its region's highest- and lowest-income households, in absolute terms, the number of its poor and working-class households far outnumbered those of the well-to-do. The lowest-income households continued to live there because Manhattan's economy, until the 1960s, provided a great many unskilled and semiskilled blue-collar and service jobs, as well as a large supply of cheap housing.

Most of the blue-collar workers employed in Manhattan, particularly the better-paid ones, commuted to their jobs from the outer boroughs or Upper Manhattan, where the new subway lines had made it possible to build better-quality housing than had been possible in the high-value land areas adjoining the business district. Nevertheless, a great many of them still lived and worked within the Manhattan business district itself. In fact, up through the 1970s, the streets and avenues within a fifteen-minute walk of the East and West Side waterfronts were still packed with unreconstructed five- and six-story tenements built on a for-profit basis by private interests for working-class families at the turn of the century.[18] Poorly built to begin with, they had suffered from decades of undermaintenance. In addition, further bolstering the working-class character of such neighborhoods as the Lower East Side and Central and East Harlem, a substantial number of subsidized low-rent high-rise housing projects had been built within them in the decades after World War II.

That, of course, was not all there was to Manhattan's housing market at the time. Throughout the last century, Manhattan's economy was undergoing continual change as its white-collar businesses expanded (and as its blue-collar ones faded). It had long been the U.S. financial capital, but very early in the century it also became the widely acknowledged front office for the nation's major corporations and the large number of specialist businesses that were drawn to them.

The top people, the families of the highest-paid employees or principals who were employed in one of these enterprises, whether in downtown's financial district or in midtown's more recently developed corporate headquarters and business services complex, resided in a handful of tightly circumscribed gold-coast enclaves such as the Upper East Side blocks that border Central Park South or, more and more, in one of the city's growing number of upmarket suburbs. But by the 1920s, the families of the office-based middle class were deserting Manhattan. At first they opted for the more desirable sections of the outer boroughs, the "subway suburbs," in Peter Derrick's felicitous phrase.[19] But after World War II and the return of peacetime prosperity, they too moved out to the suburbs.

With the collapse in the 1970s of Manhattan's blue-collar economy, the working-class neighborhoods that abutted the business district became prime candidates for recycling to new uses and users, assuming these were at hand. And such recycling quickly became amply clear. Driving this change was the increased demand for housing situated close to the business district from an upper-middle-income group that was pouring into Manhattan's workplaces as its economy entered a new phase. Earlier on, Manhattan had been merely the nation's front office, the workplace of choice of a high proportion of the headquarters operations of the kinds of big companies that made up the Fortune 500 lists. These were mainly companies that were principally focused on domestic markets. But from the 1970s on, U.S. businesses began to go global. Indeed, this was the case for major businesses in all industrially advanced countries. The global economy had been born—or more accurately, as economic historians were quick to point out, reborn.

The desire to live close to the global economy's Manhattan base of operations has grown particularly intense in the last few decades, with the result that rents and house values in the markets catering to households in this sector have skyrocketed. One of the reasons individuals working in the global economy have been able to pay these costs is that they are themselves highly rewarded. How highly? In 1970, the average wage per employee was 38 percent higher than the comparable U.S. figure. By 2000, the Manhattan "premium" had advanced to 149 percent. In Manhattan's all-important financial services sector, the comparable differential had advanced from over 86 percent to over 330 percent.

The social composition of Manhattan's residential population has shifted in response to the changing character of its workplaces. Between 1970 and 2000, the proportion of Manhattanites twenty-five years of age and older who had at a minimum graduated from a four-year college increased from 21 to 49 percent, or double the national rate and twenty-seven percentage points above that for the outer boroughs.

The response of the housing market to this demand has been swift. Many formerly working-class or lower-middle-class residential neighborhoods in such areas as the Upper West Side or the easternmost blocks of the Upper East Side—via a combi-nation of new construction and extensive rehabilitation—have been recycled into luxury housing by a market-driven process which combined locational convenience (for work as well as play), population turnover, new construction, and extensive rehabilitation. Under the influence of the expanding global economy sector, the last few decades have seen these neighborhoods grow far beyond what had long been considered their settled boundaries. Thus, the area that today is considered the Upper East Side luxury housing district covers twice the physical area and housing units it would have been described as encompassing two or so decades ago.

These developments have increasingly priced extensive portions of Manhattan's residential real estate out of the reach of what would ordinarily be viewed as lower-middle- or moderate-income households and has created greater difficulties for lower-income individuals and families. Those on lower incomes who manage to retain what must be seen as an increasingly insecure foothold in Manhattan either live in its extant downmarket neighborhoods or, if they live elsewhere, manage to remain there only because of the city's long-lived rent-regulation system or because of its still ample supply of subsidized housing, built in another era for a clientele composed of lower- and moderate income households.

Neighborhoods of Older Persons

Few neighborhoods in New York City can be said to be dominated by persons who are sixty-five years of age and older—certainly not in the same sense that the city's neighborhoods can be said to be dominated by particular racial or ethnic groups. Of course, the degree of measured domination is a function of how narrowly or widely one defines a neighborhood.

One frequently used definition is that embodied in the community-district system. At this level of geographical disaggregation, the elderly look to be widely dispersed. Measured by the proportion of population sixty-five years of age or over, the "oldest" of the twelve community districts in Manhattan is the Middle East Side's District 6, with just under 15 percent in this age group; the youngest is Lower Manhattan's District 1, with 7 percent. Because of their much smaller average household size, households headed by older persons carry a greater weight in the housing market than they do when viewed strictly in population terms. Approximately one of five of Manhattan's occupied housing units have heads of household over the age of sixty-five.

To portray the diversity of the neighborhoods in which New York's older population lives, we have divided the city into three parts: Manhattan 1, Manhattan 2, and the first ring (which includes the four outer boroughs of Brooklyn, Queens, Staten Island, and the Bronx). We separated Manhattan's neighborhoods into two divisions because the lion's share of the residents of certain parts of Manhattan—whether old or young—have as little to do with Manhattan's persona as do the residents of the outer boroughs.

Manhattan 1. Manhattan 1 includes the residential areas contiguous to or within easy walking distance of Manhattan's central business district: the Upper West Side, the Upper East Side, Greenwich Village, Chelsea, Clinton, Murray Hill, Soho, Noho, and Tribeca. Geographically speaking, Manhattan 1's neighborhoods are in the borough's southern and middle portions, reaching up to Columbia University's campus on the West Side and the medical complexes of upper Fifth Avenue on the East Side.

The real estate markets in this part of residential New York are acutely responsive to the kinds of demands for housing and neighborhood amenities that arise from the households of the growing ranks of highly educated and handsomely compensated managers and professionals employed in Manhattan's global economy sector. As of 2000, approximately one out of ten of Manhattan 1's population was over the age of sixty-five. That accounts for fewer than three-fifths of Manhattan's over-sixty-five population, not much different from their share twenty years earlier. Manhattan 1's overall population has increased by 8 percent over the last two decades, while its sixty-five-and-over population has fallen by 9 percent.

Manhattan 2. Manhattan 2 includes such neighborhoods as Harlem (East and West), the Lower East Side, Washington Heights, and Inwood. With the exception of the Lower East Side, all of Manhattan 2's neighborhoods are located in the northernmost portions of the borough. Its households for the most part occupy high-rise public housing and lower-middle-income housing projects, as well as substantial pockets of aging and poorly maintained five- and six-story tenement buildings.

As of 2000, seventy-nine thousand residents of Manhattan 2's neighborhoods were over the age of sixty-five, or one out of ten residents, accounting for 43 percent of Manhattan's total over-sixty-five population. As was the case in Manhattan 1, Manhattan 2's overall population has been increasing, while its over-sixty-five population has been dropping. And while Manhattan 1's over-sixty-five population is overwhelmingly white (86 percent), Manhattan 2's is overwhelmingly black and Latino (78 percent), which is in line with the racial composition of their respective overall populations. The majority of Manhattan 1's older population was born either in New York State or in other parts of the Northeast. The majority of Manhattan 2's older population was born either in the southern United States or in Puerto Rico.

Beyond race and nativity, though obviously related to them, there are sharp differences in the educational attainment, income, and employment of older persons in Manhattan 1 and Manhattan 2. As of 1990, 32 percent of Manhattan 1's over-sixty-five population had graduated from a four-year college or better, a rate three times higher than that for the United States. The comparable figure for Manhattan 2 was only 9 percent. And while 62 percent of Manhattan 2's older residents had not completed high school, this was the case for only 26 percent of older persons in Manhattan 1.

As might be expected from the considerable differences in their educational attainments, 27 percent of Manhattan 1's older persons were employed in 1990, compared with 12 percent in Manhattan 2. Median household income of the older persons in Manhattan 1 was three to four times greater than that of their Manhattan 2 counterparts. Home ownership among older households rose quite sharply in Manhattan 1 between 1990 and 2000, from 24 to 33 percent. By 2000, only 10 percent of Manhattan 2's older households owned their homes (or, more typically, apartments), up from 7 percent a decade earlier.

Thirty-six percent of Manhattan 1's older persons were part of (currently) married households, not that different from Manhattan 2's 34 percent. Most of the nonmarried individuals in both areas had been widowed, with a considerably smaller number having been either divorced or separated. Eighteen percent of older persons in Manhattan 2 had never married, while in Manhattan 1 the comparable figure was 14 percent. Forty-seven percent of Manhattan 1's noninstitutionalized older population lives alone, as does 38 percent of Manhattan 2's. The comparable figure for the United States as a whole is 30 percent. The much higher proportion of older persons who live alone in Manhattan reflects a stubborn fact of Manhattan life and the kind of person it attracts. Manhattan's under-sixty-five population also lives alone at much higher rates than its peers in the rest of the country and has, according to the U.S. census, for at least the last half century.

Outer boroughs. Slightly more than 80 percent of the city's older population—approximately three-quarters of a million people—lives in the outer boroughs. The total population of the outer boroughs has risen about 15 percent since 1980, while its over-sixty-five population has remained unchanged. As of 2000, outer borough whites accounted for 58 percent of its older population, considerably less than their 72 percent share ten years earlier. But in view of the advanced age profile of the outer borough's older whites, the contraction in this portion of its over-sixty-five population is bound to accelerate over the next decade. On the other hand, the growth of its minority nonwhite older population seems likely to increase enough to ensure a modest amount of net growth in the outer boroughs' overall older population.

The outer borough elderly represent too large and diverse a population to generalize easily about. We know that their better-off generational counterparts have either moved to the suburbs earlier in their family life cycles or ended up living in Manhattan 1. Outer borough neighborhoods run the gamut from prosperous and well-tended homeowner communities to physically decrepit crime-ridden areas. By comparison with those of Manhattan 1 or the country as a whole, their levels of educational attainment are modest—as of 2000 only 12 percent had graduated from college, though this was up a quite a bit from ten years earlier. However, they were somewhat more likely to have graduated at least from high school than were their Manhattan 2 counterparts. As of 2000, the median household incomes for sixty-five- to seventy-four-year-olds in the outer boroughs ranged from well below the comparable figure for the nation or for Manhattan 1 in the case of the Bronx and Brooklyn, to well above in Queens and Staten Island. Similarly, the employment rate for its over-sixty-five population was half that for Manhattan 1 and has fallen.

Of the over-sixty-five population, a considerably higher proportion in the outer boroughs was currently married than in either Manhattan 1 or 2 and a considerably smaller proportion had never been married. While these observations apply across racial and ethnic lines, outer borough elderly whites and Asians are much likelier to be currently married than are similarly aged blacks and Latinos.

The nature of the problem of social isolation among the elderly can best be seen in the neighborhoods of the outer boroughs that still have significant numbers of white households, a high proportion of which consist of widowed women who live alone. Among outer borough whites, the ratio of the older white population to the under-sixty-five white population has fallen from one out of twelve in 1950, to one out of five in 1970, and one out of four in 2000. Moreover, a high proportion of the working-age whites are themselves close to retirement. In the outer boroughs, although black, Hispanic, and Asian older persons live largely in neighborhoods where the majority of younger persons look like they do, this is hardly a guarantee against their isolation.

Older outer borough Asians and Latinos are much more likely to live with their children or other relatives than are either whites or blacks, which is also the case in Manhattan. But with the exception of Asians, a high proportion of the outer borough elderly live alone, ranging from 25 percent for Latinos to 35 percent for whites. The simple fact of living in a neighborhood in which young and old are part of the same racial or ethnic group brings no guarantee for the elderly of safe passage in their daily lives. The connection between Manhattan's economy and the outer boroughs obviously goes beyond the former's role as a tax base to pay for services consumed by the latter. Probably the more critical long-term question concerns the extent to which Manhattan's economy is able to assimilate and absorb into productive employment the young and middle-aged adults who live in the outer boroughs. Success on that score would go a long way toward improving the lives of their older population in the future simply because it would make these neighborhoods less turbulent and crime prone. Failure would do the reverse, irrespective of whatever palliative measures targeted toward the elderly can be devised.

Growing Old in a World City

World cities such as New York, which contain massive chunks of the most lucrative parts of the global economy sector, can be great places to live in for the well-to do, ambitious, and highly successful. Indeed, these are the very places to which they are drawn as they either pursue or have finally attained the top prizes generated by the world's advanced industrial economies. They are highly diverting places as well, with their rich cultural and entertainment offerings. And they are interesting, if expensive, places in which to pursue one's varied lifetime interests and to sample the sorts of psychic rewards that come from being among the rich world's movers and shakers.

However, to live this kind of life it is necessary to have a great deal of money. It is necessary, in fact, to have enough money so that money, as some might say, is no problem. However, older persons in New York City who answer this description are few in number though thicker on the ground than elsewhere. For example, of the just under 600,000 households in New York City in 2000 headed by persons sixty-five years of age and over, only 32,000 had annual incomes of $125,000 and above, which, arguably, might be considered a rough approximation of "enough" money. Thus on a citywide basis, these very high-income older households accounted for one in twenty of all older households. The comparable figure was one in ten for Manhattan as a whole; on the Upper East Side, the most affluent of Manhattan 1's neighborhoods, it was just under one in three. For the United States, less than 4 percent of older households surpassed this income mark.

The very well-off elderly, thus defined, as well as those who occupy its middling ranks—which we have generously defined as those with incomes between $30,000 and $125,000—are, by and large, able to look after themselves. The problem in a place like New York, as in virtually all big U.S. cities, is that there is a much larger and fast-growing cohort of low- and moderate-income elderly households, most of them black or Hispanic, which require a great deal of assistance. In 2000, 38 percent of all New York households headed by over-sixty-fivers had incomes below $15,000 a year, with little difference in this respect between Manhattan and the outer boroughs. The comparable national figure was a good deal lower, 27 percent. And while the share of very low-income households in the older household mix at the national level seems to have either remained the same or fallen slightly, New York's situation has worsened considerably.

What, one might ask an older person in such straitened circumstances who happens to be a resident of the Big Apple, do you gain from living in the erstwhile capital of global capitalism? Does the unique nature of Manhattan's highly dynamic, market-driven economy, which so dominates the city's daily existence, have any real significance for the way you live?

Asking such a question implies that the respondent has a choice in the matter of whether to live in New York or in another and perhaps more congenial place or, for that matter, is even interested in or capable of making such a choice. Realistically speaking, most older people, after considering the options available to them, would like nothing better than to age in place. And for reasons good and bad, though certainly understandable, they are more resistant to changing places than younger people are. The poorer they are, the fewer their choices and the greater their sense of inertia and helplessness—a particular challenge in a place like New York which, world city or not, is home to a disproportionately large number of low-income elderly and faces the almost certain prospect of even greater numbers in the foreseeable future.

But poor (or poorer) health, despite the miracles of modern medicine and its vast pharmacopoeia, is still an inevitable part of the aging process and brings in its wake a set of problems involved in ministering to the needs of the elderly that did not exist when few people survived long beyond the formal retirement age. A society such as ours will find it harder and harder to put off confronting the challenge of providing "good enough" care for the old that goes beyond such low-hanging fruit as Meals-on-Wheels and the occasional visit by a busy and bureaucratically inclined social worker.

This is obviously easier said than done. In times past, families were expected to provide care for their older members, a task immeasurably easier when the remaining lifespan of older adults was a good deal shorter than is now the case and there were more adult siblings to share the responsibilities. Many hands, as they say, make light work. And, not least, families of that bygone age had another built-in advantage: married daughters who did not work outside the home and were thus available for parental caregiving when the need arose.

It would be easy to cite other reasons modern families are either less capable or less willing to serve in loco parentis for their aging parents. And there is a further complication: the increasing number of adults who never form long-lasting relationships in or out of marriage. Parents may be able to exert some moral claim on their adult children, but what of the childless? The much greater prevalence of single never-married adults in New York's older population makes this a matter of particular local concern. Nor has there been much attention paid to the particular aging concerns of New York's large gay and lesbian communities.[20]

There is another kind of fault line visible in the system, if it may be characterized in such terms, which has developed to meet the needs of an aging population in New York and arises mainly from changes in the family structure available to the minority elderly. A high proportion of today's elderly New Yorkers are likely to be the U.S-born children of parents who came to the United States from southern and eastern Europe in the opening quarter of the twentieth century, just before highly restrictive quotas were imposed on new immigrants, particularly those—Jews, Italians, Greeks, Poles—from this part of Europe. They were raised in modest circumstances and most, it can be speculated, spent their working lives in jobs of the sort that at retirement age placed them in what would in today's terms be the lower-middle portion of the overall income distribution. Many, possibly most, of the more economically successful members of this generation moved to the suburbs and thus are no longer part of the city's elderly population. Chances are that those who didn't suburbanize, the less successful ones, had children who did better than their parents in a material sense—having enjoyed, among other advantages, the benefits of considerably higher levels of formal education.

However, in the American scheme of things, economic success and suburban-ization go hand in hand. This means that the working-class or lower-middle-class white elderly still living in the city, as they have throughout their adult lives, are now geographically separated from their offspring. All other things being equal, geographical distance creates a problem in the many situations in which an aging parent needs to reach out to an adult child for assistance.

In such situations, living in the next town or on the other side of the country is a lot different from living down the block, even with the great advances made in electronic forms of communication. However, given the widespread prevalence of intact nuclear families within this group, the social support system represented by the extended family is probably still operative in terms of the help that adult children offer their aging parents when the need arises. And the capacity to provide assistance is greater when the family unit is large than when it is small. That people of this generation and background had two to three children on average makes it easier for their adult children to share the obligation to provide support.

How, in a similar manner, would it be possible to portray the life and times of a significant group drawn from the elderly blacks in New York City, who are rapidly on their way to dominating the city's elderly population? To begin with, it is impor-tant to note that a considerable portion of these individuals were born in the U.S. South and raised in a harsh and oppressive environment of what was then a regime of legally sanctioned discrimination. They came north as young adults seeking economic opportunity and social and civic freedom in cities like New York during and after World War II as part of what has been justly called the Great Migration, whose numbers more than matched those of earlier white European immigrants. There is little question that one of the consequences of this massive relocation was an immediate improvement in their economic circumstances.

However, unlike that of white European immigrants, the upward mobility of the black migrants soon ground to a halt, and they were unable to sustain these early gains throughout their working lives. Much of this failure has been ascribed to the dramatic changes which early on began to transform the postwar economic landscape of big U.S. cities, as their blue-collar industries collapsed and a yawning disconnect opened between the skill sets of the new migrants and the requirements called for by their new growth areas. While this is undoubtedly a simplified version of what was a very complex causal chain, the result is a cohort of elderly blacks who, because of their low lifetime earnings and intermittent employment histories, are characterized by, among other negative social indicators, very high rates of income poverty.

Moreover, their children are, in the aggregate, able to offer them little in the way of support either economically or socially. This is so even though these now elderly blacks had many more children than did their white counterparts, and even though a higher proportion of their now adult children still live in the same city, or even the same neighborhood, as their aging parents. Like successful whites, better-off inner-city blacks, although there were fewer of them, moved to the suburbs. It is safe to say that the families of nonmobile blacks of this generation who have aged in the city were characterized by a high incidence of family instability, and that a great many of the children raised in such circumstances became adults who, far from being in a position to help others, including their parents, were soon heavily dependent on the not always effective or dependable resources of the local welfare state. The extent to which this is indeed the case is perhaps most poignantly indicated by recently available data from the census on the degree to which black children are being raised by (and are financially dependent on) their grandparents. While this statistic may be cited by some as an illustration of the strengths of the extended black family, it can also be as or more compellingly interpreted as an indicator of its weakness.

Since older people are so diverse in their backgrounds, interests, and resources, short of a detailed survey it is possible to answer the question with which this section began in only the most cursory manner. For example, one of the great advantages of living in a world city is said to be the greater availability of publicly accessible entertainment and cultural venues. Older persons with strong and well-developed artistic and intellectual interests—a minority, one would say, among the city's existing and emerging older population—undoubtedly place a high value on this aspect of the city's life. On the other hand, someone less educated and otherwise inclined would find the New York described and dissected in the Arts and Leisure section of the Sunday *New York Times* as, well, an intimidating snore.

This is not an example of condescension but simply an acknowledgment that who you were when younger will have a great bearing on your attitudes and preferences, not to speak of your economic situation, when you reach your more advanced years. We can realistically expect that New York City and Manhattan, because of their underlying demographics, will continue to be home to large numbers of older people for whom the issue of improved access to a rich menu of museums, libraries, and the like will take a distant second place to such mundane matters as low-priced and nutritious meals delivered at home and physical assistance in keeping medical appointments.

Certainly the fact that New York's Manhattan-based economy is increasingly synonymous with or dominated by the care and feeding of the global economy sector can be of little direct interest to older persons as a possible source of income. Few of them possess the skills or physical dexterity that employment in the global economy sector requires. The downward trend in the employment rate among older New Yorkers during the 1990s, a period in which the local economy was exceptionally strong, is indicative of the growing divergence between the skills of older locals and those sought by employers in the New York economy.

Substantial benefits nevertheless accrue to those who grow old in the Big Apple. A locality with the good fortune to attract a substantial chunk of global economy activity will inevitably possess an enhanced local tax base that could well be used to provide better than average services useful to its older residents. And beyond the additions to the local tax base, there are the blessings of philanthropy for those lucky enough to live within a community with which the philanthropist identifies.

Thus, because great fortunes are made by those who operate in the highest reaches of the global economy, it is no accident that Manhattan's hospitals and other health-care facilities disproportionately enjoy the benefactions showered on them by those so blessed, which enables them to remain great centers of medical research. Society in general benefits from this use of private wealth, but it might be of especial value to a particular subset of those prodigious consumers of medical care, the local old. Living in the South Bronx may have few obvious advantages, but this may be one not as readily available to the older residents of most other parts of the country.

One frequently cited advantage for the elderly of living in New York is that its global economy sector attracts a great many immigrants who work at jobs and for wages that native-born Americans shun. Global economy cities generate a great many below- stairs opportunities in places like hotels and restaurants, nursing homes, hospitals, restaurants, and the home- and health-care sectors.

Older persons are particularly heavy consumers of many of these kinds of services, and older persons in a place like New York benefit greatly from the presence of so many people drawn to a city where these opportunities exist in so many forms and on such a considerable scale. For the immigrants themselves, working at such low-wage jobs is not easy and often leads to difficult and contentious relationships with those they are caring for, as well as with the organizations responsible for providing the services involved. But they come nevertheless, because it is better than remaining in their countries of origin and, once here, there is always the hope of better days for themselves or their children.

Hardly least in any enumeration of the possible advantages of a place like New York for the elderly is the not so simple matter of being able to get around. Because of its size, density, and history, New York—like most other world cities—is richly endowed with public transportation systems that can, with some ingenuity, be conveniently and economically accessed by the elderly, offering them a degree of personal mobility that in most other rich world urban places are available only to people who own cars. In this respect, it is useful to note that while the transit system operates on a citywide basis, Manhattan, because of its much greater degree of residential concentration and density, is second to none among the boroughs in respect to its user-friendly public transit facilities.

Looking Ahead

What changes can be expected over the next decade in the size and characteristics of New York's older population? From a statistical point of view, predicting the size of the sixty-five-and-over population requires quantifying two principal factors: life expectancy at older ages and the migration rates among older New Yorkers.

Life expectancy among older adults can be anticipated to increase as it has been doing for the last century or so. This means that there will be more older New Yorkers in the future, and that more of them will be in the "oldest-old" category. Between 1980 and 2000, the city's sixty-five-and-over population fell by less than 2 percent, but its eight-five-and-over population increased by 58 percent and currently amounts to 13 percent of the sixty-five-and-over population.

But the dynamic factor influencing medium- and long-run changes in the city's older population has been the product of individual migration decisions. Mass immigration into New York in the decades around the turn of the last century was, of course, dominated by young people, as relatively few older persons made the journey. By midcentury, however, this large cohort and their American-born offspring, "surviving" much longer than would previously have been expected, were themselves reaching the age of retirement and producing, as already noted, a substantial expansion in the size of the city's over-sixty-five population. It was their children who moved en masse to the suburbs in the decades after World War II. A half century later, the young blacks and Latinos who moved north in this later period are becoming the majority of the city's older population as they also age in place.

But compared with that earlier generation of whites, a higher proportion of today's near and just elderly will age in place simply because their incomes are too low to allow them to move from the city. They, in effect, represent a "captive" market. The effects of this transition on the prevailing income levels of the city's older population are bound to be considerable. How considerable is suggested by the fact that as of 1990—the latest year for which these data are currently available—the median income of the city's white households headed by sixty-five- to seventy-four-year-olds was two and a half times greater than that for comparable Latino households and 78 percent above that for black households in this age group.

One way to get some guidance as to what might happen over the period from 2000 to 2010 as far as migration is concerned is to focus on the potential migration pool. Those between sixty-five and seventy-four years of age dominate migration among older persons. This can be defined as the number of persons who in 2000 were between fifty-five and seventy-four years of age; the fifty-five- to sixty-four-year-olds among them will enter their migration-prone years between 2000 and 2010, while the sixty-five- to seventy-four-year-olds will be departing them. Thus defined, the potential migration pool fell sharply between 1970 and 1990 but then stabilized at its present level of about 1.2 million persons, nearly three-fifths of whom are between fifty-five and sixty-four years of age.

This pattern characterizes both Manhattan and the outer boroughs. Short of an increase in the out-migration rate, the underlying aging process with its continued increase in life expectancy among older adults almost guarantees a slight increase in the city's over-sixty-five population in the period ahead, reversing the pattern of slight declines over the past two decades, and it almost certainly will be concentrated in the over-seventy-five age group. The chances of a surge in the out-migration rate are small, since an increasing proportion of the near elderly and the young elderly living in the city are black and Latino and, for economic reasons, are unlikely to migrate

Finally, there is a wild card as wild as one could imagine. Before the events of September 11, the city's economic future looked rosy. Since that time, however, the future of New York City may be quite different from what we anticipated. One possibility, given the threat of further acts of terrorism, is that older New Yorkers who are able to exercise some choice over where they live will move from the city in greater numbers than previously. Another is that the daily lives of older people who have little or no choice in this regard—which probably describes most of them—could be seriously affected by post-9/11 changes designed to deal with the suddenly heightened exigencies of living in a place that is a prime target for terrorist attacks.

It is impossible to predict what might happen. However, it is safe to say that 9/11 is not likely to be a once-and-for-all occurrence. The responses to the 9/11 attacks seem likely to affect the characteristics of the city's older population, as well as the quality of their lives, in ways that are unforeseeable.

Notes

1. All data cited in the text, unless otherwise noted, are from the Web site of the decennial U.S. Census of Population, www.census.gov.

2. U.S. Department of Commerce. 2000. *County Business Patterns.* Washington, DC: Government Printing Office.

3. Tobier, E. 1997. New York Revs Its Economic Engine. *Urban Land* [Urban Land Institute newsletter], October.

4. Hammack, David. 1982. *Power and Society: Greater New York at the Turn of the Century.* Part 2. New York: Russell Sage Foundation.

5. Tobier, E. 1998. The Bronx in the Twentieth Century: Dynamics of Population and Economic Change. Bronx County Historical Society Journal 35(2): 69–102.

6. Sassen, Saskia. 2001. *The Global City: New York, London, Tokyo.* Princeton: Princeton University Press.

7. An excellent overview of this very complex process is provided by Lemann, Nicholas. 1991. *The Promised Land: The Great Black Migration and How It Changed America.* New York: Knopf.

8. For an early description of this migration, see Mills, C. W, C. Senior, and R. K. Goldsen. 1950. *The Puerto Rican Journey: New York's Newest Migrants.* New York: Harper. For more recent data, see New York City Department of City Planning. 1994. *Puerto Rican New Yorkers in 1990.* New York: Department of City Planning. Before 1970, the Census Bureau collected data only on persons of Puerto Rican birth or ancestry and not, outside the Southeast, on non-Hispanic Puerto Ricans. However, beginning in 1970, the more inclusive category was adopted for enumeration purposes and the published data for that year revealed that at least a third of New York's Latino population was other than Puerto Rican.

9. Tobier, E. with W. Stafford. 1985. People and Income. In C. Brecher and R. Horton, eds. *Setting Municipal Priorities 1986*, 54–86. New York: New York University Press.

10. Brecher, C., and E. Tobier. 1977. *Economic and Demographic Trends in New York City: The Outlook for the Future.* New York: Temporary Commission on City Finances.

11. According to the U.S. Census Bureau, the median income of families headed by persons sixty-five and over rose by 66 percent in constant dollars between 1949 and 1969 and increased by another 61 percent over the next two decades. Thus, during the entire 1949–89 period, the constant dollar sixty-five-and-over median family income rose at a 28 percent faster rate than that for all families.

12. Medicare expenditure data are from the U.S. Department of Commerce, Bureau of Economic Analysis, *Regional Economic Information System, 1969–2000*; Social Security data is from Social Security Administration, Office of Policy, *OASDI Beneficiaries by State and County, 2000.* Washington DC: Government Printing Office.

13. Lee, Moon Wha. 1999. *Housing New York City.* New York: City Department of Housing Preservation and Development.

14. For a recent discussion of the SSI issue, see Greene, Kelly. 2002. Many Seniors Aren't Capitalizing on Benefits from the U.S. and States. *Wall Street Journal*, April 2.

15. A Survey of the Economics of Aging. 1996. *Economist*, January 27.

16. Stone, D. 1999. Care and Trembling. *American Prospect*, March–April, 61–66.

17. Stone, D. 2000. *Reframing Health Care Policy*. Cambridge: Radcliffe Public Policy Center, Radcliffe Institute for Advanced Study, Harvard University.

18. For a description of this process, see Tobier, Emanuel. 1988. Manhattan's Business District in the Industrial Age. In John Mollenkopf, ed. *Power, Culture, and Place: Essays on New York City*. New York. Russell Sage Foundation.

19. Derrick, P. 2001. *Tunneling to the Future: The Story of the Great Subway Expansion That Saved New York*. New York: New York University Press.

20. Some exceptions include Leduff, Charlie. 1996. Gay: Getting Old, Getting By. *New York Times*, City Section, March 31; and Ruiz, Albor. 1998. Center in Astoria Has Welcome Mat for Elderly Gays. *New York Daily News*, February 12.

4. The Health of Older New Yorkers

Daniel Weisz and Michael K. Gusmano

Introduction

Dr. Martin Luther King Jr. averred in 1966 that "of all the forms of inequality, injustice in health is the most shocking and the most inhuman."[1] Despite recent improvement in some measures of health in New York City, including life expectancy and infant mortality, significant disparities persist.

We examine in this chapter the physical health status of older persons in New York City and explore the variation in their physical health status and access to care.[2] In contrast to the perception that city residents are in worse health than other citizens, older persons in New York City are healthier than older persons in the United States as a whole. While we find reason to be optimistic about the health of older persons in Manhattan and the rest of the city, there are significant health disparities within the city that mirror the income inequalities described in the previous chapter. In New York City, as in the rest of the United States, health status varies by race and ethnicity. Compared to persons of the same age in other racial and ethnic groups, non-Hispanic blacks ages sixty-five to seventy-four have higher mortality and hospitalization rates. Among persons seventy-five years and over, however, non-Hispanic blacks have lower mortality and hospitalization rates than their non-Hispanic white counterparts. This "racial crossover" among the "older old" is consistent with findings of other studies.[3]

Recent analysis suggests that racial segregation and the geographic concentration of poverty are crucial factors in disparities of health in the United States. Indeed, there is growing recognition among public health experts and policy makers in New York City that place matters, because neighborhoods affect the health of residents, particularly vulnerable populations, including older persons. To illustrate the dramatic neighborhood-level differences in health outcomes and use of health services among older New Yorkers, we build on Tobier's framework (see Chapter 3) and contrast the health of older persons in Manhattan 1 and Manhattan 2 (the community districts in which the median household income is above or below the median for the city, respectively). We believe that such neighborhood-level analysis—by indicating neighborhoods in which programs could be developed to reduce hospital admissions—can point up opportunities to limit health-care expenditures.[4]

Health Status of Older Persons: New York City and the Nation

New York and the other world cities offer access to a host of amenities that may improve the health and quality of life of older residents. In addition to parks, cultural sites, and public transportation, there is a remarkable concentration of academic medical centers in New York City: forty-nine major teaching hospitals, eight medical schools, and an additional hundred research institutions that receive NIH grant funding.

Yet cities have been seen as sources of ill health. Rodwin notes that "from the earliest times, the city has attracted the poor and been the target of the plague, as well as war. . . . Since the city is, by definition, the place where human [population] density is greatest, it is hardly surprising that the city is [itself a factor in] disease transmission, particularly for the spread of infectious disease."[5] Even today, there are frequent claims that residents of cities suffer an "urban health penalty."[6] Studies examining a variety of health measures, including mortality rates, years of life lost, and infant mortality, provide evidence for an urban health penalty in the United States and other Organization for Economic Cooperation and Development countries.[7]

The high population density that results in cities acting as "vectors for disease transmission" is one explanation for the urban health penalty. Another contributing factor to the urban health penalty in the United States is the "white flight" out of central cities. When healthier, wealthier residents exit a city, they leave behind a larger proportion of minorities and sicker older persons.[8] Data on the migration of older persons out of New York City alone make it reasonable to assume that the health of older New Yorkers would be poorer than that of older persons in the rest of the nation. Since 1950, there has been a steady exodus of wealthier white residents and, as Tobier explains, it is the better-off ones who leave (Chapter 3).

On the other hand, the economic fortunes of older New Yorkers, like those of the city, have rebounded since 1980. The health status of older New Yorkers has followed suit. Despite the many reasons to expect poorer health among older persons in New York City compared with the United States as a whole, our examination of life expectancy among older persons suggests a different picture. In 1990, life expectancy in New York City and in the United States was virtually identical. By the year 2000, life expectancy both at sixty-five and at seventy-five was significantly higher in New York City than in the United States as a whole (Table 4.1).

Older non-Hispanic blacks in New York City have a shorter life expectancy than have older whites, but they survive longer than their counterparts nationally and the gap between races is smaller (Table 4.2).

While mortality is admittedly only one measure of health, the data are readily available, and death is the ultimate health outcome. Mortality is also correlated with morbidity, since most deaths are preceded by an illness.[9] The ten leading causes of death by age group and gender for the population of New York City in 2001 are quite similar to the national picture. Deaths due to conditions preventable by early lifestyle modification and treatable but seldom cured (diseases of the heart, which include congestive heart failure with ischemic heart disease; chronic lower-respiratory disease; cerebrovascular disorders, and malignant neoplasms) account for over 75 percent of the deaths in the sixty-five-and-over age group. Alzheimer's disease is

Table 4.1. Life Expectancy by Gender and Age: U.S. and NYC, 1990 and 2000

	Females		Males	
	U.S.	NYC	U.S.	NYC
1990				
At 65	18.9	18.8	15.1	15.4
At 75	12.0	12.0	9.4	9.7
2000				
At 65	19.3	20.1	16.2	17.0
At 75	12.3	12.9	10.1	10.8

Sources: Summary of Vital Statistics 2001, The City of New York, Bureau of Vital Statistics, NYC DHMH (www.nyc.gov/html/doh/pdf/vs/2000sum.pdf); *National Vital Statistics Reports*, Centers for Disease Control and Prevention, National Center for Health Statistics (www.cdc.gov/nchs/hus.htm).

Table 4.2. Life Expectancy by Race and Age: U.S. and NYC, 1990 and 2000

	Females				Males			
	U.S.		NYC		U.S.		NYC	
	White	Black	White	Black	White	Black	White	Black
1990								
At 65	19.1	17.2	18.7	17.3	15.2	13.2	15.3	13.2
At 75	12.0	11.2	11.8	11.4	9.4	8.6	9.5	8.8
2000								
At 65	19.4	17.7	19.9	18.8	16.3	14.2	16.9	15.3
At 75	12.3	11.6	12.6	12.5	10.1	9.2	10.6	10.2

Sources: Summary of Vital Statistics 2001, The City of New York, Bureau of Vital Statistics, NYC DHMH (www.nyc.gov/html/doh/pdf/vs/2000sum.pdf); *National Vital Statistics Reports*, Centers for Disease Control and Prevention, National Center for Health Statistics (www.cdc.gov/nchs/hus.htm).

a significant cause of death only among the oldest old (eighty-five years and over). Only a minority of deaths can be attributed to causes that are truly amenable to intervention (accidents, infectious diseases, diabetes, and hypertension). Mortality from influenza and pneumonia does increase with age. In New York City, this finding is not surprising, given the low immunization rates for flu (63 percent) and pneumonia (50 percent).[10] These immunization rates fall well below the Healthy People 2010 Initiative national target of 90 percent. Since 81 percent of the nonimmunized older New Yorkers had both health insurance and a personal physician, these low rates cannot be accounted for by lack of access to physician care.

Health Status in Manhattan and the Outer Boroughs

As Tobier explains in Chapter 3, Manhattan is the focal point of New York City's global economy. Does the stress of living in the economic heart of a world city, with its expensive housing market and vast income inequalities, lead to poorer health among older persons in Manhattan compared with those of the outer boroughs? Our analysis suggests that this is not the case.

The overall mortality rate for older persons is slightly higher in Manhattan (42.4 per thousand population) than in the outer boroughs (41.97). Age-specific death rates for the older population for Manhattan and the first ring, by age cohort and gender over the decade1989 to 1999, are shown in Table 4.3.[11]

With the exception of the eighty-five-and-over population of Manhattan, death rates have decreased over the decade 1989–1999 in all boroughs. Mortality rates in 1999 are similar in the outer boroughs and Manhattan. The rate is lower in Manhattan than in the outer boroughs among sixty-five- to seventy-four-year-olds but identical for those seventy-five to eighty-four and slightly higher in Manhattan for persons eighty-five years and older.

Examining mortality for the same age cohorts by leading causes similarly reveals a few notable differences between Manhattan and the remainder of New York City

Table 4.3. Age-Specific Mortality Rates of Persons 65+: Manhattan and Outer Boroughs, 1989 and 1999 (per 1,000 persons)

	1989		1999	
	Manhattan	**Outer Boroughs**	**Manhattan**	**Outer Boroughs**
65–74	23.6	23.9	20.9	21.4
(n)[a]	(2,529)	(10,193)	(2,066)	(8,570)
75–84	49.7	51.9	46.9	46.9
(n)	(3,342)	(13,053)	(2,939)	(12,157)
85+	114.1	131	130.9	129.3
(n)	(2,713)	(9,967)	(3,305)	(12,144)

Source: New York State Department of Health, 1990–2000.
[a] Number of deaths

using the average number of deaths for the years 1997–1999 (Table). Among the leading causes of death, heart-disease rates are lower and malignancy rates higher in Manhattan than in the outer boroughs.

Hospital admission rates represent another useful measure of health status and complement our examination of life expectancy and mortality rates. We consider total hospital admissions and hospitalization for illnesses that are among the leading causes of death (ischemic heart disease and neoplasms) in New York City for persons sixty-five years and over. Based on these measures (Table 4.5), the health of older Manhattanites does not appear to differ greatly from the health of older persons in the rest of the city. While total hospitalizations, and those for heart disease, are lower among residents of Manhattan than for the rest of the city, hospital admissions for cancer are higher among residents of Manhattan.

Self-assessed health status by borough. The New York City Community Survey, a telephone survey that collects critical neighborhood-specific information on health, represents the best source of data regarding self-reported health status of city residents. Nearly 10,000 New Yorkers were interviewed in 2000, 1,600 of whom were sixty-five and over. Only 7.3 percent of older residents of the outer boroughs who responded assessed their general health as excellent (87 of 1,196), and 39.8 percent (476) as fair or poor. Manhattan inhabitants fared a little better, with 13.1 percent (51 of 389) reporting excellent health and 37.5 percent (146) rating themselves as fair or poor. There were more individuals reporting no sick days in Manhattan (61.1 percent) than in the outer boroughs (57.4 percent). The percentage of respondents who reported experiencing eight or more days in which they felt ill during the previous year was about the same in Manhattan and the outer boroughs, 26.7 and 27.4 percent respectively.[12]

The survey indicates that there is little difference in access between Manhattan and the rest of the city. In Manhattan, 3.1 percent of older persons report "needing care but being unable to obtain it." In the outer boroughs, 3.5 percent of older persons report that this was the case. Similarly, 87.4 percent of older persons in Manhattan and 88.7 percent of older persons in the outer boroughs report having a personal physician.

Access to health care in Manhattan and the outer boroughs. Self-reports are not the only measures of access to medical care for older persons. To better understand differences in access to health-care services among older people in Manhattan and the rest of the city, we compare some characteristics of the health-care delivery and payment systems and admissions for three categories of conditions and procedures.

There are significant differences in the health-care infrastructure serving Manhattan and the outer boroughs. Of the seven academic medical centers in the area, five are in Manhattan, one in Brooklyn, and another in the Bronx. Manhattan, with about

Table 4.4. Age-Specific Mortality Rates, by Cause, of Persons 65+: Manhattan and Outer Boroughs, 1998–2000 (per 1,000 Persons)

	65–74		75–84		85+	
	Manhattan	Outer Boroughs	Manhattan	Outer Boroughs	Manhattan	Outer Boroughs
All causes	20.6	21.1	43.6	45.3	124.6	121.8
(n)[a]	(2,038)	(8,432)	(2,730)	(11,727)	(3,146)	(11,435)
Malignant neoplasms	7.4	6.6	11.5	10.1	17.7	13.3
(n)	(727)	(2,658)	(723)	(2,624)	(447)	(1,252)
Heart disease	7.0	9.1	18.6	24.1	67.1	80.1
(n)	(693)	(3,623)	(1,162)	(6,240)	(1,695)	(7,521)
Hypertensive diseases	1.1	.9	2.0	1.6	5.3	3.4
(n)	(108)	(377)	(125)	(402)	(134)	(318)
Cerebrovascular diseases	.8	.7	1.8	1.6	6.4	4.1
(n)	(81)	(283)	(115)	(412)	(161)	(381)
Chronic obstructive pulmonary disease	.8	.7	1.9	1.5	4.0	2.7
(n)	(83)	(286)	(116)	(392)	(100)	(257)
Diabetes mellitus	.7	.8	1.1	1.3	1.9	2.4
(n)	(68)	(320)	(71)	(345)	(48)	(222)

Source: New York State Department of Health, 2001.
[a] Number of deaths

Table 4.5. Hospital Admission Rates for Heart Disease and Neoplasms for Persons 65+: NYC, Manhattan, and Outer Boroughs, 2000 (per 1,000 persons 65+)

	NYC	Manhattan	Outer Boroughs
Ischemic heart disease	56.9	41.9	60.6
Neoplasms	20.4	21.5	20.1
Total hospitalizations	334.9	329.7	336.2

Source: SPARCS.

20 percent of total New York City population, is home to twenty-three hospitals and 10,870 acute care beds. The four other boroughs account for forty-two hospitals and 16,651 acute care beds. Based on the New York State Physician Licensure Re-registration Survey, 1997–1999, 37 percent of New York City active primary care physicians and 57 percent of specialists are located in Manhattan.[13] These statistics, translated to full-time-equivalent patient-care physicians by the Center for Health Workforce Studies, are shown in Table 4.6.

While it is well known that almost all the population over sixty-five has insurance coverage through Medicare, it is helpful to understand the details of this complicated plan. Hospital Insurance (Part A) helps pay for inpatient hospital care, limited inpatient care in a skilled nursing facility, home-health care, and hospice care. Part A has deductibles and coinsurance, but most people do not have to pay premiums for Part A. Medical Insurance (Part B) helps pay for doctors' services, outpatient

Table 4.6. Physicians in Patient Care: Manhattan and Outer Boroughs, 2000 (per 10,000 persons)

	Manhattan	Outer Boroughs
Primary Care	21.25	9.83
	(3,254)	(5,746)
Specialty	54.05	10.97
	(8,277)	(6,410)
Total	75.3	21.11
	(11,531)	(12,336)

Source: Manhattan: New York State Physician Licensure Re-registration Survey, New York State Department of Education, 1997–1999.
Note: Figures in parentheses = number of full-time equivalent physicians

hospital services, durable medical equipment, and a number of other medical services and supplies that are not covered by Part A. Part B has premiums, deductibles, and coinsurance that an individual must pay through another insurance plan or one of the Medicare savings programs that New York State and the federal government have created to help low-income Medicare beneficiaries with their out-of-pocket expenses, the so-called dual eligible.[14]

Medigap insurance—also known as Medicare supplemental insurance—available in ten standardized forms with different premiums and benefits, is specifically designed to supplement Medicare's benefits by paying some of what Medicare does not pay for covered services (deductibles and copayments). It may also pay for certain services not covered by Medicare. Premiums in New York City vary from $104 to more than $300 per month depending on level and details of coverage and may be paid by former employers or unions, through veteran or military retiree benefits, or out-of-pocket by beneficiaries. Medicare managed care in all its varied forms is yet another vehicle designed to fill the gaps in coverage.

There is no predictable pattern in the boroughs in the number of Medicare beneficiaries protected by hospital insurance and supplemental medical insurance as of July 1, 2000 (Table 4.7).

In Manhattan, 22.4 percent (47,853 of 213,331) of the sixty-five-and-older population is enrolled in Medicaid, that is, is dual eligible. This is only slightly lower than the 23.8 percent (187,625 of 787,650) in the other four boroughs.

Hospital admissions, by area of residence, may be interpreted as a measure of health, as well as an indication of medical service. First we examine so-called marker conditions.[15] These are conditions for which no treatment option other than hospital admission is considered appropriate. The rate of hospital admission for these conditions should not be affected by rates of supplementary insurance cover-

Table 4.7. Number of Persons 65+ Covered by Medicare Hospital Insurance (HI) and Supplemental Medical Insurance (SMI): NYC Boroughs, 2000

	HI &/or SMI[a]	HI	SMI
Bronx	121,948	110,290	113,472
Kings/Brooklyn	253,344	214,741	238,080
Manhattan/New York	185.925	170,606	169,474
Queens	252,085	228,853	237,649
Staten Island/Richmond	48,087	46,470	45,871

Source: Centers for Medicare and Medicaid Services (www.cms.hhs.gov).
[a] HI = Hospital Insurance (Medicare Part A); SMI = Supplemental Medical Insurance (Medicare Part B); &/or = unduplicated count of persons enrolled in either or both parts of the program

age or access to primary care. They include appendicitis with appendectomy, acute myocardial infarction (AMI), gastrointestinal obstruction, and fracture of the hip/femur. The rates of admission for AMI and GI obstruction are lower in Manhattan than in the rest of the city. The rates of admission for fracture of the hip or femur are virtually identical in Manhattan and the rest of the city. The rates of admission for appendicitis with appendectomy are higher in Manhattan than in the rest of the city (Table 4.7).

Next, we examine hospitalization for referral-sensitive "high-tech" procedures (cardiac operations, pacemaker implants, and lower extremity joint replacements). Because, in most cases, the failure to receive these procedures is not immediately life threatening, lower-income older persons who do not have a supplementary "Medi-gap" insurance program that covers the inpatient copays and deductibles are less likely to be hospitalized for such procedures. Given their lower level of ischemic heart disease, we are not surprised to find that cardiac operations are far less common among older residents of Manhattan than among those of the rest of the city. On the other hand, pacemaker implants and joint replacements have a somewhat higher incidence in Manhattan than in the rest of the city (Table 4.7). This finding suggests that older residents of Manhattan may enjoy greater access to these referral-sensitive procedures than do residents of the outer boroughs. We are unable to determine whether these differences are related to the greater concentration of medical resources, differences in socioeconomic status, differing insurance characteristics, or another undefined factor.

Finally, we examine hospitalization for avoidable hospital conditions (AHC). These are diagnoses for which access to timely and appropriate primary care should decrease or prevent the need for hospital admission.[16] High rates of admission for AHC among residents of an area may indicate that residents face inappropriate barriers to primary care. We find that avoidable hospitalizations are lower among older persons living in Manhattan than among those living in the outer boroughs (Table 4.7). These findings suggest that older persons in Manhattan may enjoy better access to primary care than those living in the outer boroughs. Once again, we are unable to determine whether these differences are related to the greater concentration of medical resources in Manhattan, differences in socioeconomic status, differing rates of health-insurance coverage, or perhaps another undefined factor.

Rates of hospitalization for marker conditions show no consistent pattern when we compare Manhattan and the outer boroughs. This finding is consistent with the life expectancy and mortality data that show little difference between Manhattan and the rest of the city. Despite the fact that the health status of older residents of Manhattan does not differ appreciably from that of older residents in the rest of the city, rates of hospitalization for AHC are lower and for referral-sensitive conditions are higher in Manhattan. Together, these indicators suggest that older residents of Manhattan enjoy greater access to both primary and specialty care than do older residents of the outer boroughs.

Table 4.8. Hospital Admission Rates for Persons 65+:
NYC, Manhattan, and Outer Boroughs, 2000 (per 1,000 persons 65+)

	NYC	Manhattan	Outer Boroughs
Referral-sensitive conditions			
Cardiac operations	8.0	7.6	8.1
Lower extremity joint replacement	5.9	7.0	5.7
Pacemaker implant	1.7	1.8	1.6
Marker conditions			
Appendicitis	.4	.5	.3
Acute MI	8.5	6.0	9.1
GI obstruction	3.2	2.9	3.3
Fractured hip/femur	5.1	5.3	5.1
AHCs[a]			
AHCs as percent of total admissions	19.7	17.3	20.4

Source: SPARCS.

[a] Avoidable hospital conditions, according to United Hospital Fund criteria

Health Disparities among Older New Yorkers

The data presented in the previous sections indicate that the health status of older residents of New York City has improved during the 1990s and that older New Yorkers are now healthier than their counterparts in the rest of the United States. Furthermore, we find only small differences in health status between older residents of Manhattan and those of the outer boroughs. These aggregations, however, mask enormous variations in health status within each of New York's boroughs. For example, although differences in life expectancy between older blacks and older whites are not as great in New York City as in the United States as a whole (Table 4.2), there is still a gap. Indeed there are significant racial and ethnic differences in burdens of illness and death among older persons in New York City. This is particularly true for the "younger old," under the age of seventy-five.

Non-Hispanic blacks ages sixty-five to seventy-four have a higher overall mortality rate per thousand (29.6) than have non-Hispanic whites (24.9), Asians (12.2), or Hispanics (18.2) (Table 4.8). Hospital admissions are also higher for non-Hispanic blacks than for other racial and ethnic groups.

Among persons seventy-five years and over, non-Hispanic blacks have lower overall mortality and hospitalization rates than have their non-Hispanic white counterparts. The "racial crossover" among the "older-old" cohort is a well-known phenomenon.[17] The racial crossover in health appears to be the result, in part, of a "survivor effect" among older blacks, coupled with "greater deterioration of health in old age for whites."[18]

Hispanic and Asian older persons in New York have lower overall mortality and hospitalization rates than have non-Hispanic blacks and non-Hispanic whites in both age categories. Despite the apparent health advantage enjoyed by older Hispanics and Asians in New York City, it is noteworthy that the average age of death for non-Hispanic whites is much higher than for other racial and ethnic groups. Among non-Hispanic whites, 77.7 percent of deaths after the age of sixty-five occur after the age of seventy-four. In contrast, a much smaller percentage of the deaths among older non-Hispanic blacks (62.5 percent), Asians (66.6 percent), and Hispanics (61 percent) occurs after the age of seventy-four.

What accounts for health disparities among older New Yorkers, particularly the poorer health of "young-old" non-Hispanic blacks less than seventy-five years of age? Historical explanations focus on biological and genetic factors, but recent evidence suggests that biological and genetic differences account for less than 1 percent of the excess deaths in the black population in the United States.[19] Most studies by social scientists conclude that the relationship between race and health is primarily a function of socioeconomic status (SES), including income and education.[20] Controlling for SES usually decreases the relationship between race and health. In a few studies, researchers found that racial health disparities disappear completely after controlling for SES. Yet other studies provide evidence that racial differences in health status and the use of health services remain, even after controlling for SES. As Evandrou reveals (Chapter 9), this finding is not limited to the United States. She cites studies in the United Kingdom that find significant differences in health status by ethnicity after controlling for "deprivation."

Williams and Collins argue that SES fails to fully account for racial differences in health because common measures of SES are incomplete. Most studies use income as a proxy for SES and fail to capture differences in wealth, which are larger and more difficult to measure. In addition, they argue, studies relying on SES rarely attempt to measure the effects of racism. Racism can "transform social status such that SES indicators are not equivalent across race." For example, some studies show that non-Hispanic whites receive a higher income than non-Hispanic blacks and Hispanics for a given level of education. Racism may also "restrict access to the quantity and quality of health-related desirable services such as public education, health care, housing, and recreational facilities." Finally, racism may "induce psychological distress that may adversely affect physical and mental health status."[21]

One consequence of racism with significant implications for persistent racial and ethnic disparities in health is race-based residential segregation and the geographic concentration of poverty among blacks.[22] As Williams and Collins explain, African Americans live, disproportionately, in "urban residential areas where living conditions are hostile to life and health. Unlike the white urban poor who are dispersed throughout the city, with many residing in relatively safe and comfortable neighborhoods, the black poor are concentrated in depressed central-city neighborhoods . . . where the stress of poor urban environments can lead to illness."[23] For example, they cite a recent study that found that black men between the ages of twenty-five and forty-four in Harlem are six times more likely to die than are their white counterparts across the United States.[24]

A growing body of research indicates that a neighborhood's characteristics influence the health of residents.[25] Although there is a vigorous debate about whether the relationship is causal,[26] community SES measured as median household income is strongly associated with poor health, even controlling for individual income. Similarly, neighborhood-level inequality is associated with health, violence and "collective efficacy."[27] Other recent studies find significant correlations between the characteristics of neighborhoods and the health status of their residents, even after controlling for race, education, poverty, population changes, and health-insurance coverage.[28]

The recognition that neighborhood characteristics shape the health of a neighborhood's residents led New York City to establish District Public Health Offices (DPHOs). In August 2003, New York City mayor Michael Bloomberg and Dr. Thomas R. Frieden, the commissioner of the New York City Department of Health and Mental Hygiene, announced the creation of a Bronx DPHO, one of three in New York City.[29] The city established the Community District Health Office program to address health disparities by focusing on three neighborhoods with high rates of mortality and "avoidable deaths," and developing "community-specific" approaches to improving health.

Neighborhoods and the health of older New Yorkers. There are markedly different burdens of illness and death, as well as medical service utilization rates, across the city's neighborhoods. As an approximation of neighborhoods in New York, we adopt Tobier's approach in the preceding chapter and use community districts. New York City's fifty-nine community districts, established by local law in 1975, illustrate the remarkable diversity of the city's land uses and population. They range in size from less than nine hundred to almost fifteen thousand acres, and in population from fewer than thirty-five thousand residents to more than two hundred thousand. In the analysis we present next, we contrast the health status of older residents living in the neighborhoods of Manhattan 1 with that of those living in the neighborhoods of Manhattan 2.

Compared to Manhattan 2, the population of neighborhoods in Manhattan 1 is wealthier as measured by median household income, older, and more likely to be white and non-Hispanic, and has a lower percentage of seniors below the poverty line; in the neighborhoods of Manhattan 2, residents are poorer, younger, and more likely to be non-English speaking and foreign born (see Tobier, Chapter 3).

Examination of total mortality rates by age cohort and gender over the decade 1989–1999 (Table 4.9) reveals that the populations in higher-income areas consistently experience lower mortality rates and that mortality rates have decreased over the last decade for all cohorts.

Mortality is lower for all causes in the population sixty-five to seventy-four living in wealthier areas, and lower for all causes with the exception of heart disease among the seventy-five-and-older cohort, compared with those living in poorer areas (Table 4.10).

As we did for our borough-level analysis, we examine total hospital admissions and hospitalization for illnesses that are among the leading causes of death (ischemic heart disease and neoplasm) in New York City. The investigation of hospital admissions again reveals lower rates for residents of wealthier areas (Table 4.11).

Housing, crime, water and air pollution, and a host of other "social determinants" contribute to the differences in health among older persons in living in Manhattan 1 and Manhattan 2. Nevertheless, medical care is important, particularly for older persons, and there is a great deal of concern about disparities in access to care for older New Yorkers in "underserved" areas.

Table 4.9. Mortality and Hospital Admission Rates for Persons 65+, by Race/Ethnicity: NYC, 1997–1999 (per 1,000 persons 65+)

	Mortality, All Causes		Hospital Admissions, All Causes	
	65–74	75+	65–74	75+
White Non-Hispanic	24.9	76.9	190.6	363.2
(n)[a]	(6,238)	(21,773)	(47,803)	(102,839)
Black Non-Hispanic	29.6	66.9	212.9	323.4
(n)	(3,156)	(5,252)	(22,679)	(25,404)
Asian	12.2	42.1	86.9	185.2
(n)	(455)	(907)	(3,425)	(3,990)
Hispanic	18.2	48.8	152.4	247.3
(n)	(1,597)	(2,496)	(13,358)	(12,655)

Source: SPARCS.
[a] Number of deaths

Table 4.10. Age-Specific Mortality Rates for Persons 65+, by Gender and Neighborhood Category: Manhattan, 1989 and 1999 (per 1,000 persons 65+)

	65–74		75+	
	Mhtn. 1[a]	Mhtn. 2[b]	Mhtn. 1	Mhtn. 2
1997–1999				
Male	20.3	32.6	69.9	78.5
(n)[c]	(476)	(630)	(1090)	(1076)
Female	13.5	19.8	63.2	64.1
(n)	(367)	(562)	(1883)	(1823)
1989–1990				
Male	23.9	39.8	74.7	90.9
(n)	(554)	(812)	(1190)	(1233)
Female	15.5	21.1	59.1	66.4
(n)	(481)	(682)	(1957)	(1867)

Source: New York State Department of Health 1990–2000.
[a] Manhattan 1 includes all community districts with household incomes above the citywide median
[b] Manhattan 2 includes all community districts with household incomes below the citywide median
[c] Number of deaths

When examined more closely, rates for referral-sensitive procedures, such as hip replacements or coronary revascularizations, are substantially higher in wealthier community districts across all three age cohorts; rates for "marker conditions," such as neoplasms and AMI, differ little and without any pattern with regard to age groups. These findings are consistent with the assumption that Medicare is not sufficient to guarantee access to all forms of care.

Another possible explanation for access difficulty is a structural barrier, including the lack of local primary care providers or medical specialists. The aggregate number of primary care physicians (1,225) and medical specialists (5,330) in the upper-income community districts far exceeds that in the lower income (717 and 2,538). A full explanation of these disparities is beyond the scope of this chapter, but the stark differences in hospital admissions for these conditions between the wealthier and poor areas of the city merit further investigation.

Conclusion

Older persons in New York City appear to live longer, healthier lives than do their counterparts in the United States as a whole, and the health of older residents of

Table 4.11. Age-Specific Mortality Rates, by Cause, for Persons 65+, by Neighborhood Category: Manhattan, 1997–1999

	65–74		75+	
	Mhtn. 1[a]	Mhtn. 2[b]	Mhtn. 1	Mhtn. 2
All Causes	16.6	25.5	65.5	68.8
(n)[c]	(843)	(1,192)	(2,973)	(2,898)
Malignant neoplasms	6.7	8.1	13.2	13.5
(n)	(339)	(387)	(598)	(571)
Heart disease	5.4	8.7	33.1	32.1
(n)	(275)	(387)	(1,502)	(1,352)
Influenza and Pneumonia	0.6	0.8	4.7	5.3
(n)	(28)	(40)	(212)	(225)
Cerebrovascular diseases	0.6	1.1	3.0	3.3
(n)	(29)	(52)	(137)	(138)
COPD	0.6	1.1	2.4	2.6
(n)	(32)	(51)	(109)	(109)
Diabetes mellitus	0.4	1.0	0.9	1.8
(n)	(19)	(49)	(42)	(77)

Source: New York State Department of Health, 1998–2000.

Note: Numbers in parentheses = Total population in thousands

[a] All community districts with household incomes above the citywide median

[b] All community districts with household incomes below the citywide median

[c] Number of deaths

Manhattan—New York's urban core—does not appear to differ greatly from the health of older persons in the rest of the city. These findings contrast with the more typical story of an "urban health penalty." They are particularly surprising given the extraordinary exodus of middle-class and upper-income residents from New York City during much of the postwar period. The economic expansion during the 1990s—and New York City's improved economic outlook since 1980—almost certainly contributed to these gains in longevity and health status. It will be a challenge for the city to sustain these improvements as it moves further into the twenty-first century.

Addressing the persistent disparities in health within the city represents an even greater challenge. Although the aggregate data on health status support the notion

Table 4.12. Hospital Admissions for Persons 65+, by Age, Cause, and Neighborhood Category: Manhattan, 1998–2000 (as a percentage of age cohort)

	65–74		75–84		85+	
	Manhattan 1[a]	Manhattan 2[b]	Manhattan 1	Manhattan 2	Manhattan 1	Manhattan 2
All causes	134.5	164.5	218.3	243.6	298.0	288.8
(n)[c]	(6,822)	(7,844)	(6,930)	(7,451)	(4,065)	(3,337)
Neoplasms	19.7	19.3	24.0	23.9	26.8	23.9
(n)	(1,002)	(921)	(761)	(732)	(366)	(277)
Ischemic heart disease	17.4	19.9	23.3	25.2	27.2	24.7
(n)	(884)	(949)	(739)	(770)	(371)	(285)

Source: SPARCS.

[a] All community districts with household incomes above the citywide median
[b] All community districts with household incomes below the citywide median
[c] Number of hospital admissions in thousand

Table 4.13. Hospital Admissions for Persons 65+, by Age, Type of Hospitalization, and Neighborhood Category: Manhattan, 1998–2000 (per 1,000 persons 65+)

	65–74		75–84		85+	
	Manhattan 1	Manhattan 2	Manhattan 1	Manhattan 2	Manhattan 1	Manhattan 2
Referral-Sensitive Procedures						
Coronary revascularization	9.6	7.0	10.5	7.7	5.4	4
(n)	(486)	(332)	(332)	(236)	(73)	(46)
Hip replacement	6.4	4.6	10.9	5.9	9.8	7.7
(n)	(328)	(218)	(345)	(182)	(134)	(89)
Pacemaker implant	.7	.9	2.3	2.2	4.3	4.5
(n)	(36)	(41)	(73)	(66)	(59)	(52)
Marker Conditions						
Appendicitis	.5	.4	.3	.3	.4	.2
(n)	(23)	(18)	(9)	(10)	(5)	(2)
Acute myocardial infarction	3.4	4.5	6.0	7.7	12	12.2
(n)	(175)	(215)	(189)	(237)	(165)	(141)
GI obstruction	1.8	2	3.8	3.5	6.6	7.9
(n)	(90)	(94)	(122)	(106)	(90)	(91)
Fracture hip/femur	1.6	1.3	7.8	5.3	23.6	17.6
(n)	(81)	(64)	(249)	(162)	(322)	(203)
Ambulatory Care–Sensitive Conditions	25.1	52.7	50.2	83.7	111.4	135.9
(n)	(1271)	(2516)	(1593)	(2560)	(1520)	(1570)

Source: SPARCS.

that there may be a "health advantage" to living in New York City, these data mask enormous variation in health status within the city. There are different burdens of illness and death, as well as differences in medical service utilization rates, across the city's neighborhoods. The existence of such enormous levels of poverty and ill health within the core of the wealthiest city in the world, particularly during a time of great economic expansion is, as Dr. King put it, shocking.

Recent attention by the Institute of Medicine to the issue of racial and neighborhood-level health disparities across the country, and by the New York State and city governments at the state and local levels, represents a step in the right direction.[30] The New York City Department of Health and Mental Hygiene's efforts to map neighborhood differences in health have helped raise public awareness of this issue. The establishment of District Public Health Offices has great potential for identifying innovative solutions to the problems faced by high-risk neighborhoods in New York City. It is important, however, not to be overly sanguine about the prospects for addressing these disparities in the short term. The underlying causes of neighborhood-level health inequities are complex. Along with differences in physical infrastructure, availability of services, and levels of crime, neighborhood disparities in education, wealth, and income—all of which are exacerbated and reinforced by a long history of racial segregation in housing—contribute to these health disparities. Overcoming these barriers requires sustained effort at all levels of government, working in partnership with community organizations and community residents.

Notes

1. King, Martin Luther, Jr. 1966. Address to the National Convention of the Medical Committee for Human Rights, Chicago, March 25.
2. A complete examination of mental health status would require data from outpatient settings and psychiatric hospitals. We do not currently have access to these data.
3. Johnson, Nan E. 2000. The Racial Crossover in Comorbidity, Disability, and Mortality. *Demography* 37(3): 267–283.
4. Wennberg, J. E., E. Fisher, and J. Skinner. 2002. Geography and the Debate over Medicare Reform. *Health Affairs* Web Exclusive. February 13, W96–W114.
5. Rodwin, Victor G. 2001. Urban Health: Is the City Infected? Lecture at the Millennium Festival on Medicine and the Humanities Sponsored by St. Thomas' Guy's and King's School of Medicine and Southwick Cathedral. In M. Marinker, ed. *Medicine and Humanity*. London: King's Fund.
6. Andrulis, Dennis P. 1997. The Urban Health Penalty: New Dimensions and Directions in Inner-City Health Care. In American College of Physicians. *Inner City Health Care*. Philadelphia: American College of Physicians
7. Big Cities Health Inventory. 1997. Chicago: City of Chicago Department of Public Health.
8. Greenberg, M. 1991. American Cities: Good and Bad News about Public Health. *Bulletin of the New York Academy of Medicine* 67:17–21.

9.   Fuchs, V. R., M. McClellan, and J. Skinner. 2001. Area Differences in Utilization of Medical Care and Mortality among U.S. Elderly. *NBER Working Paper* 8628. www.nber.org/papers/w8628 (accessed March 1, 2004).

10. *Influenza and Pneumococcal Resource Guide*. 2004. New York City Department of Health and Mental Hygiene. www.ci.nyc.ny.us/html/Imm/flu-ptk.html (accessed March 5, 2004).

11. The last year for which NYCDHMH released vital statistics was 1999.

12. See www.nyc.gov/html/doh/html/data/data.shtml.

13. *New York State Physician Licensure Re-registration Survey*. 1997–1999. Albany: New York State Department of Education.

14. Those eligible for the Qualified Medicare Beneficiary Program, for people with limited resources whose incomes are at or below the national poverty level; the Specified Low Income Beneficiary Program, for those whose incomes are up to 120 percent of the poverty level; and the Qualified Individual 1, for people with incomes between 120 and 135 percent of poverty level and with limited resources, do not have to pay the Medicare monthly Part B premium. The Qualified Individual 2 program is for people with incomes between 135 and 175 percent of poverty level and of limited resources; those who qualify for this program save on a portion of their Medicare Part B premium.

15. Billings, J., L. Zeitel, J. Lukomnik, and T.S. Carely. 1993. Impact of Socioeconomic Status on Hospital Use in New York City. *Health Affairs DataWatch*. Spring: 163

16. Billings, J., G. M. Anderson, and L. S. Newman. 1996. Recent Findings on Preventable Hospitalizations. *Health Affairs* 15(3): 239–249; Blustein, J., K. Hanson, and S. Shea. 1998. Preventable Hospitalizations and Socioeconomic Status. *Health Affairs* 17(2): 177–189; Weissman, J. S., C. Gatsonis, and A. M. Epstein. 1992. Rates of Avoidable Hospitalization by Insurance Status in Massachusetts and Maryland. *Journal of the American Medical Association* 268(17): 2388–2394.

17. Johnson, Racial Crossover.

18. Berkman, Cathy, and Barry J. Gurland. 1998. The Relationship between Ethnoracial Group and Functional Level in Older Persons. *Ethnicity and Health* 3(3): 175–188.

19. Cooper, Richard, and Richard David. 1986. The Biological Concept of Race and Its Application to Public Health and Epidemiology. *Journal of Health Politics, Policy, and Law* 11:97–116.

20. Lawrence, David. 2002. Which Diseases Contribute to Life-Expectancy Differences between Races? *Lancet* 360(9345): 1571.

21. Williams, David R., and Chiquita Collins. 1995. US Socioeconomic and Racial Differences in Health: Patterns and Explanations. *Annual Review of Sociology* 21:349.

22. Schulz, Amy J., David R. Williams, Barbara A. Israel, and Lora Bex Lempert. 2002. Racial and Spatial Relations as Fundamental Determinants of Health in Detroit. *Milbank Quarterly* 80(4): 677–705.

23. Willams and Collins, US Socioeconomic and Racial Differences, 356.

24. McCord, C., and H. P. Freeman. 1990. Excess Mortality in Harlem. *New England Journal of Medicine* 322:173–177.

25. Polednak, A. P. 1991. Black-White Differences in Infant Mortality in 38 Standard

Metropolitan Statistical Areas. *American Journal of Public Health* 81:1480–1482; Yen, I. H., and S. L. Syme. 1999. The Social Environment and Health: A Discussion of the Epidemiologic Literature. *Annual Review of Public Health* 20:287.

26. Kawachi, I., and T. A. Blakely. 2001. When Economists and Epidemiologists Disagree. *Journal of Health Care Politics, Policy, and Law* 26(3): 553–541; Milyo, J., and J. M. Mellor. 2003. On the Importance of Age-Adjustment Methods in Ecological Studies of Social Determinants of Mortality. *Health Services Research*, forthcoming.

27. Morenoff, J. D., R. J. Sampson, and S. W. Raudenbush. 2001. Neighborhood Inequality, Collective Efficacy, and the Spatial Dynamics of Urban Violence. *Criminology* 39(3): 517–559.

28. Cohen, Deborah A., Karen Mason, Ariane Bedimo, Richard Scribner, Victoria Basolo, and Thomas A. Farley. 2003. Neighborhood Physical Conditions and Health. *American Journal of Public Health* 93(3): 467–471; Winkleby, M. A., and C. Cubbin. 2003. Influence of Individual and Neighbourhood Socioeconomic Status on Mortality among Black, Mexican-American, and White Women and Men in the United States. *Journal of Epidemiology and Community Health* 57(6): 444–454.

29. New York City Department of Health and Mental Hygiene, Office of Communications. 2003. Mayor Michael R. Bloomberg and Health Commissioner Thomas R. Frieden Announce Launch of District Public Health Offices in Neighborhoods with Most Pressing Health Problems. Press release. August 20.

30. See www.ci.nyc.ny.us/html/doh.

5. Organizing Care for Older Persons in New York: The Social Class Vulnerabilities of a World City

David Barton Smith

How does one grow old in a city? For most older New Yorkers, the answer would be that one doesn't. One lives a full life, full of the energy of a center of such lives. For the out-of-towner, growing old or, in the language of gerontology, "aging in place" in New York City is equally absurd. It is the familiar line. The more than thirty million visitors that flood New York City each year, rubbing shoulders with its eight million inhabitants, may find it an exciting place to visit, but why would one choose to grow old in New York City?[1] Why, in particular, would one choose to remain in the city when just managing the simple tasks of daily living requires the caring and kindness of strangers? Why, when the affordability, the ample quiet space for leisurely living, and perhaps even the kindness of strangers are in more ample supply elsewhere? Some older New Yorkers do leave, but most live out their lives in the city. They do so not as a result of a logical conscious decision but as a consequence of simply continuing to live their lives.

So it is with the way care is organized for the frail older persons in New York city or anywhere else. There is no central master plan. Older persons and the informal and formal providers of their care simply invent ways to deal with the immediate circumstances they face. Their choices, however, are constrained by income, education, residence, social networks, and all the other factors that define their position in the social class hierarchy of the city. This chapter describes the large, social and economically divided, constantly evolving, complex system that cares for frail older persons in New York City. It first catalogs the more obvious pieces of that system—the people served by it, the providers that care for them, and the ways that such care is paid for. It then describes the underlying social class conflicts that have shaped the evolution of that system and threaten the long-term viability of the city itself.

The Care System

Needs and resources. The needs and resources of New York City's older persons shape the organization of care. New York City is the largest and most densely concentrated population of older persons in the United States. An estimated 901,976 persons over the age of sixty-five live in New York City, 43 percent of them with some disability or self-care limitation.[2] The "older old," the more than 99,956 persons in New York City over the age of eighty-five, account for the largest proportion of those with mobility and self-care needs and those who are residents in nursing homes. The cost of congregate housing, a group setting that provides meals and some assistance with daily living, for persons with less than $25,000 in annual income would far exceed that income and would rapidly exhaust their assets. Of householders over the age of sixty-five, 53 percent had household incomes of less than $25,000 and 18 percent had household incomes below poverty level in 2000.

How care is organized in New York reflects the extremes in wealth and poverty of its older persons. In general, income disparities are higher in New York City than in almost any other major metropolitan area in the United States. In contrast to overall income disparities in the United States, which have edged upward since 1967, income disparities have declined among older persons, reflecting shifts in public support of retirement income and Medicare.[3] Yet, income inequalities among older persons remain higher than those among the population as a whole. The Gini coefficient, the most commonly used measure of income inequality, for sixty-five-plus households in New York City was .549, and .468 for all age households in 1990. In contrast, the Gini index for the United States as a whole for sixty-five-plus households was .486, and for all age households, .408.[4]

Income disparities affect the need for services and pose challenges in the organization of care. Poor health is inversely related to income and to the cost of providing care. In the United States, it costs the Medicare program more than twice as much to provide the same benefits to older persons living in the community who are poor (also eligible for Medicaid) than it costs for those who are not poor. For those providing care for the frail older persons in congregate settings, the income inequalities in New York City are a two-edged sword. On the one hand, the majority of older New Yorkers cannot afford the cost of private congregate living arrangements. On the other hand, for many of those who can, such arrangements offer a poor substitute for the amenities, privacy, and services they can receive in their own homes.

The geographic migration effect. One cannot begin to understand the unique demands placed on the system of long-term care in New York City without understanding how that system is affected by migration patterns. When older persons leave the city, the net impact is that the city must care for a sicker, poorer population.

In general, migration rates rise at retirement age and then rise again for those over eighty years of age.[5] The so-called senior housing market is divided into two distinct segments, one catering to the "retirement peak" and the other to the "late age slope." Choices in retirement-age migration focus more on affordability and quality of life than do choices in late age migration, which are more influenced by nearness to adult children and other family members, as well as access to health services.[6]

Eight times as many older persons leave New York City as migrate to it. New York City's five counties all rank within the top fifteen in the ratio of out-of-state migration to in-migration of older persons, with Queens and Kings being second and third, outranked only by Nassau.[7] The largest interstate exchange of older persons takes place between New York State and Florida. Florida was the destination of 21 percent of New York State's older migrants, and New York in turn was the destination of 47 percent of Florida's. Many of the older migrants from Florida to New York are reverse migrants (e.g., "late age slope" migrants) during the final years of their lives. This was a common story from residents, family members, and facilities staff I interviewed in New York.

The social and economic impact of this exchange of older persons between Florida and New York is staggering. New York ranks dead last among the states by net loss in total household income, with a net loss as a result of out-migration of $3.3 billion in the household income of older persons; Florida ranks first, with a net gain as a result of in-migration of $6.5 billion per year.[8] Direct transfers from New York alone account for more than $1.8 billion of Florida's net gain. Given the generally higher income levels of New York City residents, and the fact that they account for almost half of all out-of-state migration, more than half these losses accrue directly to the city. These figures do not take into account the transfer of wealth and volunteer services, and the support of faith and cultural activities, that the added leisure of retirement brings.

Recasting this impact into the language of insurance, New York City is a victim of regional "cherry picking" and "adverse risk selection." Like the insurance practice that state insurance commissioners attempt to prevent, Sunbelt states such as Florida, and the South Florida counties of Dade, Broward, and Palm Beach, engage in unabashed predatory "regional cream skimming." Their explicit development strategy is to keep the tax rates low to encourage in-migration of older persons by offering more affordable retirement conditions, while at the same time limiting services to encourage reverse migration when older individuals have exhausted their own resources, and services such as Medicaid nursing-home care are needed.[9] Florida, unlike New York, has no state income, estate, or death taxes. Medical services, prescriptions, and groceries are exempt from Florida's 7 percent sales tax. The State of Florida's Medicaid program, which pays for almost all the long-term care for the poor, spends in comparison to New York State less per older resident ($340 vs. $2,640), and less per older Medicaid enrollee ($4,479 vs. $17,101).[10] Compared to other states, New York has the highest per capita Medicaid expenditure for long-term care and Florida has one of the lowest. In addition, Florida's long-term care expenditures are devoted exclusively to nursing facilities (94.5 percent), while 25.3 percent of New York's long-term care expenditures go for home care. Not surprisingly, Florida's elderly tend to be healthier and less impaired and to have greater financial resources.[11] An insurance plan faced with enrollment patterns similar to the elderly migration patterns that New York City faces would rapidly lose enrollment of low-risk subscribers and go bankrupt.

Broward County draws the largest number of elderly migrants from New York City to Florida and provides a useful way to illustrate the social and economic effect of this migration pattern on the city. (The next-most-popular destinations for New York City migrants are the adjoining South Florida counties of Palm Beach and Dade.) Broward County's retirement developments are a major engine driving its rapid growth and economic development. The developments spread out like the high-tide marks on a beach, divided by Interstate 95, the major artery connecting New York to South Florida. Most of the developments of the 1960s and 1970s abut each other in townships close to the shore. Many of these buildings and their inhabitants are in decline, both having aged in place. The newer developments that attract current retirees are further inland, pushing up against the Everglades. Open land for new developments has shrunk, as have the orange groves and winter vegetable farms that dominated the economy before the 1960s. As land prices have risen, developers bulldozed the older, more affordable trailer-park communities to make way for higher-priced condominiums. That forced a new wave of migration of longtime permanent residents and snowbirds who had put down roots in those developments. To put it bluntly, Broward, over time, has been cream skimming among a pool of older persons with marked differences in long-term care needs.

Developments for the more affluent have grown. Broward County offers luxury gated communities with twenty-four-hour security and roving patrols. The price tags for homes range from $300,000 to well over $1 million. In neighboring Palm Beach and Dade Counties, the prices for residences in such new luxury developments can rise to $10 million. The amenities include golf courses, tennis courts, boat-docking slips, and orange groves.

Broward offers a large stock of relatively affordable housing for the majority of New York's expatriate retirees who seek homes to match their more modest retirement budgets. Attractive manufactured homes with several baths and bedrooms in "active adult communities," with pleasant grounds with orange groves and a clubhouse, run between $30,000 and $80,000.

Mobile-home parks, at the low end of the retirement housing market, once represented a major and even dominant form of housing in some of Broward's municipalities. The homes could be purchased for $15,000 to as much as $50,000. The parks would be set up by a developer with the purchase or lease of vacant land and a modest investment in providing water, sewers, and a septic system. One could then attach a bucolic name to a few acres with palm trees and scrub and be open for business. Many of the mobile homes were settled by snowbirds who followed the winter migration south, slowly disengaging and taking up roots in their Broward County winter residences. Rising land prices, growing affluence, and the shrinkage of undeveloped land in the county now doom the mobile-home parks to extinction. The older ones began closing in the 1980s. Operators were unwilling to make the investment necessary to meet stricter housing-code standards on the homes and maintenance on facilities on which time and weather had taken their toll. For many located in the older homes, moving the trailer was not an option. The trailer owners in some parks battled back. Many had honed their skills battling landlords in New York City. They organized and won temporary legal and political victories but eventually succumbed to more powerful economic forces and their own growing frailty. One of the remaining struggles involves a mobile-home park leased on Seminole land that the tribe now plans to use to build a gambling casino complex, including a Hard Rock Café.[12]

Yet, no matter what the income bracket, the Broward County housing developments and their local municipalities struggle to deal with their residents' aging in place. Managers of the housing complexes may see the growing frailty and disorientation of a resident and notify the municipal governments, many of which have hired outreach workers, often retirees themselves, to visit and check up on residents. In many cases, this triggers a search for adult children and other relatives. Phone calls bring family members down from New York, and this often results in reverse migration.[13] Many older residents struggle not just with their growing frailty but also with the death of a spouse and with the unanticipated rising costs of living in South Florida. For those without the affluence to pay privately for their care, it is most likely to trigger a return to New York City to be close to their adult children and to take advantage of the more generous and comprehensive services that New York's Medicaid program provides for its older population.

Broward County, as a whole, struggles with the restricted resources it allocates to meet the growing needs of the most rapidly growing segment of the population, the more than thirty-five thousand over the age of eighty-five. The Area Agency on Aging reports waiting lists of more than 1,400 individuals for in-home personal care services. Thus, Broward County, like other Sunbelt destinations, skims the cream. These locales draw well and more affluent older persons as an engine for their own regional growth, attracting them with lower taxes and sometimes encouraging their return when subsidies for home care and nursing care that higher tax rates should provide prove absent. Getting the tax increases necessary to improve long-term care and supportive services for frail older persons is not a high priority on Florida's political agenda.

In summary, the cream-skimming strategy is working for Broward, and the affluence of the county's older population has grown, in part at the expense of New York City. Broward attracts more affluent retirement migration from New York City and returns late age migration of those who have exhausted their assets or ability to live independently.

Yet, in spite of the lure of the Sunbelt, more than 85 percent of New York City's older persons stay in New York. They remain a vital part of the fabric of local neighborhoods, accounting for more than their share of attendance at the city's sporting events, neighborhood restaurants, churches and synagogues, and cultural events. Just as elsewhere, most frail older persons stay where they are, tied by habit, by the comforts of navigating familiar physical surroundings, by family and friendships. They harbor a stubborn resistance to the stigma implied by retirement relocation and, as a consequence, depend on the care available in the city.

The Providers of Care

As the city's older residents age, they begin to navigate a complex network of economically segregated services. That network includes four distinct layers of increasingly more institutionalized and medicalized care: independent living or self-organized care, sheltered housing, nursing homes, and acute care hospitals.

Independent living and self-organized care. While New York City seems a hostile environment for the frail older person, as do most large urban areas, it hides a rich complex of arrangements that make independent living for many of its frail residents almost idyllic. More than 350,000 New Yorkers over the age of sixty live in naturally occurring retirement communities (NORCs). The term, coined in 1985, generally identifies apartment complexes and residential blocks where over 50 percent of the residents are fifty or older.[14] They are not apartment complexes or neighborhoods designed for this purpose. They just happen. Patterns similar to those that exist in New York City develop in any areas where new housing complexes open up, creating clusters of residents that reflect the age of the complex. Almost half the low- and moderate-income apartment buildings constructed with government assistance to families in New York City have become NORCs. There are 141 publicly supported moderate- and middle-income rental and limited-equity cooperative developments in New York City with approximately 52,761 apartment units. (The limited-equity cooperatives restrict the amount owners can receive from the sale of their apartment.) In addition, there are 240,245 cooperative or condominium apartments in nonpublicly sponsored apartment complexes in the city. Rent control applies to all buildings in New York City constructed before 1947 and to people who have been living in their apartments continuously since 1971. Tenants over the age of sixty-two who live in rent-controlled or -stabilized apartments are entitled to exemption from rental increases if they are below certain income thresholds. Not surprisingly, persons over the age of sixty-five occupy forty-one thousand rent-controlled apartments in New York City, or about 59 percent of all such apartments in the city. The median age of householders in the publicly supported housing cooperatives is fifty-four, and 28.7 percent are over age sixty-five. The cooperative ownership arrangements and the city's rent-control laws offer powerful incentives for aging in place and for the creation of NORCs.

Informal caregivers play an essential role in making all forms of independent living and self-organized care work. They make it possible for frail older persons to continue to live outside the formal care system. A survey of such providers in New York City indicates that they are most typically the daughter of the dependent older person, that they provide, on average, twenty hours of care a week, and that almost half have been providing such care for more than five years.[15] Most do so without additional paid help. They provide assistance with activities of daily living (bathing, dressing, feeding, incontinence, ambulation) and with medications. This invisible part of the health-care economy in New York City, as elsewhere, overwhelms the more visible formal one. For the country as a whole, a "midrange estimate" places the number of such informal caregivers at 25.8 million and the total value of their services at $196 billion, almost twice the amount of national expenditures for nursing-home and home-care services.[16]

For well-heeled New Yorkers, the services in NORCs are unparalleled. An apartment dweller on the Upper East Side can have dinner from an almost unlimited array of exotic restaurants delivered to their door in less than a half hour after a phone order. A solicitous doorman looks out for their welfare, assures security, and arranges transportation and the delivery of any services desired. The expertise of the world's largest concentration of medical specialists and researchers, and the stimulation of the world's largest concentration of cultural attractions, are a five-minute cab ride away. Indeed, a *Business Week* feature even promoted New York City as one of the "urban hot spots" for those seeking a retirement location where "being near the fifth hole isn't enough."[17]

For those with more limited resources who revel in the intellectual energy of the city, local groups have created inventive solutions. Morningside Gardens on West 123rd Street, for example, houses two thousand residents in six twenty-story towers on ten acres. Columbia University, Barnard College, Bank Street College of Education, the Jewish Theological Seminary, and the Union Theological Seminary, along with local churches, formed a corporation and with federal and state financial assistance built Morningside, which opened in 1957. By the mid-1980s more than half the residents were over the age of sixty-five. Morningside began experiencing all the predictable but never-planned-for problems of NORCs—the recluse whose apartment began to exude foul odors, the wandering older resident with dementia, and the aging alcoholic whose wife locked him out when he got drunk.

In 1986, the co-op governing body created Morningside Retirement and Health Services and, with some seed money from a foundation, hired a social worker to help facilitate services for residents. Those services have now expanded to include two full-time social workers, a music therapy group, a home-health aide, shopping and escort services, visits by residents in geriatrics from a local hospital, cultural field trips, a Medicare clinic for expediting residents' insurance paperwork, blood-pressure testing and monitoring, a weekly movie program, and a writing workshop. The writing workshop, conducted by Columbia faculty member and novelist

Mary Gordon, typically has about fifteen active members. Eileen Tobin, one of the workshop's early participants, published short stories in a literary magazine for the first time in 1997; in 2000, when she was eighty-five, one of her stories was published in an anthology, *Crimson Edge: Older Women Writing*. The title, as the book's editor, Sondra Zeidenstein, explains, represents the thin red line on the horizon at sunset. "But it does more than signal that the day is fading," she says; it "reconfigures the sky."[18]

For the average working person, retired teachers, social workers, and blue-collar workers with union pension plans, some of the other co-op apartment complexes in the city cannot be matched. The Penn South Mutual Redevelopment Houses lie just south of Penn Station on the West Side of Manhattan. This moderate-income cooperative complex opened in 1962. Many of the current six thousand residents moved in when it opened. More than 75 percent of the residents are now over sixty-five. "Living here is a very special thing. It's like living in a small town where everybody knows each other just a few blocks from Broadway and Greenwich Village," observed one of the more active co-op members. Just as with Morningside, the Penn South Co-op's board members saw a growing need for services to care for their aging members. They surveyed the wishes of the residents, sought funding, and recruited service partners. A program evolved that included group activities, volunteer programs, case management, and home-care coordination. The size and concentration of this older population, as well as the organizing skills of its leadership (it included retired social workers and organizers for the International Lady Garment Workers Union), attracted partners.

For example, the Visiting Nurse Service of New York saw an opportunity to find Medicare- and Medicaid-reimbursable cases while providing free care to residents through a satellite office in the Senior Center. Beth Israel Hospital opened geriatric medical practices in exchange for "free" flu shots, lectures, and screenings for the residents. St Vincent's, a psychiatric facility, also partnered with the co-op and provides cognitive assessments and more specialized mental health services to residents. In addition, the Penn South Program for seniors has been successful in getting both city and state appropriations for their activities and those of similar NORCs. The retired co-op organizers of the program have now launched new careers as consultants to other co-op housing projects both in New York and nationally and are busy developing an assisted-living expansion to serve the residents of Penn South.

The more fortunate low-income older persons have aged in place in the public housing projects located in the safer neighborhoods with more fashionable addresses. They have a strong informal network of neighborhood friends and a growing array of supportive services. The New York City Housing Authority's 346 developments and 181,000 apartment units are home to approximately 535,000.[19] The size of the operation is hard to comprehend. If it were a city, it would rank as the twenty-second largest in the United States. It is three times the size of Chicago's, the second largest. The New York City Housing Authority receives about 70 percent of its $2.4 billion in revenues from the federal government, 28 percent from tenant rents, and the remaining 2 percent from New York State. Historically, similar to public housing in many other parts of the country, it has provided homes predominantly for the working poor, with an equal mix of three income groups determined by calculating 80 percent, 50 percent, and 30 percent of the city's median income. These developments began to be built in the 1930s and were built to last. None have been torn down and they are generally well maintained. "We have served as the anchor and cornerstone in some of the lower-income neighborhoods and some, such as some of the developments on the Lower East Side, have helped revitalize the area," a housing authority official said.[20] Most who move in never leave. No new developments have been constructed since 1980. The average length of residence is seventeen years, and 34 percent, or sixty-one thousand, of the heads of households in the developments are over the age of sixty. Only 7,100 persons live in specifically designated senior housing developments. Most of the other older persons are dispersed through the family units in the Authority's developments and age in place. "There's an incredible informal network among the seniors; they look after each other and go into each other's apartments to make sure everything is okay. The apartment managers are a part of that network of services."[21]

Just as with the higher-income apartment complexes with a growing concentration of older persons, services have sprung up in response to needs. A nationally recognized senior resident advisor program began as a demonstration in 1979. It provided an advisor with a free apartment and modest salary in return for serving on call twenty-four hours a day to assist older residents with problems and coordinate services for them. The resulting program currently provides on-site services for 5,200 older persons in twenty-two developments. In addition, the Housing Authority operates 40 senior centers (of the city's 350) that provide preventive health programs and activities for older persons in its developments. Seven of the twenty-eight NORCs in the city, which are now officially recognized with state and city funds to support the organization of services, operate in the Authority's developments. The funds support outreach and social workers. Just as with the other NORCs, most have begun to develop partnerships with health-care providers for on-site services that can be covered by Medicaid and Medicare.

The home-health services covered by Medicaid, in New York State, make it possible to envision the low-income NORCs evolving into full-blown assisted-living facilities. It is the most distinctive feature of the care in New York, most of which is quite similar to that provided in other states. New York State provides the most extensive and costly Medicaid package of home-care benefits of any state. It provides both short-term home health care for patients discharged from a hospital and home-attendant care for the chronically ill. Currently about half the money spent nationally in the Medicaid program for such care is spent in New York State.

In 1998, this amounted to almost $2.4 billion, with 81 percent, or more than $1.9 billion, spent in New York City alone.[22] The Medicaid home health-care program in the city serves a frail and vulnerable population.

A recent survey estimates that 81 percent of New York City's sixty-five thousand Medicaid home health-care recipients live in its fifteen poorest neighborhoods; 40 percent live alone, 90 percent suffer from at least one chronic health condition, and 75 percent are impaired in performing at least three basic activities of daily living, such as bathing and eating.[23] "Many live in isolation and feel imprisoned in their apartments. Maybe half would benefit with assistance in getting groceries or preparing meals. Depression, alcohol abuse and suicide are common problems," an outreach worker said.[24] Those whose assets and income do not qualify them for Medicaid but who cannot afford to pay out of pocket for services represent a major impediment to the Housing Authority's developing functional full-service NORCs. As one older resident observed, "I've worked every day of my life and Mrs. Fisher never worked one. She's got a personal care aide that comes in to help her. Why can't I have one?"[25] Many could ask similar questions, particularly those who feel forced to choose between filling prescriptions and shopping for groceries.

However, the shortage of adequate affordable housing for the low-income population casts the largest shadow over all these supportive efforts. While many other urban areas in the United States face similar problems with access to affordable housing, New York City has experienced the most extreme and persistent shortage. Housing conditions in New York City have constituted an emergency under New York State law since 1950. On the Housing Authority waiting list are more than 284,000 applications for public and Section 8 housing. The waiting time for Housing Authority apartments for those who do not become special priorities (e.g., working-poor families and the homeless) now averages seventeen years. The Housing Authority also provides seventy-seven thousand families with vouchers to assist with the rental of private apartments, a system that works well if the persons eligible for vouchers live in apartments that meet the standards to qualify. It is difficult, if not impossible, to find such low-rent apartments in the current market. Federal definitions define spending more than 30 percent of one's household income for housing as excessive. The median single older household in the city, before subsidies, pays 50.7 percent of its income on housing. Thus, most of the low-income elderly live in the poorest housing in the city, buildings with growing maintenance and structural problems in neighborhoods that are no longer safe. They may have to climb six floors to a walk-up apartment that saw brighter days many years ago. For some, a stroke, a fall, or a broken hip ends the struggle to maintain their independence and the fragile network of supports they had organized around it.

Among the city's poor, many go without the care that they need. More than 13,500 received government-subsidized home-delivered meals, but the waiting lists for meals are long. For some, this single meal is supplemented with little else.

Malnutrition is widespread. Some supplement their diets by foraging in garbage bins, and a few extreme cases starve to death.[26] The visits of a senior-center outreach team uncover bleak conditions among those who are no longer able to live independently. They find a man with Alzheimer's disease left alone when his wife was hospitalized. In a squalid apartment, they find a confused woman who has not eaten for four days. Sometimes they find the dead.[27] For others, cycles of larger, more powerful forces have transformed the urban landscape.

An epidemic of fires spread through the longtime slum neighborhoods of Harlem, East Harlem, the Lower East Side, Brownsville, Bedford Stuyvesant, Williamsburg, and the South Bronx, cresting in the middle 1970s. Waves of migration and dislocations disrupted stable surrounding neighborhoods. The social dislocations spread the accompanying urban plagues of violent crime, TB, low birth-weight babies, and AIDS. The city has yet to recover from the cascading sequence of events. Public urban development policies of "benign neglect" and the resulting reallocation of fire department resources appears to have triggered this sequence of events.[28] Low-income frail elderly persons continue to be its major victims, slipping through the informal network of self- and family-organized supports and into the city's more formalized arrangements for care. Some end up in one of the city's remaining seventy-two single-room-occupancy (SRO) hotels.

The city's press for more than thirty years has chronicled the battle between older tenants on fixed incomes in these hotels and landlords seeking profits from conversions to tourist hotels or higher-priced condominiums. It is a story similar to the disappearance of the mobile-home parks in Broward County but an often more brutal one. Many of the current SROs were once reputable hotels and apartment complexes, converted to accommodate the flood of single workers into the city during and after World War II. As the demand for apartments increased in the 1970s, many hotels were converted to apartments and co-ops. There were few options for the existing tenants, often disabled or older with limited incomes. The city imposed a moratorium on such conversions in 1983, which the courts overturned in 1989. Landlords could increase their income over the rent-controlled SRO rates by conversions to tourist hotels or condominiums by more than tenfold. It was a matter of making conditions sufficiently unbearable so that people who had very little choice would leave. These existing SRO tenants cannot legally be kicked out, but as they leave or die, conversions can take place.

Until twenty years ago, tenants had fewer protections. "They weren't at all subtle back then," observed one housing advocate; "they just hired goons and kicked you out."[29] For some, the process became only a shade subtler. The SROs now range from poor but reasonably safe and clean to squalid, degrading, and dangerous. On the low end, maintenance is deferred and buildings are allowed to deteriorate. They become homes for drug addicts, prostitutes, and people with mental illness. Some SRO landlords allegedly still hire thugs to rob and terrorize tenants.[30]

Sheltered housing. New York City and New York State together provide a bewildering variety of arrangements for more formalized sheltered housing and refuge for more vulnerable older persons. In other states, such facilities are licensed as boarding, personal care, or assisted-living facilities, but the residents and the services provided are much the same. Some states also provide care to nursing-home-eligible residents in these facilities with the assistance of home-health agencies under a Medicaid waiver program. In New York State, there are three kinds of licensed facilities that provide such care: adult homes, enriched housing, and assisted-living programs operated within either an adult home or an enriched housing setting. The licensed adult homes provide housing, meals, and some limited social activities and personal care to residents. Of the fifty-one adult homes licensed in the city, forty are for-profit operations and the remainder nonprofit. About half mix more than 25 percent discharged psychiatric hospital patients with frail older persons.

In addition to the adult homes, there are nine enriched housing programs located in subsidized, nonprofit, low-income complexes that provide a somewhat similar array of services for their older apartment dwellers. Ten of these licensed facilities have Assisted Living Programs (ALPs) approved for payment by the state Medicaid program and designed to provide care for nursing-home-eligible residents in conjunction with a licensed home-health agency; their total capacity is 1,056. The ALP units are entitled to Medicaid payments equivalent to half the nursing Medicaid rate for particular types of patients, in addition to the Supplemental Security Income (SSI) payments. For a typical resident in an ALP unit, a "Physical A" (a patient needing relatively routine and inexpensive physical care), the facility receives a Medicaid payment of $59.65 per day. Altogether, these licensed facilities in New York City have a capacity for 9,327 residents. The average size is 141 beds. They range in size from a 427-bed proprietary adult home located on Staten Island to an eleven-resident enriched housing arrangement operated by a nonprofit in Manhattan. In general, the facilities in the city are larger than ones located upstate and in other parts of the country. They rely almost exclusively on either private payments by residents or SSI payments. Few facilities serve both the private and SSI populations. The current SSI rate in New York for adult-care facilities is $27 a day.

The licensed adult homes that rely on public payments cover the full range of conditions. Some manage through the energy and dedication of their staff and residents to create clean, warm, lively communities in spartan surroundings, places where no adult child would feel bad about leaving a parent. Others, particularly those whose residents are mostly psychiatric patients, rival the snake pits of the early twentieth century. One of the worst is a for-profit home, housing 360 mentally ill residents, that remains open despite a decade of horror stories.[31] In 1989, two residents of the home died under mysterious circumstances, one padlocked in a closet. In 1993, a decomposed body was found wedged behind a basement freezer. In 2000, the Health Department ordered the evacuation of residents on the first floor after an inspection found soiled linen, vermin infestation, and badly damaged walls and ceilings. In

2001, the Health Department conducted an inquiry into the assembly-line prostate operations on twenty-four residents involving questionable appropriateness and consent. The urologist performed the surgery at one of the city's only remaining small for-profit hospitals, in which he had an ownership interest. In April 2002, the *New York Times* published a three-part series detailing similar abuses and the failure to adequately regulate the city's adult homes.[32]

In addition, a largely invisible unlicensed segment offers privately paid arrangements for older persons who can afford them. Those operating in this segment describe their facilities as assisted living or senior residential housing. They operate as part of the private apartment market in New York City and target higher-income frail older persons. Monthly fees that include rent, meals, and some services in the unlicensed private facilities range between two and six thousand dollars. Eighteen of these unlicensed facilities responded to a telephone survey in the fall of 1999.[33] They had a total capacity of 2,020 units. The average number of apartment units in these unlicensed facilities was 112. They have provided such care for an average of about ten years and overall operate at 88 percent of capacity. Thirteen of the eighteen responding facilities were nonprofits, and the remainder were for-profit operations. Most observers in 1999 forecasted explosive growth of this segment of the market from the many planned conversions of hotels and apartment buildings and new construction in progress. Some residences have the look and feel of luxury hotels. Atria West Side, a recently converted residential hotel on the Upper West Side of Manhattan, for example, offers a penthouse lounge and terrace gardens with spectacular views of the Manhattan skyline. Amenities include a theater with surrounding sound and parlors with fireplaces. Residents can, for a price, rent spacious, high-ceilinged apartments with two bedrooms, two baths, a full kitchen, and private terraces with a skyline view. However, in an accommodation to the city's rent-control laws, about a third of the facility's inhabitants are tenants who predate the acquisition and conversion by Atria. These include couples with children and middle-aged professionals. Thus, Atria West Side offers, through no intention of its own, perhaps one of the only intergenerational assisted-living facilities in the country.

At the other extreme, services now coordinated under New York City's Department of Homeless Services provide shelter for the poorest and most desperate of the city's older inhabitants.[34] Its Division of Adult Services manages forty-four temporary-accommodation shelters with a capacity for over 7,500 persons. The department directly operates eight of these shelters, and the remainder are operated under contract by nonprofit social service organizations. Seventy-nine percent of those in these shelters are male. The average age is forty-three. Alcoholism, drug addiction, and mental health problems figure prominently in this population, but many operators believe the older persons in the mental health population need most of the same assistance as those over sixty-five years and frail cared for in the other settings. For those living on the streets, the department operates nine drop-in centers, eight of which are under contract with nonprofit social service providers that offer social services, meals, and showers. Seven outreach teams, six under contract with nonprofit social service organizations, attempt to provide services to those living on the streets and in other public places. The objective of all these efforts is to transition this population to more permanent housing arrangements. In addition to the licensed adult homes and enriched housing mentioned earlier, the dwindling number of SRO hotels houses some of the older persons in this population. Landlords renting to a homeless individual can also receive a one-time rent bonus and Section 8 subsidies up to what is defined as the fair market rate.

Those who slip through the cracks of all these sheltered housing arrangements end up filling the emergency rooms of the city's hospitals. Many for whom little can be done have impaired and declining mental and physical status. Those who have had successful lives blend in with those who have lived marginal ones, sharing the universal human experiences of aging, illness, suffering, and death. They are all too often assigned the label GOMER (Get Out of My Emergency Room) or other pejorative terms by the frustrated young interns and residents who attend to them.[35] They wait together either to be admitted to the hospital, pending nursing-home placement, or to be moved directly from the emergency room to a nursing home.

Nursing homes. There are 185 licensed nursing homes in New York's five boroughs, with a total of 43,897 beds for those who, largely for medical reasons, cannot be cared for in the less restrictive settings. These facilities provide twenty-four-hour skilled nursing supervision and care. They range in size from the 816-bed Jewish Home and Hospital in the Bronx and the 775-bed Coler Memorial public facility on Roosevelt Island to a 35-bed proprietary one on Staten Island. The average size is 237 beds. Ownership of the city's nursing homes is split between proprietary (51 percent) and voluntary operations (44 percent). Seven facilities operated by the city make up the remainder. The 43.7 beds per one thousand population over sixty-five in the state contrasts with 52.7 in the United States as a whole, and 29.1 in Florida. In 1997, the average occupancy rate was 98 percent, higher than for any other state. There were 50,433 Medicaid-eligible older New Yorkers who received care in these nursing homes in fiscal year 1997–1998 at an average cost of $40,239 and a total cost of $2.031 billion.[36] Unlike most other states, Medicaid payments to nursing homes in New York compare reasonably to private rates. Concentrations of Medicaid and private residents in different facilities reflect more the composition of the service area rather than selective facility admitting practices.

Acute care hospitals. There are seventy-four licensed acute hospitals in New York's five boroughs, with a total of 31,428 beds and an overall occupancy in the second quarter of 1998 of 69.5 percent. This means there are 4.26 acute hospital beds per one thousand people in the city. The bed-population ratio and the occupancy rate in the city are slightly higher than the overall national figures (4.00 hospital beds per one thousand and an occupancy rate in 1998 of 65 percent). New York's older persons were discharged from acute hospitals 298,712 times during 1998 with an average length of stay of 9.37 days. This translates into 297 discharges and 2,784 total days per thousand older persons. The hospital discharge rate for New York City's older residents is 20 percent below the national rates (297 vs. 365 per thousand), but their average length of stay is 51 percent higher than the national average (9.37 vs. 6.20).[37] As a result, New York City's older persons had a rate of hospital days per thousand 30 percent higher than the national rate (2,784 vs. 2,149). In other words, New York City's older persons are less likely to be admitted to a hospital but stay longer and fill more acute hospital beds. About half return to their homes, with 14 percent of these receiving home-health care.

Almost all of New York City's seventy-four acute care hospitals are owned by nonprofit voluntary organizations. The only significant exceptions are the eleven public hospitals operated by the city's Health and Hospitals Corporation, which continue to play a unique and vital role in the city's health system. This contrasts to the southern and western regions of the United States, where for-profit hospitals have a large, if not dominant, presence. The dominance of nonprofit ownership in New York reflects the history of hospital development in the Northeast and Midwest, and the city's own distinctive aversion to for-profit health care. Only five small marginal proprietary facilities are currently licensed as hospitals in the city. Major teaching hospitals and medical centers have expanded by acquiring hospitals, which created considerable consolidation of ownership in the last decade.[38] The city's hospitals struggle with growing financial problems, with 61 percent reporting operating losses in 2000, eleven of thirty-six studied by the United Hospital Fund in jeopardy of closing, and another nine facing financial problems that placed them at risk of such a fate.[39]

Paying for Care

While costs of care for the frail older persons in New York City are high, New Yorkers as a whole have ample resources (Table 5.1). The average income of residents sixty-five years and over is more than $25,000, and their average net worth is approximately $311,000. These resources pay for living expenses and for medical care and personal assistance not covered by health insurance. If these combined costs exceed their income, they can liquidate their assets by selling their home or dipping into savings. The federal Medicare program pays out an average of more than $9,000 a year in New York City to help with the cost of medical care covered under this program for both physician and hospital expenditures. For low-income persons and those who become indigent because of the cost of their care, the state Medicaid program spends an average of almost $19,000 per person. Most of these Medicaid dollars cover nursing-home and home-care costs not covered by the Medicare program. Family members also chip in to help cover the costs of this care and informally provide much of it themselves. Excluding savings and the support of adult children and other family members, a total of $37,500 per older New York resident helps to cover their living expenses, personal care expenses, and medical costs. The city alone, excluding the suburban counties in its metropolitan area, represents an "elder-care market" of almost $40 billion. Only a few of the most affluent counties in the United States and few of the most affluent countries in the world can come close to matching this level of resource provision per older resident.

This seeming affluence however, masks two persistent unresolved conflicts in the financing of care.

The first conflict is that paying for care blends funds for living expenses with health-insurance payments. Pensions, Social Security, and SSI payments for low-income older persons work differently than health insurance. Insurance typically pays for rare, unpredictable, catastrophic events, not for other services individuals want, which pits the interests of the individual against those of the insurance company and creates what insurance companies call a "moral hazard." Also, to make insurance affordable, plans must limit what they will pay for and whom they will pay. Typically, no similar constraints limit what individuals can do with their own retirement income. As a result of the concern about abuse of public funds, health-

Table 5.1. Resources for Paying for Care for Persons 65+: NYC, 1998

	Total Persons 65+[a]	$ per Person	Total (in $ billion)
Income and Assets[b]			
Income	1,005,227	25,205	25.3
Net worth[c]	1,005,227	311,000	312.6
Health Insurance			
Medicare[d]	846,364	9,000	7.6
Medicaid[e]	246,712	18,716	4.6

[a] Claritas estimates, 1998.

[b] Bureau of Economic Analysis estimates, age corrected by Federal Reserve 1998 Survey of Consumer Finance (Kennickell, Starr-McCluer et al. 2000. Federal Reserve Board Bulletin 86, January: 1-29.

[c] Net worth: "City Estimates for Households," Federal Reserve 1998 Survey Adjusted for Age and Household Size, *Ibid*

[d] Medicare: July 1998 Medicare total elderly enrollment and Average Adjusted Per Capita Cost for New York City's Counties, Health Care Financing Administration files

[e] Profile-FY 1998-99, NYC, All Aid Categories for Persons 65+, New York State Department of Health (www.health.state.ny.us/nysdoh/medstat/medicaid_profiles/99/ demographic/99cal65.htm)

insurance payments are usually more generous than those that cover routine living expenses for the indigent.

For example, the New York State Medicaid Program pays nursing homes between $118 and $244 a day for care. In contrast, an adult home that cares for a person who just needs board, room, and personal care gets $27 a day. (In calls to higher-cost kennels in Manhattan, we found that this was half the typical cost per day for boarding a dog.) As a result, the pooling of resources that cover living and medical expenses is fraught with complications. For example, health insurance will pay for board and care in a hospital or a nursing-home setting but not in one's own home. On the other hand, food stamps and Section 8 low-income rent subsidies can help support persons living independently but cannot be used to defray their costs in a health facility.

The blending of health care and day-to-day living in the same formal setting also creates tensions between those providing and receiving care. These decisions go beyond the accounting problems of figuring out who should pay for what and into the problems of who is qualified to provide what kind of services and who decides what is purchased. With one's own money, an individual is free to decide what to eat, where to live, and whom to hire to provide assistance at home. However, in a health-related institutional setting, a physician (or maybe an insurance company) decides what medications patients should take, whether they should be hospitalized, and what care they should receive during such a hospitalization. What happens when health care and day-to-day living take place in the same setting and one has to make decisions about how to allocate a common pool of dollars? Who is in charge? These are not new conflicts, but when these different purposes are addressed in a common setting they are certainly heightened. As one moves from costs covered by one's own income and assets, to costs covered as a beneficiary of an insurance plan, to costs covered by direct charitable and public subsidies of providers, control shifts from the recipient of these services to the provider. One moves from a simple market transaction to a more complex set of relationships and expectations.

The second conflict involves the inequitable distribution of income and assets. Private housing and health-services complexes target their developments to people with average income and wealth, since they usually have no problem paying for them, but income and assets, of course, are not equally distributed. As noted earlier, income disparities are particularly large in New York City's older population. The need for care tends to be inversely related to income, and this further exacerbates the impact of these disparities on care. Some argue that this consistent inverse relationship between income and health status is, in part, a consequence of the burdens placed on social networks and social cohesion by inequality.[40] If this is the case, certainly frail older persons, with their greater dependence on such networks, are the most vulnerable. They are perhaps the canaries in the coal mine.

The Persistent Class Conflicts Embedded in the Organization of Care

These problems in the financing of care are not new. From the city's beginnings, the organization and financing of care for frail older persons has reflected a less visible class conflict over the nature of that care. This has involved a fundamental conflict over its purpose, its organization, and the role of government in the regulation and financing of such care.

Purpose. Well into the twentieth century, public debate about how to care for frail older persons was submerged in the debate over how to deal with the poor. Medicine could offer little that could make any difference, and families informally provided most of the day-to-day care needed. Frail older persons represented only a tiny fraction of the population. In 1900, only one-tenth of 1 percent of the population of the United States was over the age of eighty-five, now considered an age above which a large proportion of long-term care services are provided. In 2000, the proportion of the population over eighty-five had grown more than sixteenfold to 1.6 percent and is projected to reach 4.6 percent, or almost twenty million, by 2050.[41] The poor, however, of which frail older people once represented only a small fraction, have always been a concern. The debate on how to handle the indigent hinged on how much government should focus on attempting to eliminate, or at least ameliorate, the problems of poverty and how much on simply controlling it. The prevailing position was that efforts to alleviate poverty might well attract an even greater concentration of poor, and so one should focus on control. Throughout New York City's four-hundred-year history, the fear that beggars, petty thieves, the homeless, and unruly mobs would inundate the city focused concern on policing the poor. Those fears helped shape care for the frail older persons, as well.

Organization. A second related conflict involved whether to organize such care around "outdoor" or "indoor" relief. Support for indoor relief—providing care in an institution—is based on an assumption that residents and their care can be better controlled in such a setting. Outdoor relief involves providing financial support so that recipients can purchase what they need for themselves, or directly providing food, fuel, and personal assistance in the recipient's own home. In other words, should care be institutionalized or deinstitutionalized? The answer to this question reflected the purpose of such care and the relationship between those providing the services and those receiving them. If those who are to receive care are considered dangerous or destructive to themselves or to the social fabric of a community, then it is likely that communities will choose to provide care through indoor relief. If the recipients of such care are seen as members of a community, then the balance shifts toward the more sympathetic, more attractive, and less stigmatized treatment provided by outdoor relief.[42]

The conflict over indoor as opposed to outdoor relief, however, was also a conflict over cost. The advantage of indoor relief was that you could restrict the numbers receiving care through the capacity of the institution and thereby control cost. However, per recipient, outdoor relief is far cheaper. For example, in Massachusetts in 1889, the average cost of keeping a pauper in an almshouse was $180 per year and the average cost for each "outdoor" pauper was $40 per year.[43] Thus, simply shifting paupers from indoor to outdoor relief reduced the cost per person to less than one-quarter of the previous cost. In 1950, a similar conclusion was reached by the Municipal Hospital System in New York, which found that shifting hospital patients to their newly established home-care program (e.g., outdoor relief) not only would relieve the overcrowding of the hospitals but also would cost only an average of $2.66 per day, approximately one-fourth the cost of general care on the wards of the municipal hospitals.[44] Mayoral candidate John Lindsay even argued, in 1964, for a dramatic expansion of nursing-home beds on such grounds, noting that the cost of care in the more institutionalized municipal hospital settings was $48 per day versus only $15 dollars a day in nursing homes, or less than one-third the cost.[45] While the costs of the services involved in computing such ratios have grown by a factor of more than ten, similar arguments have been made more recently about the "savings" one could accrue by shifting care from skilled nursing homes to home care or assisted-living settings, but the remarkably similar ratios of the relative costs quoted rarely prove cost effective under more rigorous examination.[46]

Outdoor relief, however, while more attractive to the recipient and not limited by the physical capacity of a building, makes controlling the costs and the number of recipients of such care more difficult. The fear has always been that such outdoor relief would encourage more recipients of care and end up costing far more. The concern is that such benefits, rather than substituting for care provided indoors and saving money, would greatly expand the cost by expanding use to those now receiving such care informally from family members. Medicaid officials in many states today refer to this as the "woodwork problem," a reference to the way new beneficiaries, attracted by the less restrictive benefits, come out of the woodwork. They argue that the expansion of benefits for home-health services will increase the overall cost of long-term care for the Medicaid program and point to New York State's experience with expanded benefits.

Often, however, the choice between indoor and outdoor relief has had less to do with what was more cost effective or compatible with prevailing beliefs and more to do with calculating how the costs of such care could be shifted onto other parties. For example, states assumed responsibility for the chronically mentally ill population at the end of the nineteenth century. Local officials saw this as a golden opportunity to shift to the state hospitals the cost of caring for older persons housed in local almshouses.[47] The population in state psychiatric hospitals and the average age of residents rose dramatically in the first three decades of the twentieth century.[48] This flow was reversed in the 1960s and 1970s, partly as a result of the advantages Medicare and Medicaid offered the state in shifting the financial burden onto the federal government by moving this older psychiatric population to nursing homes and to adult homes, where medical costs of care would be reimbursable through the Medicare and Medicaid programs.[49]

Public role. What should the role of government be in providing, financing, and regulating care for frail older persons? Should it be a matter of limited public concern best left to the resources of the individuals and their families? Is this just another good or service best left to the market, or part of a broader public responsibility to provide some level of security to citizens in old age? Such questions have risen to the surface only in the wake of periodic disclosures of financial abuses and sub-standard treatment of older persons that have sparked outrage. Most of the time, however, the predominant view has been that government's role should be one of last resort, discouraging and controlling pauperism. Perhaps such periodic political outbursts over the conditions of care for frail older persons are inevitable given the tensions over the purpose and organization of such care. In any event, these cycles of scandal, reform, and neglect are interwoven into the history of care in New York City, as they are across the nation as a whole.

The Institutional Migration Effect: The Growth of Private Market Assisted Living

All these recurring conflicts over the financing of care, and over its purpose, organi-zation, and the role of government in it, came to a head in the 1990s. A combination of trends converged—growing affluence; an increasing proportion of two-salary households among adult children; the growing medicalized and institutional char-acter of nursing homes, in part reflecting their growing dependence on the Medicaid program; a more development-friendly political environment in the city; and rising consumer expectations for more control and choice—and created a dramatic growth of unregulated private pay facilities designed to cater to this emerging market.

Assisted living as it emerged in the 1990s aggressively targeted the growing pri-vate late-age market within New York City much the way South Florida had targeted the city's affluent retirement market in earlier decades. It offered residents their own private homelike apartments, greater choice, more autonomy, and the illusion of upper-class status with amenities such as black-tie waiters and lobbies with glass chandeliers at prestige addresses—rather than the relegation to the almshouse that older persons and their adult children continue to associate with the nursing home. They were also able to offer such accommodation at a price that was usually lower than the more costly care for nursing-home residents in more regulated facilities. In contrast to nursing homes, which had difficulty acquiring capital to renovate or replace aging physical plants, assisted-living developers enjoyed seemingly unlimited access to capital through private investors, real estate investment trusts, and stock in rapidly expanding publicly traded assisted-living companies. Low interest rates and rising prices in the New York City real estate market made such investments particularly attractive. What had been small regional "ma and pa" operations, such as Sunrise Assisted Living and Kapson Senior Quarters, were suddenly transformed into rapidly expanding publicly traded national corporations.

Assisted living in the 1990s was viewed by many of its developers less as another layer of care for the aging than as a direct challenge to the existing organization of such services. It emphasized resident empowerment, choice, and the ability, through services organized around the residents' individual needs, to age in place. These new private market assisted-living facilities did not just compete with a segment of the traditionally organized continuum of care. They attempted to feed off the entire continuum. This trend was similar to the Florida geographic migration effect described earlier. Like the geographic cream skimming, the assisted-living institutional version of cream skimming attracted people with higher incomes who could afford private rates and required less care. When private pay assisted-living residents run out of money or become unprofitable to care for, they are discharged. As a result, hospitals, nursing homes, and the traditional continuum of services face caring for an increasing share of indigent patients that cost more. The private assisted-living facilities absorb the profits, and the more traditional providers of health care absorb the increasing losses. A cream-skimming double-death spiral of geographic (retirement age) and institutional (late age) migration has begun to accelerate.

The Future of Care in New York City

The emergence of private market assisted living in New York is at the intersection of the conflicting forces shaping health and housing policies in the United States. It is in the eye of the looming storm. Nursing-home occupancy levels have dropped, as has the number of private pay patients, and nursing homes have become increasingly dependent on Medicaid. The growth of private market assisted living raises new and troubling questions about social class, the nature of communities, and, ultimately, the kind of society we want to become.

The pessimistic scenario is that the institutional migration effect produced by the growing ascendancy of private assisted living combined with the geographic migration effect will return the organization of care for older people in the city to its nineteenth-century status. Hospitals and nursing homes that have cared for all income segments of the population will return to their nineteenth-century role as institutions exclusively serving the indigent. Private duty nurses and physicians will care for upper- and middle-income persons in their own homes as they did during the nineteenth century. Public and voluntary hospitals will revert to their almshouse roots, providing care for the poor. The shocking conditions that plagued the eighteenth- and nineteenth-century almshouses will return on a larger scale.

The optimistic scenario is that the current transformation reflects a more general change in the organization of care, offering greater control and choice to residents and their family members, that will cut across all care provided to older persons regardless of income. Perhaps the yearning for community created by the September 11 destruction of the World Trade Towers, the end of the bull market, and revelations of corporate abuses will have a salutary effect in shaping more common solutions. The quality of life, if not the viability of New York City itself, hangs in the balance between these pessimistic and optimistic versions of the future.

Notes

1.   Better Business Bureau of New York City. 2002. A Visitor's Guide to New York; Boyer, R., and S. D. Savageau. 1987. *Retirement Places Rated.* Chicago: Rand McNally.

2.   U.S. Census, 2000. Summary File 3 http://factfinder.census.gov: Age by Sex (page 8), Age by Types of Disability for Bronx, Kings, New York, Queens and Richmond County (page 41) (accessed May 1, 2005).

3.   Masumura, W. T. 1996. Moving up and down the Income Ladder. *Current Population Reports.* U.S. Census Bureau. Washington DC: Government Printing Office, 70–56; Jones, A. F., and D. H. Weinberg. 2000. The Changing Shape of the Nation's Income Distribution, 1947–1998. *Current Population Reports.* U.S. Census Bureau. Washington DC: Government Printing Office

4.   Computed from U.S. Census, 1990. Summary File 3: Household Income in 1989 (page 80); Age of Householder by Household Income in 1989 for Bronx, Kings, New York, Queens and Richmond Counties (page 86), http://factfinder.census.gov (accessed May 1, 2005).

5.   Warnes, A. M. 1992. Age-related Variation and Temporal Change in Elderly Migration. In A. Rogers, ed. *Elderly Migration and Population Redistribution*, 38. London: Belhaven Press.

6.   Kallan, J. E. 1993. A Multilevel Analysis of Elderly Migration. *Social Science Quarterly* 74(2): 403–419.

7.   Computed from U.S. Census, 1990, and Longino, C. F. 1995. *Retirement Migration in America.* Houston: Vacation Publications.

8.   Longino, *Retirement Migration in America*, 85.

9.   Berry, B. M., and J. C. Henretta. 1996. *The Florida AHEAD Respondents: Characteristics of Florida's Elderly Population Aged Seventy and Over. HRS/AHEAD Working Paper 96–039.* Ann Arbor: Population Studies Center, University of Michigan.

10.   Holahan, J., J. Weiner, and S. Wallin. 1998. *Health Policy for the Low Income Population: Major Findings from the Assess the New Federalism Case Studies.* Washington DC: Urban Institute (www.urban.org/url.cfm?ID=308044).

11.   Berry and Henretta, *The Florida AHEAD Respondents.*

12.   Vise, D. D., and E. Bolstad. 2000. Seminoles Plan Gaming Resort for Hollywood. *Miami Herald,* July 6.

13.   Smith, D., and J. Apt. 1994. A Community Health Assessment for Broward County, Florida: North and South Broward Hospital Districts. Consulting report to the North and South Broward Hospital Districts. Philadelphia.

14. Hunt, M., and G. Gunter-Hunt. 1985. Naturally Occurring Retirement Communities. *Journal of Housing for the Elderly* 3(3/4): 3–21.

15. Levine, C. 2000. *A Survey of Caregivers in New York City: Findings and Implications for the Health Care System*. New York: United Hospital Fund.

16. Arno, P. S., and C. Levine. 1999. The Economic Value of Informal Care Giving. *Health Affairs* 18(2): 182–188.

17. Baig, E. C., and T. Reiss. 1998. When a Home near the Fifth Hole Isn't Enough. *Business Week*, July 20, 98.

18. Haberman, C. 2000. Joy and Anger as a Career Takes Flight. *New York Times*, April 7.

19. New York City Housing Authority Fact Sheet. 2001. New York City Housing Authority.

20. Author interview #60, 2001. Author files.

21. Ibid.

22. New York State Department of Health. 2000. Medicaid Profile—Ffy 97–98. Albany: New York State Department of Health.

23. Hokenstad, A., M. Ramirez, Kathryn Haslanger, and Kathleen Finneran. 1998. *Medicaid Home Care Service in New York City*. New York: United Hospital Fund.

24. Author interview #59, 2001. Author files.

25. Ibid.

26. Goodnough, A. 1994. Old in New York, and Struggling; The Neediest Cases: An Array of Troubles Affect the Elderly Poor. *New York Times*, December 4.

27. Ibid.

28. Wallace, D., and R. Wallace. 1998. *A Plague on Your Houses: How New York Was Burned Down and National Public Health Crumbled*. New York: Verso.

29. Siegal, N. 1998. Checkout Time? As S.R.O. Owners Make Way for Tourists, Long-Term Tenants Say They're Left in the Lurch. *New York Times*, November 22.

30. Lobbia, J. A. 1997. Thugs Say Landlord Paid Them: A Slumlord Saga, Continued. *New York Times*, April 29.

31. Levy, C. J., and S. Kershaw. 2001. Inquiry Finds Mentally Ill Patients Endured "Assembly Line" Surgery. *New York Times*, March 18. New York State fined Leben Home and forced a change of administrators. It is still open, but operating under new management and a new name—Queens Adult Care Center.

32. Clifford, J. L. 2002. Voiceless, Defenseless, and a Source of Cash. *New York Times*, April 30.

33. Rudder, Cynthia, and David B. Smith. 2000. Survey of Assisted Living in New York State New York: Nursing Home Community Care Coalition of New York State.

34. New York City Department of Homeless Services. 2001. About the Department: Adult Services Fact Sheets, Single Adults for Fy 1999. New York: Department of Homeless Services.

35. Leiderman, D. B., and J.-A. Grisso. 1985. The Gomer Phenomenon. *Journal of Health and Social Behavior* 26(3): 222–232.

36. New York State Department of Health. Medicaid Profile-Ffy 97–98.

37. Hall, M. J., and J. R. Popovic. 2000. 1998 Summary: National Hospital Discharge Survey. Hyattsville, MD: National Center for Health Statistics, 6; New York State

Department of Health. 2001. *SPARCS 1998 Annual Report*. Albany: New York State Department of Health.

38. Cantor, J., K. Haslanger, Anthony Tassi, Eve Weiss, Kathleen Finneran, and Sue Kaplan. 1998. *Health Care in New York City: Service Providers' Response to an Emerging Market*. Washington DC: Urban Institute.

39. United Hospital Fund. 2001. *United Hospital Fund Reports Severe Financial Problems at NYC Non-Specialty Voluntary Hospitals*. Press release. New York: United Hospital Fund.

40. Wilkinson, R. G. 1996. *Unhealthy Societies: The Affliction of Inequality*. London: Routledge; Auerbach, J. A., and B. K. Krimgold, eds. 2001. *Income, Socioeconomic Status, and Health: Exploring the Relationships*. Washington DC: National Policy Association.

41. Federal Interagency Forum on Aging-Related Statistics. 2000. *Older Americans 2000: Key Indicators of Well-Being*. Washington DC: Federal Interagency Forum on Aging-Related Statistics, 56.

42. Lowell, M. C. R., C. R. Henderson, Robert D. M'Gonnigle, Levi L. Barbour, F. B. Sanborn, and Issac P. Wright 1900. Public Outdoor Relief. *American Journal of Sociology* 6(1): 90–104.

43. Ibid., 99.

44. *New York Times*. 1950. Home Care "Saves" 29 City Hospitals. January 6.

45. Lindsay, J. 1964. *A White Paper on New York City's Crisis in Health Care Facilities: A Program of Positive Action and Progress*. Typescript. Temple University Library HealthPAC Archives, Philadelphia.

46. Weissert, W., M Chernew, and R. Hirth. 2001. Beyond Managed Long-Term Care: Paying for Home Care Based on Risk of Adverse Outcomes. *Heath Affairs* 20(3): 172–180.

47. Grob, G. N. 1994. Mad, Homeless, and Unwanted: A History of the Care of the Chronic Mentally Ill in America. *Psychiatric Clinics of North America* 17(3): 541–548.

48. Sutton, J. R. 1991. The Political Economy of Madness: The Expansion of the Asylum in Progressive America. *American Sociological Review* 56(5): 665–678.

49. Mechanic, D., and D. A. Rochefort. 1990. Deinsitutionalization: An Appraisal of Reform. *Annual Review of Sociology* 16:301–327.

6. The Housing of Older New Yorkers

Kenneth Knapp

Introduction

Perhaps the single most important element that helps define a city's quality of life is its housing. It is not just a source of shelter, but also a major component of household wealth, especially for older persons, who have higher ownership rates than do younger persons, and the vast majority of whom own their homes free of mortgage obligations.[1]

"Housing, like all issues of modern urbanization, is complex," Patricia Pollak wrote in 1995.[2] Housing in New York City, one of the oldest cities in the United States and the most populous and most economically and culturally diverse, is no exception. More than 400,000 residents live more than twenty stories above street level; 600,000 live on ground floors. About 1.2 million live in buildings comprising one hundred or more units; nearly 1.4 million reside in single-unit structures. Of the city's eight million residents, 65 percent are renters. Some renters live in rent-controlled or rent-stabilized apartments, some in public housing, others in unregulated free-market residences. There is variety among homeowners, too—they live in conventional owner-occupied homes, private cooperatives and condominiums, or regulated units.[3]

This chapter provides a summary of the housing of older New Yorkers.[4] Among the features of housing discussed are tenure, regulation status, type of structure, housing costs, and measures of housing quality.

I discuss housing in New York City as a whole and in each of the city's five boroughs—the Bronx, Brooklyn, Manhattan, Queens, and Staten Island—with a focus on a comparison of the core of the city, Manhattan, to the others.[5] While such a comparison is instructive, there are often great disparities of housing conditions within each borough. Since these disparities often reflect disparities in household incomes of different areas within boroughs, sub-borough areas have been selected for analysis based on median household income.[6] Within each borough, sub-boroughs with the highest and lowest median household incomes are compared (Table 6.1). Staten Island has only three sub-boroughs, and data for these are not presented (incomes across these three are higher and less variable than is true citywide).

The median income in New York City is $45,000. Although Manhattan has a lower median income ($52,243) than Staten Island's ($66,000), and one virtually equal to that of Queens ($51,200), this figure conceals great disparities across the sub-boroughs of Manhattan. Of the fifty-five defined sub-boroughs across all five boroughs, the four wealthiest are in Manhattan: the Upper West Side, Stuyvesant

Table 6.1. Residents Who Are White and Median Household Income: NYC, Boroughs, and Selected Sub-Boroughs, 2000–2002

| | | Median household income | | |
| | | | Age 65+ | |
	White %	**All**	**Owner**	**Renter**
NYC	45	$45,000	$35,160	$14,544
Boroughs				
Bronx	30	32,000	25,000	13,000
Brooklyn	41	40,800	30,000	12,200
Manhattan	54	52,243	64,400	14,086
Queens	44	51,200	35,424	19,800
Staten Island	78	66,000	35,000	18,892
Selected Sub-Boroughs[a]				
Morrisania/East Tremont (Bronx)	22	18,000	16,272	9,804
Throgs Neck/Co-op City (Bronx)	61	52,600	21,300	10,800
Bedford Stuyvesant (Brooklyn)	7	28,000	34,301	14,944
Flatlands/Canarsie (Brooklyn)	38	61,000	38,000	15,476
East Harlem (Manhattan)	25	23,000	16,000	9,600
Upper East Side (Manhattan)	87	104,200	70,100	21,932
Astoria (Queens)	57	41,525	28,600	20,232
Bayside/Little Neck (Queens)	65	67,000	42,000	17,600

Source: Percent White -- Census 2000 data accessed through InfoShare, and U.S. Census Bureau, County and City Data Book: 2000, (13 Edition), Washington DC; Median Income -- NYC HVS (2002).

[a] Within each borough, the sub-borough with the lowest median household income is listed first, followed by that with the highest median household income. Staten Island sub-boroughs are not shown because it has only three sub-boroughs. Incomes in Staten Island are generally higher and less variable than for NYC as a whole.

Town/Turtle Bay, Greenwich Village/Financial District, and the Upper East Side—richest of all, with a median income of $104,200. On the other end of the spectrum, East Harlem, poorest in Manhattan ($23,000) and ironically the northern neighbor of the Upper East Side, is the city's third-poorest neighborhood. The Lower East Side/Chinatown, Central Harlem, and Washington Heights/Inwood, all in Manhattan, also are among the city's poorest neighborhoods.

Income disparities are not nearly as wide in the Bronx—unfortunately for its residents. Five of the city's six poorest sub-boroughs are in the Bronx (Manhattan's East Harlem being the exception), which has the lowest median income ($32,000) among the five boroughs. Eight of the ten sub-boroughs defined for the Bronx have median incomes below the citywide level. In contrast, narrow income disparities are good news if one lives in Queens. Only two of twelve sub-boroughs in Queens, Astoria ($41,525) and Jackson Heights ($44,200), have incomes below the median for New York City; the other ten all have higher incomes than the two wealthiest sub-boroughs in the Bronx, Riverdale/Kingsbridge and Throgs Neck/Co-op City.

Forty-five percent of New Yorkers are white.[7] For the most part, income disparities across boroughs and sub-boroughs mirror racial disparities. Staten Island, the highest-income borough, has the highest proportion of white residents (78 percent); the Bronx, the poorest borough, has the lowest (30 percent). In each borough, the percentage white is lower in poor than in wealthy sub-boroughs—although in Queens and Staten Island, racial disparities are not as great. As with incomes, racial disparities are greatest in Manhattan: of the wealthy Upper East Side, 87 percent is white (nearly double the proportion for New York City), compared to only 25 percent in East Harlem.

Whites, then, are clustered in the city's better neighborhoods, while nonwhites frequently are not as privileged. Part of the explanation for the clustering by race is, for most, an unfortunate residual of historical housing policy—many of the city's first housing projects were explicitly developed for either blacks or whites, and those developed for the latter group according to this "separate-but-equal" rationale were invariably not equal, but superior to those of the former—superior in both quality and location.[8]

Tenure and Regulation Status

The vast majority of older Americans would like to stay in their current homes for as long as possible. The American Association of Retired Persons found that well over 90 percent of all persons age sixty-five and over express this desire.[9] Older homeowners who own their dwellings outright, as most do, may be in a much better position than renters to age in place.[10]

Homeownership represents a certain amount of control not enjoyed by renters (delete the preceding), not only over one's desire to age in place, but also over long-term availability of space, central heating and air conditioning, structural soundness, and other widely desired housing features. Moreover, the home is not simply a shelter, but an entry into and continuous access to a desired community, one that provides the household its preferred combination of schools, parks, public services, and lifestyle opportunities. Lastly, buying a home is a financial investment—the single largest investment most people ever make. A very large percentage of the total wealth of most Americans age sixty-five and over is represented by their home equity.

Tenure. Nationwide, ownership is nearly twice as common as renting—about 65 percent of all householders own their homes, about 35 percent rent.[11] Ownership rates in metropolitan areas are slightly lower than the national average.[12] The prevalence of homeownership in New York City, though, is well below both the national and metropolitan area averages—in America's biggest city, renters outnumber homeowners two to one, just the opposite of what is found at the national level (Table 6.2).

Citywide, ownership is more common among older (49 percent) than among younger residents (33 percent), a pattern echoed in each borough. Manhattan has the lowest incidence of homeownership among the boroughs (21 percent). Although this figure is not much lower than the overall rate in the Bronx (22 percent), the rates among those sixty-five and over in Manhattan (29 percent) are considerably lower than those of the same age group in the Bronx (40 percent)—so the similarity in the overall rates between the two boroughs is due to the Bronx's age profile, which

Table 6.2. Residents Living in Owner-Occupied Units: NYC, Boroughs, and Selected Sub-Boroughs, 2002

	All %	Residents 65+ %	Residents <65+ %
NYC	34.79	48.82	33.03
Boroughs			
Bronx	22.21	39.67	20.41
Brooklyn	31.11	42.77	29.71
Manhattan	21.35	28.66	20.38
Queens	48.27	66.01	45.80
Staten Island	70.41	79.15	69.23
Selected Sub-Boroughs[a]			
Morrisania/East Tremont (Bronx)	7.54	21.59	6.32
Throgs Neck/Co-op City (Bronx)	75.05	70.96	75.89
Bedford Stuyvesant (Brooklyn)	22.06	33.69	20.40
Flatlands/Canarsie (Brooklyn)	60.12	76.22	58.46
East Harlem (Manhattan)	8.40	14.70	7.65
Upper East Side (Manhattan)	37.04	46.61	35.57
Astoria (Queens)	20.22	57.32	15.75
Bayside/Little Neck (Queens)	70.17	83.31	68.25

Source: NYC HVS (2002).

[a] Within each borough, the sub-borough with the lowest median household income is listed first, followed by that with the highest median household income. Staten Island sub-boroughs are not shown because it has only three sub-boroughs. Incomes in Staten Island are generally higher and less variable than for NYC as a whole.

is the city's youngest. Homeownership in Staten Island is quite high (70 percent), higher even than the national average.

Disparities between rich and poor neighborhoods are evident from Table 6.2; the gap in terms of homeownership is extremely wide in each borough, but greatest in the Bronx, where less than 8 percent of residents in Morrisania/East Tremont own their homes, compared to 75 percent in high-income Throgs Neck/Co-op City.

Renters are not necessarily in worse shape than homeowners. This truism is clearly borne out in the case of the Upper East Side, where the rate of homeownership (37 percent) is little higher than the city average, and where the rate among those age sixty-five and over (47 percent) is lower than for the same group citywide. Homeownership in a very high income area such as the Upper East Side, where the average home value is close to $1 million, clearly means something different than homeownership in even the richest sub-borough in the Bronx—Throgs Neck/Co-op City—where the average home value is $168,000.[13] Affording a home in the Upper East Side is beyond the means of most New Yorkers, and renters in this and other high-income sub-boroughs are likely to be much better off financially than are many homeowners in poorer areas of the city.

Regulation status. Many low- and middle-income renters receive direct or indirect rental subsidies through their residence in public housing or Mitchell-Lama apartments. Two essential features distinguish these types of residences.[14] First, tenant eligibility is limited to those with incomes below a certain threshold, usually expressed as a percentage of the median income for the New York metropolitan area. Second, rents are kept below a certain percentage of a tenant's income. Mitchell-Lamas are privately owned developments that receive tax and other incentives in return for charging below-market rents, and public housing is owned and operated by the New York City Housing Authority. Some public housing developments in New York City are supported by New York State or federal financing, others are not.

Renters of all income levels have access to indirect rent subsidies through New York's rent-control and rent-stabilization laws (see the chapter glossary). In essence, rent increases and other aspects of rental lease agreements in these regulated apartments are restricted to those established by New York City's Rent Guidelines Board, whose annual public hearings on the matter are typified by the wailings of landlord and tenant groups, the former arguing for higher, the latter for lower rent increases.

About 54 percent of older renters in New York City live in rent-regulated apartments (Table 6.3—"stabilized" includes both rent-controlled and stabilized units), 5 percent live in Mitchell-Lamas, and 20 percent live in public housing. Thus, nearly 80 percent of older renters in the city are protected by some form of rent ceiling. One in five, though, pay market rents.

The regulation status of the rental apartments of older residents in the Bronx and Brooklyn are similar to the citywide pattern, but in Queens, and especially in Staten

Island, a much higher percent of older renters live in unregulated, market-rent apartments (36 and 55 percent, respectively). Among older renters in Staten Island, the proportion that lives in stabilized apartments is roughly half that of the entire city. Manhattan's older renters are much likelier than older renters in the other boroughs to live in public housing (28 percent) or stabilized apartments (60 percent), and much less likely to pay market rents (6 percent). This is fortunate for older Manhattanites, as the median market rent in their borough ($2,400/month) is dramatically higher than that in any other borough (second highest is Queens, $900/month).[15]

Homeowners, too, have access to lower-than-market-priced dwellings via Mitch-

Table 6.3. Regulation Status of Rental Apartments as a Percent of Renters 65+: NYC, Boroughs, and Selected Sub-Boroughs, 2002

	Stabilized %	Mitchell-Lama %	Public Housing %	Unregulated %
NYC	53.72	5.12	20.29	20.87
Boroughs				
Bronx	56.74	5.55	22.24	15.47
Brooklyn	51.24	5.18	19.50	24.09
Manhattan	59.57	6.23	28.47	5.74
Queens	50.56	3.63	9.66	36.16
Staten Island	28.33	1.47	15.30	54.89
Selected Sub-Boroughs[a]				
Morrisania/East Tremont (Bronx)	39.97	0.00	55.18	4.85
Throgs Neck/Co-op City (Bronx)	51.87	23.50	7.92	16.71
Bedford Stuyvesant (Brooklyn)	26.05	0.00	39.76	34.20
Flatlands/Canarsie (Brooklyn)	13.55	0.00	41.60	44.85
East Harlem (Manhattan)	16.95	6.95	74.26	1.83
Upper East Side (Manhattan)	57.72	11.96	24.12	6.21
Astoria (Queens)	60.73	3.20	21.41	14.66
Bayside/Little Neck (Queens)	6.87	0.00	0.00	93.13

Source: NYC HVS (2002).

[a] Within each borough, the sub-borough with the lowest median household income is listed first, followed by that with the highest median household income. Staten Island sub-boroughs are not shown because it has only three sub-boroughs. Incomes in Staten Island are generally higher and less variable than for NYC as a whole.

ell-Lama cooperative developments. City-sponsored Mitchell-Lama co-ops provide middle-income families with an affordable homeownership option through tax exemptions, lower-interest mortgages, and limited developer profits. Some such developments have shared supervision by New York City's Housing Preservation and Development (HPD) and the federal Department of Housing and Urban Development (HUD); others are supervised by the state Division of Housing and Community Renewal.[16] (The glossary provides more details for this and the other regulation types shown in Table 6.4.)

About 5 percent of older homeowners in New York City live in regulated Mitchell-Lamas—the rate is much higher in Manhattan (17 percent) than in any other borough except the Bronx (14 percent). Thus, as with renters, older homeowners in Manhattan receive a greater degree of insulation from free-market forces than is true in the other boroughs.

Older homeowners in Manhattan are much likelier to reside in private co-ops (64 percent) and condos (13 percent) than those in any of the other boroughs. The conventional type of owner-occupied dwellings—for the most part one- or two-family homes—are much more prevalent among older homeowners in the other boroughs, ranging from 72 percent in the Bronx to 93 percent in Staten Island.

All older homeowners in the poorest sub-boroughs of the Bronx (Morrisania/East Tremont) and Brooklyn (Bedford Stuyvesant) live in conventional housing—none live in co-ops or condos.[17] Just the converse is found in East Harlem, Manhattan's poorest area, where none of the older homeowners live in conventional housing, and where eight in ten live in Mitchell-Lamas. As for Queens, most live in conventional housing, and there is little difference between the poorest sub-borough (Astoria, with 85 percent in conventional housing) and the richest (Bayside/Little Neck, 76 percent).

Co-ops are, perhaps not unexpectedly, prevalent in the Bronx's highest-income area—not called Throgs Neck/*Co-op City* for nothing[18]—where 36 percent of older owners live in Mitchell-Lamas. In Manhattan's Upper East Side, 83 percent of older homeowners live in private co-ops, 9 percent in private condos.

The distribution across regulation-status types, then, for older renters and homeowners in Manhattan is quite different than that found in the other boroughs. In Brooklyn, Queens, and Staten Island, there is relatively little disparity in the regulation status between rich and poor areas, while disparities are greater within the Bronx, and especially within Manhattan.

As is true nationwide, older residents in New York City are likelier than younger residents to be homeowners. Homeownership in New York City is low by national standards, and is lowest in Manhattan. But in Manhattan, older renters and owners are likelier than in the other boroughs to live in regulated housing, providing them with more protection against the market forces that might otherwise threaten a widely held desire to age in place. There is a positive correlation between ownership rates and median income across sub-boroughs.

Table 6.4. Regulation Status of Homeowner Dwellings: Distribution of Homeowners 65+ in NYC, Boroughs, and Selected Sub-Boroughs, 2002

	Conventional	Private Co-op	Private Condo	Mitchell-Lama Co-op
	%	%	%	%
NYC	72.79	17.81	3.99	5.41
Boroughs				
Bronx	72.48	9.23	4.41	13.88
Brooklyn	85.34	9.68	0.32	4.65
Manhattan	5.19	64.43	12.92	17.46
Queens	79.41	15.78	3.38	1.44
Staten Island	93.08	1.74	5.17	0.00
Selected Sub-Boroughs[a]				
Morrisania/East Tremont (Bronx)	100.00	0.00	0.00	0.00
Throgs Neck/Co-op City (Bronx)	59.46	4.51	0.00	36.04
Bedford Stuyvesant (Brooklyn)	100.00	0.00	0.00	0.00
Flatlands/Canarsie (Brooklyn)	97.87	0.98	1.16	0.00
East Harlem (Manhattan)	0.00	18.75	0.00	81.25
Upper East Side (Manhattan)	2.41	82.97	9.24	5.38
Astoria (Queens)	84.66	8.26	7.08	0.00
Bayside/Little Neck (Queens)	75.87	22.77	1.36	0.00

Source: NYC HVS (2002).

[a] Within each borough, the sub-borough with the lowest median household income is listed first, followed by that with the highest median household income. Staten Island sub-boroughs are not shown because it has only three sub-boroughs. Incomes in Staten Island are generally higher and less variable than for NYC as a whole.

Housing Conditions

To provide some background for the living arrangements of older New Yorkers, this section begins with a review of main structural types: one- or two-family homes, multi-unit buildings equipped with elevators, and walkups. Housing characteristics associated with the health and safety of residents are analyzed based on HUD's housing quality standards for bathroom facilities, food preparation and refuse disposal, space and security, thermal environment, structural soundness, overall sanitary conditions (such as rodent infestation), and other conditions. For each of these, HUD establishes minimum levels of acceptability for housing programs it sponsors or manages.[19]

Type of building structure. Building structures may be divided into three categories: one- or two-family homes; multiunit buildings equipped with an elevator; and walkups, which are multi-unit buildings without elevators (see the glossary).

In New York City, 41 percent of older residents live in one- or two-family homes, 43 percent in multi-units with elevators (Table 6.5). The remaining 16 percent live in walkups, which means they must climb stairs to access their dwellings. In many other cities in the United States, it is not uncommon for older persons to move to a new home because they could no longer manage the stairs of their previous dwelling. Moving to homes without stairs is not an option for many older New Yorkers because such homes are relatively scarce.

While rent stabilization makes housing affordable to many older (and younger) residents who might otherwise not be able to live in the city, these stabilized housing units are often in walkup buildings. This largely underappreciated problem will not disappear soon, considering that New York's population is aging along with the rest of the country (and developed world). The problem is most acute in Brooklyn, where nearly one in four older persons lives in a walkup. Nearly one in five older Manhattanites lives in a walkup—70 percent of whom do not live on the first floor.

Even these figures underestimate the necessity for older New Yorkers to climb stairs every day just to enter their homes. First, many buildings of all structural types have steps leading to their entrances, and these are often equivalent to a full flight of stairs. Second, two-family homes are almost always two-story buildings or higher, and the family living on the upper floors must use stairs to access their dwellings. Last, many one-family homes have stairs within them, too, although this is less compelling a difficulty than that faced by residents whose use of stairs simply to *access* their homes is inescapable.

One- or two-family homes are much more common in Queens (63 percent of older residents) and especially in Staten Island (89 percent) than in the other boroughs. Within the boroughs, there are differences between poor and rich areas in terms of housing structure, but no clear pattern emerges. In the Bronx, for example, a disproportionate number of older residents in poor Morrisania/East Tremont live in walkups; in Throgs Neck/Co-op City, a much higher percentage lives in one- or two-family homes. In Queens, nine in ten older residents in affluent Bayside/Little Neck live in one- or two-family homes, compared to just four in ten in less well-off Astoria. Disparities in structural type between the rich and poor sub-boroughs of Brooklyn are similar to those in Queens.

In Manhattan, borough of great disparities, we find common ground between rich and poor, white and black, rather mundanely, in the breakdown by type of build-

Table 6.5. Distribution of Residents 65+ by Type of Building Structure: NYC, Boroughs, and Selected Sub-boroughs, 2002

	One- or two-family home %	Multi-unit equipped with elevator %	Walkup[a] %
NYC	40.70	42.9	16.40
Boroughs			
Bronx	34.10	50.53	15.37
Brooklyn	38.50	37.28	24.21
Manhattan	0.42	81.01	18.57
Queens	62.79	26.79	10.41
Staten Island	88.69	7.83	3.48
Selected Sub-Boroughs[b]			
Morrisania/East Tremont (Bronx)	20.01	55.66	24.33
Throgs Neck/Co-op City (Bronx)	46.12	46.03	7.85
Bedford Stuyvesant (Brooklyn)	25.31	36.41	38.28
Flatlands/Canarsie (Brooklyn)	84.48	12.53	2.99
East Harlem (Manhattan)	0.00	88.22	11.78
Upper East Side (Manhattan)	1.15	85.37	13.49
Astoria (Queens)	42.12	36.10	21.78
Bayside/Little Neck (Queens)	91.58	0.76	7.66

Source: NYC HVS (2002).

[a] A walkup is a multi-unit dwelling without an elevator. See the Appendix under "Structures, Types of Building" for more details.

[b] Within each borough, the sub-borough with the lowest median household income is listed first, followed by that with the highest median household income. Staten Island sub-boroughs are not shown because it has only three sub-boroughs. Incomes in Staten Island are generally higher and less variable than for NYC as a whole.

ing structure. About nine in ten older residents of both East Harlem and the Upper East Side live in multi-units equipped with elevators, and nearly all the rest live in walkups. Yet, there are other neighborhoods in Manhattan in which the percentage of walkups is considerably higher. In Central Harlem, for example, over 20 percent of older persons live in such buildings.

Kitchen and bathroom facilities. While international cultural differences ultimately determine whether certain housing features should be considered basic or optional, in many developed countries, access to complete bathroom and kitchen facilities is considered fundamental to adequate housing.

Indeed, these facilities are so widespread in the United States as to be a disappointment for those looking for differences between old and young, or between rich and poor. Nearly 100 percent of occupied dwellings in the country have complete kitchen and bathroom facilities. New York City is no different.[20]

Dwelling space. Privacy, comfort, and health are more attainable if living space is adequate. Although cramped quarters and overcrowding may impair quality of life, "adequate" does not necessarily mean large. Excessive space may increase the burdens of home maintenance, utility bills, and distance to be traversed, and these may be especially problematic for older persons.[21]

One common measure of space is rooms per person—that is, the number of rooms in a dwelling divided by the number of persons living in it. Nationwide, this ratio is greater for older than for younger persons, meaning that older persons generally have more space. Among older person, homeowners have more space than do renters. Older persons, both homeowners and renters, have more space than do their younger counterparts.[22]

These patterns are largely echoed throughout New York City—older residents have more space than do younger ones, and owners have more space than do renters. Contrary to what might be expected, space in Manhattan (1.3 rooms per person) is generous compared to the other boroughs, with the exception of Staten Island (1.5). However, when space is analyzed by tenure, a different story emerges. Specifically, among older residents, homeowners in Manhattan have more space (2.0 rooms per person) than do homeowners in the other boroughs; in contrast, older renters in Manhattan have *less* space (1.8) than do renters living outside Manhattan.[23]

Another difference between Manhattan and the other boroughs is that in the others, space for older homeowners is considerably greater in rich than in poor sub-boroughs, but in Manhattan, space is only slightly greater for Upper East Side residents than for those in East Harlem (2.5 vs. 2.3 rooms per person). This pattern generally holds for renters—there is virtually no difference between the richest and poorest sub-boroughs in Manhattan. In Queens, older renters in Astoria, the poorest sub-borough, actually have more space than do homeowners (1.9 vs. 1.5).

One reason older residents tend to have more space than younger persons is that a much higher percentage lives alone. Space in Manhattan might be considered unexpectedly high, but this is very likely because a greater percentage of older Manhattanites lives alone than is true in the other boroughs (see Chapter 2).

Structural soundness and maintenance deficiencies. Structural soundness and the overall condition of a building certainly have an impact on the health and safety of residents. The condition of the buildings in one's surrounding neighborhood, while not endangering health and safety directly, also affect quality of life.

About 5 percent of New York's occupied housing stock is considered dilapidated—that is, it does not provide occupants with safe or adequate shelter.[24] City-wide, the percentage is lower among older (3.1 percent) than younger residents (5.4 percent), and lower among homeowners (1.6 percent for those age sixty-five and over) than among renters (4.5 percent).

Both these trends hold for all boroughs except Staten Island, where the percentage in dilapidated buildings is actually higher among older homeowners (3.3 percent) than among older renters (2.1 percent). Although a higher percentage of older residents in the Bronx lives in dilapidated buildings (5.5 percent) than do those of the other boroughs, this is much more a reflection of the quality of its renter- than its owner-occupied housing; while 8.2 percent of older renters live in dilapidated buildings in the Bronx, only 1.4 percent of older homeowners do, which is less than half the New York City average and more favorable than the percentages for older owners in Brooklyn and Staten Island.

There is a noticeable difference between owners and renters in Manhattan: a smaller percentage of older homeowners (1.2 percent) lives in dilapidated buildings than do those in any other borough, but the percentage of older renters that do so (4.3 percent) is second highest. Not surprisingly, a much smaller percentage of the residents of richer than of poorer sub-boroughs lives in dilapidated structures. Nearly one in four residents in the Morrisania/East Tremont area of the Bronx lives in a dilapidated structure, the highest rate of any sub-borough in New York. As throughout the city, older residents in this sub-borough are less likely than younger residents to live in dilapidated buildings. Even so, more than one in five older renters lives in dilapidated buildings.

While dilapidated buildings pose a threat to the safety and well-being of those who live in them, the condition of the surrounding buildings in these neighborhoods also affects quality of life. Buildings with windows boarded up to protect against weather or entry are unsightly and reflect negatively on a neighborhood's quality. About 13 percent of all New Yorkers say their neighborhood contains boarded-up buildings. A smaller percentage of older New Yorkers (9 percent) reports the same, and this is true among both renters and owners in every borough. The percentage in Manhattan (16 percent) is second highest among the boroughs (Brooklyn's is 18 percent). Among poor sub-boroughs, Bedford Stuyvesant in Brooklyn has by far the largest percentage—44 percent for older homeowners, 62 percent for older renters.

Table 6.6 shows the percentage of residents who reported four or more of seven maintenance deficiencies: heating equipment breakdowns; additional heating required; rodent infestation; toilet breakdowns; water leakage from outside unit; crack/holes in walls, ceilings, or floors; and broken plaster/peeling paint.[25] About 7 percent of all New Yorkers report four or more such deficiencies. The percentages are generally much lower for older than for younger New Yorkers, across all boroughs and sub-boroughs, and lower for homeowners than for renters. As might well be expected, residents in poor neighborhoods report the highest incidence of maintenance deficiencies—18 percent in Morrisania/East Tremont in the Bronx, 9 percent in Bedford Stuyvesant in Brooklyn, and 7 percent in Manhattan's East Harlem.

To summarize, housing conditions are generally better for older than for younger New Yorkers—few report maintenance deficiencies, fewer live in dilapidated homes,

Table 6.6. Distribution of Residents Living Alone, by Age and Gender: NYC, Boroughs, and Selected Sub-Boroughs, 2002

	All Ages	Age 65 and over		
		All	Female	Male
	%	%	%	%
NYC	12.47	35.04	42.40	23.53
Boroughs				
Bronx	10.71	38.73	44.35	29.75
Brooklyn	9.98	35.43	41.94	24.63
Manhattan	24.14	45.24	52.93	32.13
Queens	9.09	28.46	36.68	16.95
Staten Island	8.73	24.16	31.60	13.39
Selected Sub-Boroughs[a]				
Morrisania/East Tremont (Bronx)	12.19	58.93	63.87	49.94
Throgs Neck/Co-op City (Bronx)	17.70	48.34	60.42	29.31
Bedford Stuyvesant (Brooklyn)	13.07	34.75	39.06	27.18
Flatlands/Canarsie (Brooklyn)	7.93	35.47	39.45	29.02
East Harlem (Manhattan)	16.80	48.84	49.13	47.92
Upper East Side (Manhattan)	29.98	47.69	60.52	26.42
Astoria (Queens)	13.61	37.59	47.93	21.44
Bayside/Little Neck (Queens)	6.92	18.46	26.71	9.48

Source: NYC HVS (2002).

[a] Within each borough, the sub-borough with the lowest median household income is listed first, followed by that with the highest median household income. Staten Island sub-boroughs are not shown because it has only three sub-boroughs. Incomes in Staten Island are generally higher and less variable than for NYC as a whole.

fewer in neighborhoods with boarded-up buildings. That older residents have larger living quarters in terms of rooms per person largely reflects the higher incidence among the aged of living alone. Virtually all have complete kitchen and bathroom facilities located in their dwellings. Although most live in either multi-units with elevators or one- or two-family homes, many older New Yorkers live in walkups and must use stairs to access their homes.

While it has not been discussed here, New Yorkers, young and old, generally have access to sufficient heating and cooling equipment in their homes, although renters are somewhat worse off than are homeowners in this regard.[26] Indeed, for almost every measure of housing quality, older renters fair less well than do homeowners. This, in combination with their higher housing costs relative to income, discussed next, strongly suggests that older renters—in what might justifiably be called the renter-occupied capital of the United States—are an especially vulnerable group.

Housing Costs

Most Americans sixty-five and over are either retired or work part-time, and their economic security depends not only on their income and wealth, but also on their ability to meet ongoing housing costs. High costs make it much more difficult for many older persons to buy groceries and other nonhousing goods or services such as transportation, vacations, health care, and medicines. Homeowners may defer home repairs, or may be unable to pay property taxes. Tenants may be evicted for nonpayment of rent.

The largest component in a renter's housing costs is, of course, the contract rent; total housing costs include utilities, if paid separately from the rent. Monthly housing costs for renters are highest in Manhattan ($1,156/month), and lower for older than for younger renters in all five boroughs.[27]

Total monthly costs of homeowners include mortgage payment, utilities, taxes, and other expenses.[28] Since owners' monthly costs include payments on outstanding mortgages, they might be expected to have higher costs than renters, and this is true for the general population. Monthly housing costs for homeowners are highest in Manhattan ($2,019), and higher in each borough than for renters. As is true for renters, costs for older homeowners are lower than costs for those who are younger. This is because a larger percentage of older homeowners has paid off its mortgages.

Although housing costs, for both older owners and older renters, are generally lower than those of younger New Yorkers, the gap between old and young is wider among owners than among renters. Housing costs of older homeowners are less than 60 percent of those paid by younger owners throughout the city, whereas housing costs for older renters are typically 75 percent of those paid by younger renters.

Expressed as a percentage of median income, however, the situation faced by older renters appears much less favorable (Table 6.7). For older renters citywide, 35 percent of household income goes toward housing costs. The percentage is lower among older owners (24 percent), and this pattern holds across the five boroughs, although the gap between older owners and renters is quite small in the Bronx. The gap is comparatively wide in Staten Island, where housing costs for older renters (39 percent of household income) are highest among the five boroughs.

Analysis by sub-borough shows that the general pattern of higher housing costs for older renters than for older homeowners does not always hold. For example, in both Brooklyn's poor Bedford Stuyvesant and in Manhattan's high-income Upper

Table 6.7. Residents Reporting Four or More Maintenance Deficiencies[a]: NYC, Boroughs, and Selected Sub-Boroughs, 2002

	All %	Residents 65+ %	
		Owner	Renter
NYC	7.42 %	0.54 %	0.64 %
Boroughs			
Bronx	14.72	0.00	42.11
Brooklyn	7.96	0.98	24.37
Manhattan	8.82	0.00	29.90
Queens	2.65	0.40	15.33
Staten Island	2.56	1.17	14.02
Selected Sub-Boroughs[b]			
Morrisania/East Tremont (Bronx)	18.03	0.00	18.00
Throgs Neck/Co-op City (Bronx)	3.94	0.00	0.00
Bedford Stuyvesant (Brooklyn)	9.30	10.82	8.61
Flatlands/Canarsie (Brooklyn)	1.89	1.29	5.83
East Harlem (Manhattan)	6.78	0.00	10.86
Upper East Side (Manhattan)	3.50	0.00	4.15
Astoria (Queens)	2.13	0.00	2.74
Bayside/Little Neck (Queens)	2.29	0.00	1.91

Source: NYC HVS (2002).

[a] See the Appendix under "Deficiencies, Maintenance" for details.

[b] Within each borough, the sub-borough with the lowest median household income is listed first, followed by that with the highest median household income. Staten Island sub-boroughs are not shown because it has only three sub-boroughs. Incomes in Staten Island are generally higher and less variable than for NYC as a whole.

East Side, expenses expressed as a percentage of household income are greater for older homeowners than for older renters (Table 6.8). Expenses are higher for older homeowners in these two very different areas because of the way their older residents are distributed by the regulation status, as discussed earlier. In Bedford Stuyvesant, 40 percent of older renters live in public housing (Table 6.3), which is considerably higher than the 20 percent across New York City who do so. This has a large downward impact on the average costs to older renters in that sub-borough. In the Upper East Side, too, relatively few renters face market rents—only 6 percent, compared to the New York City average of 21 percent. Aside from these exceptions, older homeowners in New York City must allocate a smaller percent of their incomes to meet housing costs than do older renters.

It was noted earlier that absolute housing costs are lower for older than for younger New Yorkers of both tenure types. Another important pattern that emerges from the figures in Table 6.8, though, is that when expressed as a percentage of income, costs are *greater* for older residents citywide and in all five boroughs except Queens, where there is virtually no difference between younger and older homeowners. Analysis of the selected sub-boroughs reveals that this overall pattern holds for renters, but not for homeowners. Indeed, in only one, the Upper East Side in Manhattan, are housing costs as a percentage of household income higher for older homeowners (49 percent) than for younger (16 percent). In all the other selected sub-boroughs, there is either near equality between the percentages for younger and older homeowners, or the inequality points in the direction opposite the general pattern.

In sum, housing costs are especially burdensome for older renters in New York; although exceptions to the rule exist in some areas of the city, these exceptions do not appear to be related to the relative wealth or poverty of an area. While it can be said that older New Yorkers are generally more burdened than are younger residents by high housing costs, and that this is true for both renters and homeowners, older homeowners in many areas of the city appear to be no more burdened than are younger homeowners, and in many cases they are even less burdened.

Conclusion

In general, the housing conditions of older New Yorkers contribute positively to their quality of life. Even though homeownership—widely valued as a source of financial security and control over one's living environment—is quite low by national standards, a higher percentage of older than younger residents own their homes. Older residents also enjoy better housing conditions than younger residents generally do—fewer live in dilapidated buildings or in dwellings with severe maintenance deficiencies. Virtually all have complete bathrooms and kitchens, adequate heating and cooling equipment, and other basic housing features. Fewer live in cramped quarters, fewer in undesirable neighborhoods.

Table 6.8. Median Monthly Housing Costs
as a Percent of Income by Tenure and Age: NYC, 2002[a]

	Owner		Renter	
	Age 65+	< 65	Age 65+	Age< 65
NYC	23.62	21.68	35.10	25.10
Boroughs				
Bronx	33.23	22.87	34.40	27.00
Brooklyn	26.39	24.76	37.10	25.80
Manhattan	20.63	16.81	33.20	22.60
Queens	22.40	22.43	36.90	25.00
Staten Island	21.48	18.88	38.80	24.00
Selected Sub-Boroughs[b]				
Morrisania/East Tremont (Bronx)	11.57	39.42	34.80	32.20
Throgs Neck/Co-op City (Bronx)	35.45	19.38	62.80	22.80
Bedford Stuyvesant (Brooklyn)	32.74	30.64	29.90	20.50
Flatlands/Canarsie (Brooklyn)	26.39	28.11	34.60	26.00
East Harlem (Manhattan)	22.42	24.22	35.60	28.20
Upper East Side (Manhattan)	49.46	15.67	33.10	20.00
Astoria (Queens)	26.47	35.82	41.60	24.00
Bayside/Little Neck (Queens)	16.42	18.07	71.90	31.80

Source: NYC HVS (2002).

[a] Excludes households with no cash rent, zero or negative income, monthly costs equal to 100% or more of current income, and mortgage payment not reported. See the Appendix for more details of housing costs by tenure.

[b] Within each borough, the sub-borough with the lowest median household income is listed first, followed by that with the highest median household income. Staten Island sub-boroughs are not shown because it has only three sub-boroughs. Incomes in Staten Island are generally higher and less variable than for NYC as a whole.

There are important exceptions to these general findings. Housing affordability is a major issue among all New Yorkers,[29] but older New Yorkers are especially at risk. Older renters fair even less well, not just in terms of housing affordability, but in terms of housing quality. Those living in the city's poorest neighborhoods are worse off yet; up to one in four in some areas live in quarters unsafe for human habitation. Most vulnerable of all are older New Yorkers living alone, the vast majority of whom are women.

Glossary

Condominium. A condominium (condo) is a building or development with
individually owned apartments or houses. The owner has his/her own deed,
and very likely, his/her own mortgage on the unit. The owner also holds a
common or joint ownership in all common areas and facilities that serve the
project—land, roofs, hallways, entrance elevators, etc.

Cooperative. A cooperative (co-op) is a building or development owned by
its shareholders and organized as a corporation. Ownership of shares in
the corporation entitles each shareholder to hold the lease for one or more
apartments (houses). If the person or persons owning the cooperative shares
also occupies the unit, the cooperative unit is considered owner occupied.

Housing Costs, Monthly—Owner. Housing expenses of homeowners as used
in this chapter are analogous to the total expenses of renters (called
"gross rent"). Total monthly housing expenses of homeowners include the
following:

1. Monthly Mortgage or Loan Payment. This is the amount paid to the lender or
    lenders for the mortgage(s) or loan(s) outstanding on the apartment (house).
    It includes payments for principal and interest, real estate taxes, fire and li-
    ability insurance, and mortgage insurance, if they are part of the mortgage
    payment.
2. Maintenance Fees, Monthly Condominium or Cooperative. These apply only
    to owner-occupied condominiums or cooperatives. Some or all of the fol-
    lowing may be included in condominium or cooperative maintenance fees:
    real estate taxes; fire insurance; other hazard insurance; payments on the
    underlying building mortgage; salaries of maintenance employees; heating
    expenses; utilities; and reserves for major repairs, maintenance, etc.
3. Fire and Liability Insurance. The monthly cost of the insurance if paid sepa-
    rately from the mortgage or cooperative/condominium maintenance fee.
4. Real Estate Taxes. The monthly real estate taxes paid.
5. Utilities. Monthly electricity, gas, water, and sewer expenses.

Housing Costs, Monthly—Renter. Housing costs of renters were calculated as
the monthly gross rent, which is the contract rent plus the cost of utilities
(electricity, gas, and water and sewer) and other fuels (oil, coal, kerosene,
wood, etc.) if paid by the renter in addition to rent.

Plumbing Facilities. A housing unit has complete plumbing facilities if it has hot
and cold piped water, a flush toilet, and a bathtub or shower. All facilities
need not be located in the same room, but all must be in the unit.

Regulation Status. Regulation status definitions as used in this chapter have been
divided into those applicable to homeowners and those to renters, as follows:

Regulation Status—Owners

1. Owner, Conventional. Privately owned houses or buildings *not* part of a co-operative or condominium building or development. This category includes owner-occupied single-family houses, living quarters that are part of commercial or industrial buildings, and all other types of owner-occupied units not in cooperatives and condominiums.

2. Mitchell-Lama Coop. Units constructed under the New York State or New York City Mitchell-Lama cooperative program. The purpose of the program is to enable moderate- and middle-income families to secure decent affordable housing through limited-equity cooperative ownership. The mechanisms employed to keep both the initial down payment and monthly carrying charges within the means of middle-income families, to which the program is restricted, are tax exemption, state- or city-provided low-interest mortgages, and limited developer profit. In certain instances, federal subsidies are combined with the state and local measures to achieve the program's objectives.

3. Private Coop/Condo. Privately owned cooperative or condominium units not constructed under the New York State or New York City Mitchell-Lama program. A portion of the units in this category may have benefited from some other type of government assistance (e.g., J-51, 421A).

Regulation Status—Renters

1. Stabilized. Rent-controlled and rent-stabilized apartments have been lumped together in this chapter, but these are subject to different regulations. Controlled units are subject to the provisions of the Rent Control Law and Regulations, which have jurisdiction over occupied private rental units. All increases in rent are set and must be approved by New York State's Division of Housing and Community Renewal. The following units are classified as rent controlled: units in buildings with three or more units constructed before February 1, 1947, where the tenant moved in before July 1, 1971, or units substantially rehabilitated prior to January 1, 1976, under the provisions of J-51, which were initially occupied by the current tenant prior to January 1, 1976; units in buildings with one or two units constructed before February 1, 1947, which were initially occupied by the current tenant prior to April 1953. Some controlled units may remain in buildings converted to cooperatives or condominiums. There are additional provisions not covered here. Under law, all rent-controlled apartments that are voluntarily vacated after June 30, 1971, are no longer subject to the jurisdiction of the Rent Control Law. If the unit is in a building with fewer than six units, it becomes decontrolled; if the unit is in a building with six units or more, it becomes rent stabilized.

The stabilized category is divided into two parts: units built pre-1947 and units built in or post-1947. The following units are classified as pre-1947 stabilized units: units in buildings with six or more units constructed before

February 1, 1947, where the current tenant moved in on or after July 1, 1971; units decontrolled prior to July 1, 1971, under the luxury or vacancy decontrol provisions of city rent regulations, unless the current tenant moved in after the effective date of a cooperative or condominium conversion (if any). The following units are classified as post-1947 stabilized: units in buildings with six or more units which were constructed between 1947 and 1973 or after 1974 if the units received a 421-a or J-51 conversion tax abatement that is still in effect (some previously tax-abated units are no longer rent stabilized after the expiration of tax benefits) and the current tenant moved in prior to a cooperative or condominium conversion (if any); units in buildings occupied prior to 1974 under the Mitchell-Lama program which have been "bought out" of the program. In addition, some housing units subject to regulation by virtue of various governmental supervision or tax-benefit programs are subject to rent-regulatory status pursuant to section 2521.1(k) of the Rent Stabilization Code.

2. Mitchell-Lama Rental. Rental units in buildings constructed under the provisions of article 2 of the Private Housing Finance Law (PHFL) are classified as Mitchell-Lama Rental. The Mitchell-Lama program is primarily housing for moderate- and middle-income tenants; therefore, occupancy is restricted to households meeting certain income limitations. The mechanisms employed to keep rents at affordable levels include tax exemption, state- or city-provided low-interest mortgages, and limitations of return on equity. In certain instances, federal subsidy programs are combined with the state and local assistance measures to achieve the program's objectives. Rents are directly regulated; adjustments are based on changes in operating costs, debt structure, and profitability in the particular project and must be approved by the appropriate state or city agency. Certain Mitchell-Lama projects were refinanced under 223F, National Housing Act, and rents are regulated by the U.S. Department of Housing and Urban Development (HUD).

3. Public Housing. Rental units in structures owned and managed by the New York City Housing Authority are classified as Public Housing. Only households with specified low- or moderate-income levels may qualify as tenants. The Authority regulates rentals and terms and conditions of occupancy. Private housing leased by the Authority is not classified here as Public Housing. In this chapter, other regulated rental apartments have been included in the "public housing" category; these include: (a) unit is in a building that received a subsidy through a federal program which requires HUD to regulate rents in the building; (b) unit is in a building constructed under article 4 of the PHFL and still covered by the provisions of the article; (c) unit is located in a building originally intended as commercial loft space, is occupied as rented residential space, and has its rents regulated by the New York City Loft Board.

4. Unregulated Rentals. Apartments rented according to market rates, and not regulated in terms of permissible rents.

5. In Rem. In Rem units have been excluded from all tabulations in this chapter. These are units located in structures owned by the City of New York as a result of an in rem proceeding initiated by the city after the owner failed to pay tax on the property for three or more years for one- and two-family dwellings, or one or more years for a multiple dwelling. Though many of these units in multiple dwellings had previously been subject to either rent control or rent stabilization, they are exempt from both regulatory systems during the period of city ownership.

Subsidy, Rent. A rent subsidy refers to whether the federal, state, or local government pays part of the householder's rent either to a member of the household or directly to the landlord under the following programs:

1. Under the federal Section 8 certificate or voucher program, the government pays part of the rent for low-income families and individuals. The tenants pay approximately 30 percent of their household income for rent, and the Section 8 program pays the difference between the tenant's payment and a fair market rent.

2. The Public Assistance Grant is made up of the Basic Grant and Shelter Allowance. The Shelter Allowance is meant to be used for the payment of rent. If the rent is higher than the Shelter Allowance, the tenant must pay the remainder of the rent with the Basic Grant.

3. A Senior Citizen Rent Increase Exemption is for persons age sixty-two and above living in rent-controlled, rent-stabilized, or Mitchell-Lama units. For tenants with incomes below a threshold amount, the city pays the difference in monthly rent resulting from increases that raise rent to more than one-third of income.

4. Any other federal, state, or city housing-subsidy program.

Notes

For their extremely helpful comments, suggestions, and guidance, the author thanks two of his colleagues at the ILC-USA, Kottai Gnanasekaran and Charlotte Muller; Frank Braconi, director of New York City's Citizens Housing and Planning Council; and especially Michael Gusmano, coeditor of this book. Bob Callis of the U.S. Census Bureau's New York City Housing and Vacancy Survey also was very helpful. Dhiman Das provided exceptional research assistance, above and beyond the call of duty. Much of the glossary is taken verbatim from U.S. Census Bureau, *New York City Housing and Vacancy Survey: 2002* data.

1.   Muller, Charlotte, Kottai Gnanasekaran, Kenneth Knapp, and Irena Dushi. 2002. *Older*

Homeowners and Renters in Six U.S. Cities: Housing and Economic Resources. ILC Working Paper, International Longevity Center–USA.

2.   Ibid.

3.   "Unit" is defined in the chapter glossary, as are many other terms used in this chapter. Figures tabulated from *New York City Housing and Vacancy Survey: 2002* microdata (hereafter NYC HVS). 2002. Washington, DC: U.S. Census Bureau.

4.   Throughout this chapter, "older" refers to persons age sixty-five and over.

5.   Each of the five boroughs corresponds to a county in the State of New York. The names of the counties differ from the borough names for Brooklyn (Kings County), Manhattan (New York County), and Staten Island (Richmond County).

6.   Citywide, there are 55 sub-boroughs: the Bronx has 10; Brooklyn, 18; Manhattan, 10; Queens, 14; and Staten Island, 3. Roughly equivalent to the community districts discussed in other chapters of this book, "sub-boroughs" are defined in the glossary.

7.   That is, white only (not white and another race). Blacks represent 26 percent of the city's population, and the remaining 29 percent of the population are American Indian, Asian, of Pacific Island decent, some other race, or a mixture of two or more races. Hispanics can be of any race. (Data for sub-boroughs are from Census 2000, accessed through *InfoShare*, and U.S. Census Bureau, *County and City Data Book: 2000.* 13th ed. Washington DC.

8.   Plunz, Richard. 1990. *A History of Housing in New York City: Dwelling Type and Social Change in the American Metropolis.* New York: Columbia University Press.

9.   American Association of Retired Persons. 2000. *Fixing to Stay: A National Survey of Housing and Home Modification Issues.* Washington DC: AARP, 24–25. The percentage refers to those respondents who *strongly* or *somewhat agreed* with this statement: "What I'd really like to do is stay in my current residence for as long as possible."

10. About 80 percent of older homeowners have no mortgage. U.S. Census Bureau. 2001. *American Housing Survey for the United States.* Washington DC.

11. The rate of homeownership in the United States reached a record high of 67.2 percent in mid-2000. Eggers, Frederick J. 2001. Homeownership: A Housing Success Story. In Susan M. Wachter and R. Leo Penne, eds. *Housing Policy in the New Millennium: Conference Proceedings.* Washington, DC: U.S. Department of Housing and Urban Development.

12. U.S. Census Bureau, 1999. *American Housing Survey for the United States.* Washington, DC.

13. Tabulations of NYC HVS data.

14. These are more fully described in the glossary.

15. Tabulations of NYC HVS data.

16. Information from http://nyc.gov (accessed February 2004).

17. The sample size involved in the tabulations of the NYC HVS data here does not allow us to conclude with certainty that 100 percent of the residents live in conventional housing—it is likely that a very small percentage lives in other housing types.

18. Of all residents of Mitchell-Lama co-ops in NYC, 35 percent live in Co-op City. Tabulations of NYC HVS data.

19. *U.S. Code*, Title 42, §1437.

20. U.S. data are from U.S. Census Bureau, *American Housing Survey for the United States*; those for New York are from tabulations of NYC HVS microdata. See the glossary for more details.

21. Muller et al., *Older Homeowners*.

22. U.S. Census Bureau, *American Housing Survey for the United States*.

23. Tabulations of NYC HVS data.

24. All related figures are from tabulations of NYC HVS data. See the glossary for more details.

25. See the glossary for more details.

26. Muller et al., *Older Homeowners*.

27. Figures in this section are from tabulations of NYC HVS data.

28. For homeowners, monthly housing costs are the sum of all mortgage payments, real estate taxes, property insurance, utilities, water and sewer charges, garbage collection, and so on. See the glossary for more details.

29. Schill, Michael H., and Glynis Daniels. 2003. State of New York City's Housing and Neighborhoods. In *Economic Policy Review: Policies to Promote Affordable Housing. Proceedings of a Conference Cosponsored by the Federal Reserve Bank of New York and New York University's Furman Center for Real Estate and Urban Policy* 9(2). June.

7. Lifestyle Patterns, Social Networks, and Use of Formal Services in New York: The Impact of Ethnicity, Class, and Culture on Older People

Marjorie H. Cantor

A major objective of supportive services for older persons is the maintenance of a positive quality of life. Although this goal is rarely defined as such, factors that contribute to a positive quality of life for an older person include economic security, adequate health care, suitable housing and environmental conditions (including personal and household safety and adequate transportation), and meaningful roles and relationships. An additional and crucial component as people get older and face the potential of increased frailty is the nature and extent of the social care they receive.

What is meant here by social care? The term is often used synonymously with social services, but the concept is much broader and encompasses both informal and formal care, which exist side by side. Although purely medical and health-care services may be involved, usually the assistance is of a social nature, addressing three major kinds of needs: first, opportunities for socialization and self-actualization, such as those provided at senior centers; second, assistance with everyday tasks of daily living, usually provided by the informal system augmented by the formal system; and third, help with more personal care, necessitated by illness or disability.[1] This last type of assistance is sometimes the provenance of family but increasingly involves formal home-health services. The goal of social care is to augment individual competency rather than increase dependency.

How does the system work? Perhaps it can best be illustrated through a system model as shown in Figure 7.1. The social support system is made up of a series of concentric circles, each containing a different type of support element, ranging from informal at the center to formal at the periphery. The older person is at the core of this model, interacting with each of these circles at varying times according to particular needs. Although each of these elements usually operates independently, at times they interact, illustrating the concept of a broad-based social support system.

In the outermost circle, farthest from the older person, are the political entities, such as federal, state, and local legislatures responsible for determining social policy and entitlements. Somewhat closer, in the next circle, are the governmental and voluntary agencies that execute these economic and social policies. These bodies provide the services mandated under laws such as the Social Security Act and the Older Americans Act, or those dictated by community need. Organizations in the two outer rings are clearly the formal part of the support system.

Figure 7.1. The Social Care System of Older Persons: A Model

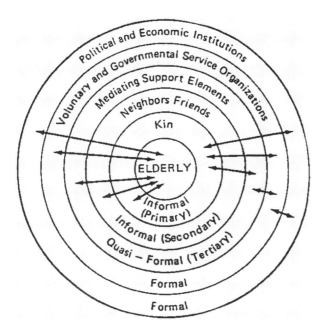

Source: Cantor, Marjorie. 1977. "Neighbors and Friends: An Overlooked Resource in the Informal Support System." Paper presented at the Thirtieth Annual Meeting, Gerontological Society, San Francisco.

Still closer, between formal organizations and kin and significant others, are the nonservice and quasi-formal organizations. Often called mediating structures, such groups can serve as a link between the older person and the broader community and may provide direct help at times of emergency need. Included in this circle are religious organizations; ethnic, cultural or social groups; and neighborhood and block associations; as well as individuals who help older people informally, such as storekeepers, mail carriers, building personnel, and even bartenders.

Finally, closest to the older person and most directly involved in day-to-day life are the individuals who comprise the two innermost circles, the informal system of family, friends, and neighbors. These significant others interact most frequently with older people, are turned to first when instrumental and emotional support are needed, and comprise the broad base of the social support system both in the United States and around the world. By placing the older person at the center and informal care as the closest of the circles, it is clear that changes in the status of older persons and in the availability of informal care have a crucial effect on the other elements of the social care system.

Although older people may receive help from family, community, or tertiary groups, they also often provide considerable help to other generations in the kinship system, as well as to friends and neighbors, demonstrating the reciprocity of informal social care. And increasingly, older persons are active on the political scene, influencing legislation that affects younger generations as well as their own. Thus, the interdependence of generations across the life cycle, represented in the model by bidirectional lines that cross the concentric circles, is crucial to the operation of the Social Care Model. The holistic nature of the social care system is further underscored by the fact that members of the informal and formal systems perform many of the same services, either concurrently or in seriatim. And most important, with its notion of concentric circles and interrelationships among them, the model emphasizes the interrelatedness of the informal and formal care components, both of which are necessary for a responsive care system.[2]

All research and service experience regarding the care of older persons points to need as their primary motivation for turning to assistance, whether from the informal or formal system. I have no quarrel with this finding. But on closer examination of our research findings in New York, it became clear that there are other contextual factors that, in conjunction with need, play an important role in whether or not an older person actually receives assistance. Key among these are ethnicity, class, and culture. The nature of social care and the relative roles of informal and formal supports are particularly germane in light of the demographic changes that are altering the societal landscape, including the decline in extended families, the dispersion of children in response to employment and career opportunities, the continued entrance of women into the labor force, and the increasing racial and ethnic diversity in the U.S. population and particularly in New York. This chapter attempts to shed light on these issues, using New York City as a point of departure.

During the past twenty years, there have been two major studies of the urban older persons of New York. The first, "The Elderly in the Inner City of New York," was completed in 1970. The second, "Growing Older in New York in the 1990s," was a replica of the first, providing an updated picture of older New Yorkers and allowing comparisons across a twenty-year period in which services for older persons had expanded considerably.[3]

Both studies had representative samples and covered a wide range of topics, including demography, social networks, and use of formal services. But perhaps the most significant aspect of the research was its cross-cultural nature, allowing an examination of the similarities and differences among the three major groups of older New Yorkers— white, African American, and Hispanic older persons.

This chapter mainly reports on findings from "Growing Older in New York in the 1990s," the more recent of the studies, with references as appropriate to the earlier study. "Growing Older" involves a probability sample of all noninstitutionalized persons sixty-five and over based upon the Medicare lists provided by the Health Care Financing Administration (since 2001, the Centers for Medicare and Medicaid Services), stratified by age and ethnicity. Minority older persons and the very old were oversampled to insure sufficient numbers of these groups for statistical analysis, resulting in a sample of 1,570 individuals. Louis Harris and Associates conducted interviews in the home in the language of the respondent. Comparisons with the 1990 census suggested that the respondents were highly representative of all New Yorkers sixty-five and over.

Several major findings run through both studies.

1. There is tremendous diversity among the older persons of New York, although certain themes are common to all ethnic groups.
2. Older people are not abandoned by their families, and informal social networks are as strong in 1990 as in 1970.
3. Older people and their families have strong preferences for sources of assistance, and these preferences operate in a hierarchical compensatory manner, with family seen as the first source of assistance, followed by friends and neighbors. Formal sources are turned to only when the informal system is not present or cannot provide the required help
4. The concept of social care and the social care system are vital to an understanding of how older people receive assistance to meet a variety of needs. "Social care" is defined broadly to include the myriad of informal and formal activities, as well as personal support services, which taken as a whole support the efforts of older persons to maintain the greatest degree of personal independence and self-sufficiency. Furthermore, the system of social care involves individual support components such as family and friends, and assistance from community, social agencies, and government.
5. According to older persons, New York City is a positive environment for older people, and the positive feelings are if anything even stronger today than in 1970. Not only do neighborhoods contain the needed services, but also the city itself offers rich cultural life and transportation.

I now turn to the role of ethnicity, class, and culture as contextual factors in the provision of social care.

The Importance of Race and Ethnicity in U.S. Society

Race and ethnicity have been factors in U.S. life since the country's founding. Despite the prevalence of anti-immigrant sentiment, the accepted view has been that the strength of America was as a melting pot, where people from all over could merge their distinctive ethnic and cultural identities and become Americans. Currently this view has been challenged, and there is growing recognition that the United States is in reality a culturally pluralistic society in which there is a pull toward assimilation and at the same time an attempt to maintain ethnic and cultural identity. As a result, we have seen a broadening in ethnic studies to include the effects of common culture, religion, and group identity, as well as race and class, on behavior and social norms. In line with this thinking, Mark Brennan and I in our recent book *Social Care of the Elderly: The Effects of Ethnicity, Class, and Culture* present case studies of Jewish, Latino, and African American older persons, each chosen to illustrate the impact of culture, ethnicity, and class and their effects on the provision of social care.[4] The following sections summarize our findings.

Jewish Older Persons

The older Jewish population of New York and their children form a substantial proportion of the white population and, in many respects, serve as a prototype of future white older persons. They are mainly native born and relatively well educated. They tend to be middle class and generally have higher socioeconomic status and a higher median income than do older New Yorkers as a whole, although a small but not insubstantial group have poverty or near poverty incomes (see Tables 7.1 and 7.2). The relatively better economic circumstances of many Jewish older persons seems to mitigate and even postpone the onset of frailty, and they report better health than many of their peers. It is interesting to note that, among men, Jews seem to survive into old age, and as a result Jewish older persons are more likely to be still married and living with spouses but rarely with children. However, there is a higher proportion of old-old among Jewish persons compared to older persons in general; 40 percent are eighty or older.

Informal social networks are greatly influenced by factors such as group history, culture, class, and level of acculturation. Previous research has suggested that the African American and Latino minority elderly have somewhat different social networks and patterns of assistance than their white peers have.[5] In examining the family life of Jewish elderly, it therefore seems most appropriate to limit comparisons to those older New Yorkers whom they most resemble, their non-Jewish white peers.

With respect to the informal social networks of New York City's Jewish older persons, several points are important (see Table 7.3). Although most Jewish older persons have at least one living child, they have on average fewer children than their peers and their children are more dispersed. Approximately one-third of the Jewish children live within the five boroughs, with 13 percent within walking distance of their parents (in both cases a far smaller proportion than is found with respect to other white older persons, as well as among black and Latino older persons). About one-fourth live in the surrounding suburbs and could reach their parents in one or two hours. But 41 percent of Jewish children live beyond the New York metropolitan area, requiring time and expense to return to assist a parent. As a result, there is less face-to-face contact in the case of Jewish older persons than in other groups and their children and more reliance on the telephone and perhaps e-mail. Children are therefore far less likely to provide hands-on assistance with tasks of daily living than is the case with other older persons. However, they are just as likely to respond at times of illness or crisis, and in line with the relatively affluent circumstances of

Table 7.1. Demographic Characteristics of Jewish and All NYC Respondents 65+, 1990

	Jewish NYC Respondents 65+ (n=335) %	All NYC Respondents 65+ (n=1,570) %
Age		
65–69	17.3	30.0
70–74	19.4	29.6
75–84	46.0	31.1
85+	17.3	8.4
Gender		
Female	56.1	60.1
Male	43.9	39.1
Marital status		
Married	51.3	43.1
Widowed	39.7	37.5
Divorced or separated	4.2	9.8
Never married	4.5	8.7
Nativity		
U.S.	62.7	69.6
Foreign born	35.5	28.3
Education		
8th grade or less	19.4	14.4
Some high school	11.9	16.1
High school graduate	29.9	28.8
Some college	14.3	11.9
College graduate	10.7	5.5
Postgraduate	9.6	6.7
Self-perceived health		
Excellent	17.3	13.0
Good	37.6	41.4
Fair	31.6	32.2
Poor	12.8	10.6
Living arrangements		
Alone	40.6	39.4
With spouse	49.9	41.7
With others (not spouse)	9.9	18.8

Source: Cantor, M. H., and M. Brennan. 2000. *Social Care of the Elderly: The Effects of Ethnicity, Class, and Culture.* New York: Springer.
Note: This source applies to all tables in this chapter.

Table 7.2. Economic Characteristics of Jewish and All NYC Respondents 65+, 1990

	Jewish NYC Respondents 65+ (n=335) %	All NYC Respondents 65+ (n=1,570) %
Socioeconomic status		
High	15.3	11.8
Medium high	10.7	7.9
Medium	28.4	17.5
Medium low	31.8	37.4
Low	13.8	25.4
1989 income		
$6000 or less	6.3	14.0
$6001–$8500	7.2	11.0
$8501–$10,000	6.0	6.2
$10,001–$15,000	15.3	14.2
$15,001–$25,000	14.6	14.0
$25,001–$35,000	9.0	8.5
$35,001–$50,000	8.7	5.4
$50,001 or more	11.1	3.9
Average income	$26,345	$18,921
Median income	$20,001	$13,751
Poverty level		
At or below poverty	10.0	20.4
Near poverty (101%–150%)	19.5	22.6
Over 150% poverty	70.5	57.0
Sources of income (independent items)		
Social Security	96.7	92.5
Interest or dividends	74.0	54.8
Pensions	45.4	50.7
Wages/salaries/commissions	17.3	14.2
Supplemental Security Income	8.4	12.6
Family or friends	5.4	6.5
Other	5.4	4.7
Perception of economic well-being		
Cannot make ends meet	2.1	5.2
Just manage to get by	33.4	44.4
Enough money with a little extra	35.2	31.6
Money not a problem	28.1	16.7

many Jewish children, the flow of money is likely to be from parents to children (but for parents in need, the Jewish children are just as responsive as are children of other older persons.).

While spouse and children form the core of informal care, friends and neighbors often play an important secondary role. Jewish older persons were as likely as other older white persons in the city to report having one or more close friends and were as likely to know one or more neighbors well. But Jewish older persons reported knowing more of their neighbors.

Thus, Jewish older persons have both resources and needs arising from the higher proportion of old-old and the greater geographic dispersion of children and their less frequent provision of hands-on assistance.

How does culture and group identity act to temper these needs and provide pathways to formal service utilization in the case of Jewish older persons? Most important are the culturally based attitudes among Jewish older persons regarding the role of family and community. In this respect, several themes are worth noting. The first is the centrality of the family in Jewish life, reflecting the long history of persecution of Jews and the role of the family as a place of joy and refuge in a hostile world, as well as maintaining connections between generations and preserving Jewish heritage.[6] A second theme is the high value in Jewish culture placed on both intellectual pursuits and professional and business attainment.[7] In their efforts to support the aspirations of their children, Jewish older persons feel strongly about maintaining their independence and not becoming a burden on them, even if this means geographic separation and sometimes loneliness.[8] The third theme is the strong sense of community in Jewish tradition.

The sense of marginalization among Jews over the centuries has underscored the cultural norm of self-help, including the responsibility of each person to the larger community, and in return the community's responsibility to help those in need.[9] A present-day testament to the historic emphasis on community is the widespread array of services sponsored by the Jewish community in New York. These values, combined with a respect for knowledge and professional skills, have meant that the stigma of turning outside one's family for help is not part of the Jewish cultural landscape. And in fact a higher proportion of Jewish older persons evidenced a willingness to turn to the formal system or rely on themselves than was the case among their peers (see Table 7.4).

The greater use of health and in-home services, including nursing homes and senior centers, by Jewish older persons would appear to stem from an amalgam of objective needs (i.e., greater age, children more dispersed and less likely to provide hands-on assistance) and cultural attitudes and values mutually cherished by older and younger generations of Jews. But, as we will see in the case of the family-centered Latino older persons, cultural norms regarding help from outside the immediate family can also serve as a barrier to turning to the formal system.

Table 7.3. Informal Social Networks of Jewish and Non-Jewish White NYC Respondents 65+, 1990

	Jewish Respondents 65+ (n=335)	Non-Jewish White Respondents 65+ (n=512)
Average number of children[a]	1.6	1.9
Respondent has at least one:		
Spouse[b]	51.3	38.5
Child	80.0	75.0
Sibling	72.8	71.3
Other relative in NYC[b]	56.7	40.6
Friend/confidant	37.3	37.1
Neighbor known well	62.7	67.4

[a] p<.01, one-way analysis of variance
[b] p<.001, Chi-square test of significance

Latino Older Persons

During the 1980s, the number of Latinos sixty-five and over in New York increased by 60 percent, with Latinos comprising nearly 10 percent of the older persons of the city by 1990.[10] In the past, the largest group of Latinos in New York was from Puerto Rico. In recent years, however, sizable numbers of new immigrants from the Dominican Republic and Central and South America, as well as Cuba, have resulted in considerable diversification of the Latino population. Most New York Latinos, regardless of origin and level of acculturation, are severely economically disadvantaged, struggling in old age on limited or poverty-level incomes, and many report their health as poor or at best fair (see Tables 7.5 and 7.6).

It has often been assumed that minority older persons live in extended family households and therefore have someone at home to help at times of need. However, over one-third of Latino older persons in the sample lived alone, and the number of live alones has risen since our first study in 1970, from 25 to 37 percent, and is likely to continue to rise. The remaining two-thirds are about equally divided between those living with a spouse and those living with children in an extended family household.

Although the traditional extended family among Latinos may be on the wane, the Latino community continues to maintain a strong family-centered informal support system, and most older Latinos are well-integrated into such networks and receive considerable assistance from younger members of the kin system.

Table 7.4. Extent of Formal Services Use in Past Year of Jewish and All NYC Respondents 65+, by Type of Assistance, 1990

	Jewish Respondents 65+ (n=335) %	All NYC Respondents 65+ (n=1,570) %
Entitlements		
Social Security	16.7	19.1
Medicare	22.7	18.2
Medicaid	3.6	4.6
Department of Social Services	6.5	6.4
In-home services		
Home care (all types)	14.9	10.3
Visiting nurse service	11.9	6.8
Health services		
Nursing home	3.0	1.2
Veterans Administration /VA hospital	5.4	7.4
Emergency room	21.2	19.8
Inpatient hospital	18.8	16.8
Local community services		
Senior center	20.0	17.3
NYC Department for the Aging	6.6	5.5
NYC Housing Authority	5.1	5.2
Police department	9.0	7.5
Rabbi/minister/priest	8.4	9.2

Networks of Latino older persons are therefore more kin centered and less broad based than those of either white or black older persons. Compared to their black or white peers, Latino older persons have the most children on average, the most living nearby, the most frequent contact with children, and the most hands-on help with tasks of daily living. In addition, many older Latinos report the presence of a spouse, and as a group, Latino older persons had larger networks of other relatives in New York than did their white or African American peers. But in accordance with the emphasis on kin as the mainstay of the informal network, Latinos were the least likely of the older persons to report having a friend or knowing neighbors well (see Table 7.7). Thus, if family members are unable or unwilling to provide needed assistance, older Latinos have fewer compensatory options than do white or black older persons. Furthermore, their often limited English makes turning to community-based agencies more problematic.

Table 7.5. Demographic Characteristics
of Latino NYC Respondents, by Place of Origin, 1990

	Total (n=337)	Puerto Rico (n=192)	Dominican Republic (n=47)	Cuba (n=25)	Other (n=73)
	%	%	%	%	%
Age					
65–69	21.1	22.4	25.5	20.0	15.1
70–74	23.4	25.5	21.3	28.0	17.8
75–84	42.1	39.1	44.7	36.0	50.7
85+	13.4	13.0	8.5	16.0	16.4
Gender					
Male	37.4	34.4	44.7	28.0	43.8
Female	62.6	65.6	55.3	72.0	56.2
Marital status					
Married	33.8	31.3	44.7	40.0	31.5
Widowed	38.6	42.7	31.9	32.0	34.2
Divorced or separated	20.2	19.8	14.9	24.0	23.3
Never married	6.2	5.2	6.4	4.0	9.6
Refused/not sure	1.2	1.0	2.1	0.0	1.4
Self-perceived health					
Excellent	7.4	6.3	10.6	4.0	9.6
Good	36.5	35.9	36.2	44.0	35.6
Fair	40.7	43.2	38.3	44.0	34.2
Poor	14.8	14.6	14.9	8.0	17.8
Refused/not sure	0.6	0.0	0.0	0.0	2.7
Length of residence[a]					
20 years or less	14.2	3.1	34.0	16.0	30.1
21–30 years	21.1	10.9	34.0	40.0	32.9
31–40 years	19.0	21.4	10.6	32.0	13.7
41–60 years	27.9	40.1	12.8	12.0	11.0
61 years or more	14.2	21.4	2.1	0.0	8.2
Refused/not sure	3.6	3.1	6.4	0.0	4.1
Language at home[b]					
Spanish only	72.0	64.9	87.2	80.0	78.1
Spanish and English	17.0	20.9	10.6	12.0	12.3
English only	11.0	14.1	2.1	8.0	9.6

Note: Totals equal 100%.

[a] p<.001, Chi-square test of significance

[b] p<.05, Chi-square test of significance

Table 7.6. Socioeconomic Characteristics of Latino NYC Respondents 65+, 1990

	Total (n=337)	Puerto Rican (n=192)	Dominican (n=47)	Cuban (n=25)	Other (n=73)
	%	%	%	%	%
Education					
8th grade or less	58.8	57.3	68.1	60.0	56.2
Some high school	11.0	14.4	4.3	8.0	8.2
High school graduate	13.6	17.7	4.3	12.0	9.6
Some college	3.3	2.1	0.0	12.0	5.5
College graduate	0.9	0.5	0.0	0.0	2.7
Postgraduate	0.9	0.0	0.0	0.0	4.1
Refused/not sure	11.6	8.3	23.4	8.0	13.7
Hollingshead SES group					
High (I)	10.4	6.8	21.3	8.0	13.7
Medium high (II)	4.2	4.2	0.0	8.0	5.5
Medium (III)	5.9	4.7	4.3	8.0	9.6
Medium low (IV)	35.3	38.5	31.9	32.0	30.1
Low (V)	44.2	45.8	42.6	44.0	41.1
1989 income					
$6000 or less	38.9	33.9	48.9	28.0	49.3
$6001–$8500	19.0	21.4	14.9	28.0	12.3
$8501–$10,000	8.3	8.3	0.0	12.0	12.3
$10,001–$12,500	3.6	5.2	0.0	0.0	2.7
$12,501–$15,000	3.9	5.7	2.1	0.0	1.4
$15,001–$25,000	4.5	4.2	2.1	12.0	4.1
$25,001–$35,000	0.9	0.5	2.1	4.0	0.0
$35,001–$50,000	0.9	0.5	0.0	4.0	1.4
$50,001 or more	0.0	0.0	0.0	0.0	0.0
Refused/not sure	20.2	20.3	29.7	12.0	16.4
Poverty level					
At or below poverty	56.9	50.3	81.8	45.5	63.9
Near poverty (101%–150%)	28.3	32.7	9.1	31.8	26.2
Over 150% poverty	14.9	17.0	9.1	22.7	9.8

Note: Totals equal 100%; mean income is based on midpoints of income categories.

In line with the strong cultural preference for family-centered assistance, only 43 percent of the Latino older persons in New York City turned to one or more community agencies during the year previous to being interviewed (Table 7.8), a significantly lower proportion than was found among white and black older persons (58 and 57 percent respectively).

Perhaps even more sobering are the findings regarding the underutilization of needs-based entitlements. Despite the fact that virtually all older Latinos (85 percent) were living on or near poverty-level incomes, they were the least likely of the three major ethnic groups to utilize needs-based entitlements such as Supplemental Security Income (SSI) and food stamps. The only exception was that Latino older persons were somewhat more likely than African American or white older persons to utilize Medicaid. It would appear that health is an area in which government assistance is sanctioned, while needs-based income-enhancing entitlements pose more barriers for many impoverished older Latinos.

Table 7.7. Informal Social Networks among Latino NYC Respondents 65+, by Place of Origin, 1990

	Total (n=337) %	Puerto Rico (n=192) %	Dominican Republic (n=47) %	Cuba (n=25) %	Other (n=73) %
Spouse	33.8	31.3	44.7	40.0	31.5
Child[a]	78.6	81.3	83.0	52.0	78.1
Mean[a]	(2.8)	(2.6)	(3.8)	(1.5)	(3.1)
Sibling-living	73.0	69.3	83.0	72.0	76.7
Mean in NYC[b]	(1.5)	(1.4)	(2.6)	(1.1)	(1.2)
Other NYC relative[a]	47.5	43.2	74.5	44.0	42.5
Mean in NYC[a]	(3.5)	(3.5)	(5.7)	(2.6)	(2.2)
Confidant	39.8	39.6	36.2	48.0	39.7
Mean	(0.6)	(0.6)	(0.5)	(0.7)	(0.6)
Friend/confidant	27.3	29.2	17.0	36.0	26.0
Mean	(0.4)	(0.4)	(0.2)	(0.4)	(0.4)
Neighbor known well	47.2	47.9	44.7	44.0	47.9
Mean	(1.6)	(1.7)	(1.6)	(0.9)	(1.5)
No components	3.0	3.1	2.1	4.0	2.7

[a] p<.01 standard deviation
[b] p<.05 standard deviation

Table 7.8. Types of Formal Services Used by Latino NYC Respondents 65+ in Past Year, by Place of Origin, 1990

	Total (n=337) %	Puerto Rico (n=192) %	Dominican Republic (n=47) %	Cuba (n=25) %	Other (n=73) %
Entitlements					
Social Security	13.1	14.1	10.6	12.0	12.3
Medicare	11.9	9.9	6.4	20.0	17.8
Medicaid	8.0	7.3	2.1	8.0	13.7
Long-term care services					
Home care (all types)	12.2	13.6	12.8	8.0	9.7
Visiting nurse service	4.2	4.2	2.1	0.0	6.8
Veterans Administration /VA hospital	3.0	4.7	2.1	0.0	0.0
Nursing home	0.0	0.0	0.0	0.0	0.0
Government agencies					
Department of Social Services	7.7	6.3	6.4	20.0	8.2
NYC Housing Authority	6.2	6.8	4.3	4.0	6.8
NYC Department for the Aging	3.9	4.7	2.1	0.0	4.1
Police department	3.6	3.1	2.1	0.0	6.8
Socialization/recreation					
Senior center (past month)	8.9	10.9	2.1	12.0	6.8
Religious					
Priest/minister/rabbi	5.3	2.6	6.4	12.0	9.6
Spiritualist	0.3	0.0	0.0	0.0	1.4

Note: Independent items, totals do not equal 100%.

The reason for the low service use on the part of older Latinos has been the subject of considerable speculation (see Table 7.8). Some suggest that the strength of the informal system and the cultural mores against turning outside the kin network except in situations of severe distress has provided an alternative resource system.[11] Others have hypothesized that negative cultural attitudes regarding the use of the formal system, along with the institutional barriers created by that system (particularly those involving language and lack of cultural sensitivity), militate against the use of community services.[12] The size of our sample and the richness of our data set allowed us to examine the relative importance of both these hypotheses as explanations for low use of formal services on the part of Latino older persons.

We used a hierarchical regression model to test the importance of cultural barriers as opposed to alternative resources. Our findings suggest that both alternative resources and cultural and institutional barriers have an impact on service use, but neither alone provides a sufficient explanation (see Table 7.9).

Rather, the strength of the informal family-oriented system and the institutional barriers to negotiating the formal system interact to limit the ability of older Latinos to utilize those services that exist. However, as the needs for assistance increase and become more complex, and the capacities of the family are overreached, some alternative to sole dependency on family resources must be provided. Thus, both older and younger members need pathways to services that are culturally sensitive and acceptable.

Our findings suggest that in strong ethnic communities such as the Latino and the newer Asian American communities, neighbors, friends, clergy, and community leaders are essential as pathways to service, offering knowledge, support, and even intervention to assure that the cultural barriers—whether within the kin network or in the services themselves—are bridged. Only through such pathways can the strengths of the family system be combined with the facilities of the broader community to the benefit of older Latinos and similar immigrant groups. It should be noted that as pressures of acculturation increase among the younger members, the need for a partnership between the informal and formal systems will be even more urgent.

African American Older Persons

We turn now to older African Americans of New York City and a major question in ethnic studies: the relative importance of race and class in affecting lifestyles, social networks, and the use of community services.

In New York City, the number of blacks over the age of sixty-five increased by 30 percent between 1980 and 1990, and blacks now account for about 17 percent of the city's older persons. Although African Americans were among the city's earliest arrivals, their history has been one not of assimilation and increasing opportunities but of economic and racial exploitation and barriers to the opportunity structure of the society.

Nevertheless, many of today's older blacks were active in the civil rights struggles of the 1950s and 1960s, and we are seeing the results of those struggles in the emergence, for the first time, of a substantial group of black older New Yorkers with moderate retirement incomes. This does not mean that African American older persons as a group are well off. Rather, the vast majority suffers from higher levels of poverty, poorer health, and lower levels of education than do their white peers, and they are only marginally better off than Latino older persons. But the appearance of a group of moderate-income black older persons, mainly employed in unionized skilled blue-collar occupations, civil service, or business, or as teachers, nurses, or social workers, allows the first glimpse of how more equality in education and occupations during the working years can affect the quality of life in retirement, as well as intergenerational patterns of assistance.

To address this question, the African American sample of "Growing Older in New York in the 1990s" was divided into two groups: older persons reporting incomes from poverty to 150 percent of poverty (n=218) and those reporting incomes over 150 percent of poverty (n=83). A group of white older persons (n=483) with the same median incomes were used for comparison purposes to gauge the relative effects of race and income on social care. Although income and class are not synonymous in this analysis, income is used as a proxy for the more inclusive concept of social class. What are some of the differences we found?

Older African Americans as a group have an average age of 73.7, with one-third seventy-five and over. Low-income blacks were significantly older on average compared to both moderate-income blacks and moderate-income whites. Among low-income blacks, nearly two-thirds were seventy-five or older, while among moderate-income blacks and whites only half are seventy-five plus. As in all populations of older persons, women outnumber men, but this is especially true among older African Americans. Again, class differences are evident—low-income blacks were overwhelming female (73 percent), while among the moderate-income blacks and whites there was a more equal division by gender. Marital status also differs according to income. Among older African Americans as a group, women are twice as likely as men to be widowed (61 to 29 percent). Given the relative age and gender differentials, it is not surprising that low-income blacks were the least likely to be currently married and more likely to be widowed, while the proportion still married among the moderate-income blacks and whites was approximately the same (about half), and only one-third were without a spouse as a member of their informal network.

On average, black older persons reported 9.6 years of education, somewhat less than white but more than Latino older persons. However, the proportion of black older persons with more than an eighth-grade education has increased substantially over the past twenty years. Still, within-group differences are considerable. While 43 percent of low-income blacks reported an eighth-grade or less education, only 25 percent of the moderate-income blacks had such minimal education. Among moderate-income whites, only 17 percent had an eighth-grade education or less.

Table 7.9. Multiple Regression Analyses on the Number of Formal Services Used by Latino NYC Respondents 65+ (n=337), 1990

	Analysis Stage							
	One		Two		Three		Four	
	b	(R²)	b	(R²)	b	(R²)	b	(R²)
Alternative resources								
Social network size	.00	(.00)			-.00	(.00)	.02	(.00)
Network interaction	-.15ª	(.01)			-.11	(.01)	-.07	(.01)
Instrumental support satisfaction	-.03	(.00)			-.03	(.00)	.01	(.00)
Emotional support satisfaction	-.01	(.00)			-.02	(.00)	.06	(.00)
Number of ways children help	.03	(.00)			.03	(.00)	.01	(.00)
Neighbor involvement help	.20ª	(.04)			.20ª	(.04)	.18ª	(.04)
Cultural barriers								
Length of NYC residence			.10	(.01)	.07	(.00)	-.01	(.00)
Language spoken at home (English)			.08	(.00)	.07	(.00)	.11	(.00)
Connection to formal needs-based entitlements			.16ª	(.02)	.14ᵇ	(.02)	.16ª	(.02)
Personal characteristics								
Age							.06	(.01)
Gender (female)							-.15ª	(.01)

Education level				-.01 (.00)
Living alone				.03 (.00)
Living with spouse				.04 (.00)
Place of origin:				
Puerto Rico				-.04 (.00)
Dominican Republic				-.08 (.01)
Cuba				.01 (.00)
Income adequacy				.07 (.00)
Extent of need				
Perceived number of needs				.31[a] (.11)
Activity limitations				-.13 (.00)
Depression				.29[a] (.05)
Multiple R=	.22	.17	.27	.51
R²=	.05	.03	.07	.26

[a] p<.01 standard deviation
[b] p<.05 standard deviation

With respect to higher education, the differences between low- and moderate-income blacks are even sharper—7 and 18 percent respectively. Again, moderate-income whites were far more likely to report college or postgraduate education. Thus, the educational differentials between whites and blacks, though narrowing since 1970, are clearly present and are a major factor in the income disparities among white, black, and Latino older persons.

In line with their higher socioeconomic status, moderate-income white and black older persons are the most likely to report being in relatively good health, with approximately two-thirds of both groups reporting their health as good or excellent. On the other hand, more than half the low-income blacks perceived their health to be only fair or poor (see Table 7.10).

Finally, living arrangements, like other socioeconomic variables, reflect class/income status. Contrary to general assumptions, most of New York's black older persons do not live in extended family households. In fact, two out of five (42 percent) live alone, and about one-fourth live with a spouse. Only one-third live with others, mainly children or fictive kin. And it was the low-income blacks who were more likely than moderate-income blacks to live alone (49 and 29 percent, respectively). However, African American older persons, regardless of income, were more likely than were white older persons to be living in extended households with children and grandchildren but without a spouse. And as expected, the prevalence of such households was greatest among low-income blacks, compared with moderate-income blacks and whites (36, 23, and 11 percent respectively). Of these combined households, most are headed by older women and represent a sharing of resources in the face of poverty and other social ills. A further illustration of the crucial role played by many of these older women is that 17 percent of black older persons were solely responsible for the care of grandchildren, a higher proportion than that found among white and Latino older persons.

In summary, it is clear that with respect to basic demographic and socioeconomic variables there are decided differences between low- and moderate-income black older persons and that middle-class black older persons are more similar to their middle-class white peers. It is important to note, however, that moderate-income blacks probably do not have the economic reserves of their white peers and that, given the severe social problems facing many minority families, moderate-income black older persons are called upon more often to share their resources than is the case among whites with similar incomes.

Given the sociodemographic difference between the vast majority of older blacks who have low incomes and the much smaller group of older blacks who have moved into the middle class. are there differences, as well, in the nature of their informal supports? The extent of the network and the amount of interaction among members determine the effectiveness of informal networks in providing social care. Here the strong cultural values of black America with respect to family and church make class differences less sharp. Given the findings regarding marital status previ-

Table 7.10. Characteristics of Low- and Moderate-Income Black and Moderate-Income White Respondents 65+: NYC, 1990

	Low-Income Black (n=218)	Moderate-Income Black (n=83)	Moderate-Income White (n=430)
	%	%	%
Age (years)[a]			
65–69	18.3	27.7	25.3
70–74	18.8	24.1	23.3
75–84	46.3	39.8	42.6
85+	16.5	8.4	8.8
Average age (sd)[b]	77.1 (7.1)	74.4 (6.6)	75.2 (6.5)
Gender			
Male	26.6	55.4	48.1
Female	73.4	44.6	51.9
Marital status			
Married	15.6	48.2	55.8
Widowed	56.4	34.9	30.9
Divorced	8.7	4.8	4.2
Separated	11.9	4.8	1.4
Never married	7.3	7.2	7.7
Education			
8th grade or less	42.6	24.6	16.9
Some high school	25.4	28.3	16.3
High school graduate	24.5	30.9	30.4
Some college	4.4	7.4	15.6
College graduate	1.5	4.9	7.9
Postgraduate	1.5	3.7	12.9
Average years education (sd)[b]	9.2 (3.2)	10.7 (3.2)	12.3 (3.7)
Self-perceived health			
Excellent	9.3	16.9	22.0
Good	38.4	47.0	43.9
Fair	34.3	32.5	27.8
Poor	18.1	3.6	6.3

[a] p<.05 standard deviation

[b] p<.001 standard deviation

ously mentioned, it is not surprising that low-income blacks were the least likely to report the presence of a spouse in their network (16 percent), as compared with approximately half of moderate-income blacks and slightly more among moderate-income whites (48 and 56 percent, respectively). Findings with respect to the relation between income and presence of at least one child in the network are similar to that regarding spouses. As was true for their white and Latino counterparts, the vast majority of New York's African American older persons have at least 1 living child (76 percent), and the average number of children living was 2.9. However, low-income blacks were more likely to be without a living child in their social network than were moderate-income black and white older persons (28, 18, and 21 percent, respectively). The greater likelihood of being without a spouse in the household or a living child to assist as needed would appear to place low-income blacks at a disadvantage compared to their moderate-income peers.

But this disadvantage is compensated for in the case of low-income blacks by the number of children, their location, and the amount of assistance. Both low- and moderate-income black older persons with children have more children on average than do moderate-income whites, 2.1 and 2.4 as compared with 1.8 in the case of moderate-income whites. Thus, black older persons as a group have larger numbers of children capable of assisting them at times of need (see Table 7.11).

But equally important from a care perspective are where the children live and what kind of assistance they provide. In general, the children of white older persons are more geographically dispersed than are the children of the black or Latino older persons of the city. But among black older persons, there are differences in residential patterns according to income levels. The children of low-income blacks are more likely to live nearby, either within walking distance or within the five boroughs of New York. On the other hand, children of moderate-income blacks and whites are more dispersed and more likely to live in the suburbs surrounding the city (18 percent in both cases), or to live beyond the metropolitan area (about 40 percent). Among low-income older blacks, only 13 percent of children live in the suburbs and about 30 percent live beyond the metropolitan area.

Children of the low-income black older persons not only live closer but also are more likely to be in face-to-face contact with their parents once or more per week—50 percent, as compared to about 40 percent in the case of moderate-income blacks and whites. Among the latter groups, face-to-face contact is more likely to occur once or twice a month. In compensation, children of moderate-income blacks and whites are in touch with their parents more frequently by phone. Thus, social class has its effect on the location of children, as well as on the amount and form of interaction between parents and children. And in all these respects, the low-income black older persons are the most advantaged. About nine out of ten older people receive assistance from children, and there were no differences in the receipt of help among low- and moderate-income black and moderate-income white older persons, underscoring the fact that helping parents is a strongly held cultural norm for all.

Table 7.11. Presence of Social Networks among Low- and Moderate-Income Black and Moderate-Income White Respondents 65+: NYC, 1990

	Low-Income Black (n=218)	Moderate-Income Black (n=83)	Moderate-Income White (n=430)
	%	%	%
Spouse[a]	15.6	48.2	55.8
Children			
At least one living[b]	71.6	83.1	79.1
Average number (sd)[a]	2.1 (2.3)	2.4 (2.3)	1.8 (1.4)
Sibling in NYC[a]	57.3	63.9	75.1
Other relative in NYC	53.2	62.7	50.0
Confidant (any)	66.1	71.1	64.2
Friend/confidant	44.5	55.4	41.6
Neighbor known well	62.4	66.3	67.2
Average network size (sd)	12.9 (21.8)	10.3 (7.6)	11.2 (17.7)
Number of support elements[a]			
One	9.8	2.4	3.0
Two	22.0	16.9	12.9
Three	29.9	16.9	29.0
Four	25.7	32.5	26.6
Five	11.7	25.3	22.7
Six	0.9	6.0	5.8

[a] p<.01 standard deviation

[b] p<.05 standard deviation

There are significant between-group differences in the types of assistance provided by children. Financial help was the most frequently reported type. Moderate-income black and white older persons were the most likely to receive such assistance in the form of gifts, while low-income black older persons were more likely to report direct monetary assistance from children. As we found in our research in general, as parents' needs increase, children respond with greater assistance. Thus, in the case of the poorer black older persons, the sharing of economic resources between generations is much more likely than among moderate-income blacks or whites. Although the likelihood of providing assistance at times of illness or other crisis was not related to income, when it comes to assistance with tasks of daily living (such as shopping, cooking, housekeeping), low-income black older persons were far more likely to receive such help from children than were their moderate-income black or white peers.

The greater amount of hands-on help in the case of low-income blacks prob-ably reflects the proximity of children, more sharing of households, and the greater vulnerability of lower-income older persons with respect to health status and economic resources. This is not to suggest that the children of moderate-income black or white older persons are not responsive to their parents' social care needs but rather that the configuration of social networks, the frequency of contact, and the type of assistance seems to be clearly influenced by class. Middle-class older blacks are more similar to middle-class older whites with respect to the nature of informal social care than they are to the much larger and much more vulnerable low-income black older persons.

Just as class affects the size and nature of informal supports among the African American elderly of New York, class in combination with need impacts the use of formal community services. Among older blacks, 57 percent turned for assistance to one or more community services in the past year, and there was no difference in the likelihood of turning to the formal sector in the case of low-income blacks, moderate-income blacks, or moderate-income whites, although there was a dif-ference in the number and type of agencies turned to. Low-income blacks used significantly more formal services on average (1.4) compared to moderate-income blacks and moderate-income whites (1.1). Reflecting their greater economic and social vulnerability, low-income blacks were more likely to report turning for help to the Medicaid Office, Department of Social Services, Public Housing Authority, and in-home services, including home care and the Visiting Nurse Service, than were their middle-class black or white peers. On the other hand, moderate-income blacks were the most likely to utilize the services of the Veterans Administration, including the VA hospital. This latter finding probably reflects the important role the military played for this cohort of black elderly as an avenue of training and eco-nomic security, and many middle-class blacks continued to use the benefits available to them as veterans. Finally, given the historical role played by the black church as a community-organizing force, particularly with respect to social support and problem-solving resources, black elderly in New York, regardless of income/class, were significantly more likely than were their moderate-income white peers to turn to their minister for assistance.

Differences between the characteristics of older New York African Americans in poverty and those in the rising middle class along a variety of socioeconomic and social care variables underscore the heterogeneity of the older black population of the city and the importance of recognizing differences as well as similarities in policy planning and program implementation. But the existence of middle-class black older persons, more similar to their white peers than to low-income older blacks, illustrates how the opportunity structure of earlier years affects the nature and quality of life in old age. Thus the extent of equal opportunities with respect to education and occupations will clearly affect whether or not there will be a continuing rising middle class in future cohorts of black and other minority older persons.

Conclusions

The foregoing case studies of Jewish, Latino, and black older persons underscore the diversity of the older population of New York City. But equally important, they suggest that ethnicity, class, and culture interact to shape lifestyles and patterns of social care, and that attention to all three is necessary to understand the great variety of older people and how they live in New York and elsewhere. Furthermore, in policy planning and program development for older people, it is essential to recognize this diversity and the vital role played by ethnicity, class, and culture in older people's response to, and their ability to access, health and social services. How best to insure that the great variety of older people from differing economic strata, ethnic and cultural backgrounds, and family structures obtain the assistance needed is a major challenge for policy makers and providers in the coming years as the size and heterogeneity of the older population increases. Several themes have emerged from the study of older New Yorkers germane to this challenge. The first pertains to minimizing barriers to service.

There is a need for culturally sensitive programming, recognizing the strengths and preferences among various communities of older persons and their families. Furthermore, there is a need to reinforce shared values across generations and communities in our service delivery. Not only ethnicity and culture are involved, but also social class is an important factor. Most importantly, as we saw in the Latino case study, we must insure that there are adequate pathways to basic entitlements. To develop these vital connections, we must address issues of language and crippling bureaucracy. Clearly, language can be a crucial barrier to utilization of services, and programs must be sensitive to and aware of how they get their messages across. Because older Latinos, as well as the elderly of other newly arrived immigrant groups, often have difficulties with the English language, it is essential that there be bilingual staff and that forms and informational material about services and entitlements be translated into several languages, such as Spanish, Chinese, Korean, Russian—whatever language is spoken by the targeted population of a program or service. Additionally, any announcements regarding services or benefits should appear in the foreign language press, radio, and television to insure that the targeted groups are reached.

Older people of all groups studied talked about the difficulty of dealing with the bureaucracy when attempting to obtain information about eligibility for entitlements or the too often torturous process of securing entitlements. Particularly for low-income, foreign-born, and older persons with minimum education, there may be a need for translators and expediters between the older persons and the services and bureaucracies. While family members, especially children and grandchildren, are an obvious source of such assistance, the increasing dispersion of children and the growing numbers of Latino, black, and white older persons who live alone suggest that many may not have anyone nearby to act as an intermediary in dealing with complex organizations with their myriad rules and regulations. Even for well-educated, English-speaking older persons, dealing with governmental programs such as Medicare and Social Security, as well as hospitals and medical personal, can be daunting and frustrating. Thus, reaching out and simplifying procedures and information is essential if older people are to successfully negotiate the formal service system. In addition, we need to find those key individuals in the community who can serve as pathways to services. Adult children, neighbors, ministers, doctors, and community leaders all need information about services available to the older persons with whom they interact. Fortunately, the Care Givers Initiative under the Older Americans Act has finally recognized the role of caregivers and their needs. This is a wonderful beginning, as community agencies across the country are reaching out to provide information, social support groups, respite services, and pathways to securing concrete assistance. But the need for more social adult day-care and home-health assistance is vital if the caregiving initiatives are to succeed.

A second theme running throughout the three case studies is the importance of family and the relative roles of kin and the formal system in providing social care. First and most important, to provide adequate care for older people, both systems must continue to operate and must be partners in the provision of social care. Neither can do it alone. Families are not abandoning their older members, but pressures on families are growing, particularly in this period of uncertainty and economic downturn. As we move forward in the twenty-first century, the growing number of older persons coupled with increases in the number of working women and changing family structures will require new responses to social care on the part of families and communities. Furthermore, advances in health care have resulted in older persons living longer, with the onset of frailty occurring later in the life span. As a result, serious incapacity has been pushed into the late eighties and nineties, and family caregivers are more frequently in their sixties and seventies, sometimes suffering from illnesses themselves.[13] Thus, the role of the formal system as a partner and backup for family care is growing in importance at the very time we are seeing funding cuts at the local, state, and federal levels. The family in its broadest sense will remain important, but it cannot continue to act without more assistance. As we have noted, all three groups of older persons studied indicated a need for more assistance, particularly in home services necessary to maintain independence. What is needed is a clearly articulated partnership between family and community so that together they can meet the needs of future older persons. To insure such a partnership will involve, as we have seen, changes in attitudes about the appropriateness of assistance outside the family system, as well as recognition on the part of professionals of the vital role played by the families in the lives of older persons.

Finally, there is the theme of diversity and the recognition of the need for a variety of types of assistance and opportunities to meet the heterogeneity of older persons and their needs. As we welcome the increasing numbers of young older persons as the baby boomers enter the aging cohorts, community-based programs need to be more clearly targeted to the differing age cohorts and the diversity in income and educational levels. For the oldest old, needs for medical care, in-home supportive services, and a variety of living/care arrangements (including assisted living, adult day care, and institutional care) will become even more important in light of the increased age at which frailty is projected to occur. The need for supportive community-based services for such older persons will become an even more serious policy issue, particularly as it is projected that 80 percent of women, the traditional caregivers of older persons, will be employed. Furthermore, in the absence of an adequate long-term care system in the United States, it is important to recognize that many relatively well-off middle-class older persons, white, black, or Latino, may become poor overnight when faced with serious illness, requiring both familial and community assistance to allow them a decent quality of life in old age.

For younger older persons of all ethnic, class, and cultural backgrounds, the community will need to consider how to meet their educational and recreational needs and most importantly provide them with productive roles in society, whether through continued employment if desired or opportunities for meaningful volunteerism. Such opportunities are important not only for the well-being of older persons, but also for the good of the broader community. Retired and with time on their hands, they can be a valuable source of volunteer assistance. Further, they often need assistance to connect with the cultural and educational institutions of the community. Senior centers and other community agencies such as naturally occurring retirement communities face the challenge of becoming attuned to the interests of younger older persons—offering creative programming, including computer literacy, hands-on art and music experiences, and forums for political and civic discussions. Even if one suffers from chronic illness, one's mind does not stop, and we are challenged to help older people of all backgrounds age successfully and contribute according to their skills and abilities.

Thus, the opportunities for partnership are many. The policy and program challenges of the future require that both the frail and the well elderly have the supports and opportunities necessary for a quality old age, and that we recognize ethnicity, class, and cultural considerations as vital in the structuring and operation of services and role opportunities. By appreciating the importance of these factors, the formal sector will be better prepared to fulfill its role as a partner with families in providing social care to the current and future generations of older persons.

Notes

1. Brody, E. M., and S. J. Brody. 1981. New Directions in Health and Social Supports for the Aging. In M.A. Lewis, ed. *The Aging: Medical and Social Supports in the Decade of the 80s*, 35–48. New York: Fordham University Third Age Center; Cantor, M. H. 1975. The Formal and Informal Social Support Systems of Older New Yorkers. Paper presented at the International Congress of Gerontology, Jerusalem, Israel.

2. Cantor, M. H. 1989. Social Care: Family and Community Support Systems. *Annals of the American Academy of Political and Social Sciences* 303:99–112; Cantor, M. H. 1991. Family and Community: Changing Roles in an Aging Society. Donald P. Kent Award Lecture. *Gerontologist* 31:337–346.

3. Cantor, M. H., and B. Gurland. 1993. *Growing Older in New York City in the 1990s: A Study of Changing Lifestyles, Quality of Life, and Quality of Care*. 5 vols. New York: New York Center for Policy on Aging, New York Community Trust.

4. Cantor, M. H., and M. Brennan. 2000. *Social Care of the Elderly: The Effects of Ethnicity, Class, and Culture*. New York: Springer.

5. Ibid. 1993. *Family and Community Support Systems of Older New Yorkers*. Vol. 4 of Cantor and Gurland, *Growing Older in New York City*.

6. Climo, J. J. 1987. Older Persons Parents and Adult Children in the Aging Revolution. *Reconstructionist* 53:9–13.

7. Rosen, E. J., and S. F. Weltman. 1996. Jewish Families: An Overview. In M. McGoldrick, J. Giordano, and J. K. Pearce, eds. *Ethnicity and Family Therapy*, 611–629. 2d ed. New York: Guildford Press.

8. Glicksman, A., and T. Konopecky-Cox. 1994. Jewish Aged in the United States: Sociodemographic and Socioeconomic Characteristics. In Z. Hard, D. Biegel, and D. Guttman, eds. *Jewish Aged in the United States*, 23–45. New York: Springer.

9. Rubentstein, R. L. 1994. The Aging in Elderly Community: Community, Cultural, and Life-Course Factors. In Z. Hard, D. Biegel, and D. Guttman, eds. *Jewish Aged in the United States*, 61–79. New York: Springer.

10. Hanreider, B. D. 1992. The Older Population in New York City: Changes in Race, Hispanic Origins, and Age, 1980–1990. New York: City of New York Department for the Aging.

11. Rodriguez, O. 1987. *Hispanic and Human Services: Help-Seeking in the Inner City*. Bronx, N.Y.: Hispanic Research Center, Fordham University.

12. Rodriguez, *Hispanic and Human Services*; Wallace, S. P., K. Campbell, and C. Lew-Ting. 1993. Structural Barriers to the Use of Formal In-Home Services by Older Latinos. *Journal of Gerontology: Social Sciences* 49:253–263.

13. Manton, K. G., L. S. Corder, and E. Stallard. 1997. Chronic Disability Trends in Elderly United States Populations. *Proceedings of the National Academy of Sciences* 94:2593–2598.

8. Aging, Health, and Social Services in London

Anthony M. Warnes

Introduction

This chapter has two aims: to present a summary of the social, demographic, and health profiles of older people in London; and to identify some key issues concerning services for older people that require the attention of city government and welfare administration.

London lies in the southeast of Great Britain, at the center of the United Kingdom's largest concentration of population and its most prosperous and dynamic commercial region. As that of a world city and of the nation's capital, London's economy has an exceptional concentration of commerce, financial and legal services, and professional government employees. In comparison to the rest of the United Kingdom, London's population has a strong overrepresentation of people of working age, and among them unusually high shares of people with high incomes and high occupational status. Generally, its older population is also relatively prosperous and healthy (certainly as compared with the former coal-mining and heavy industrial regions of the country). Within the administrative area of the Greater London Authority, however, and particularly in the inner districts, there are concentrations of low-income and multiply deprived older people, and a rapidly increasing number in the minority ethnic groups, many of whom have had a lifetime of disadvantages.

As with any world city, there are alternative definitions of London's geographical extent and several levels of government and administration. Until 1965, the city was governed by the London County Council and by many metropolitan boroughs (the second tier of local government). The London County Council's area extended about ten kilometers from the center and approximated the built-up area in 1890; this same area is now generally known as Inner London. From 1965 until 1986, the Greater London Council provided the strategic local government function for a larger area, with an average radius of twenty kilometers from the center, approximating the built-up area of 1939. The added ring around the former London County Council area is now generally known as Outer London. Within the Greater London Council, thirty-two London boroughs were created, most by amalgamating two or three of the old metropolitan boroughs. These boroughs (and the Corporation of the City of London for the central "square mile" financial district) provide the normal British local government services (education, public housing, road maintenance, social services), and they survived the dissolution by Margaret Thatcher of the Greater London Council in 1986. The Greater London Council area has now become the territory of the Greater London Authority, which took up its powers on July 3, 2000.[1]

The built-up area of course continued to expand during the twentieth century, but in an unusual way. During the late 1940s, a green belt approximately ten kilometers wide was created around London. In the green belt, there have been very strong restrictions on development—agricultural land has been protected. As a result, housing and population growth have taken place beyond, in a ring forty to sixty kilometers from the center throughout the Home Counties, that is, the counties that surround and are contiguous to London. For some purposes, statistics are collected for an Outer Ring that bisects some of the Home Counties to form the Outer Metropolitan Area. The Greater London Council plus the Outer Metropolitan Area comprises the London Metropolitan Area. Remarkably, even by the 1980s, many of the areas of fastest population and housing growth were well beyond this zone and sixty to eighty kilometers from the center.[2]

While the birth rate has remained low since the early 1970s, London's economic dynamism, progressive increases in real incomes, and other factors have led to a high rate of household fission, that is, the division of the population into an ever greater number of smaller households (and an increasing number of second homes). This, in turn, has reinforced the strong inflation of both land and property prices. The shortage of low-cost or affordable housing is now a major problem in the city, and one of the many manifestations of increasing income and wealth and health inequalities in London, as throughout the United Kingdom.

Not only does London's population size differ according to the area definition that is used (in 2002 the GLA had 7.36 million people, the London Metropolitan Area well over 12 million, and London and the Home Counties nearly 17 million), so also do the demographic, social, and health characteristics of the city. For example, the inner area has a relatively low share of elderly people, while many parts of the periphery, particularly along the North Sea and English Channel coasts, have unusually high shares of older people (Table 8.1). Another contrast is that Inner London has high concentrations of low incomes, multiple deprivation, and high rates of HIV/AIDS, drug-related deaths, and infant mortality, whereas Outer London and most of the towns and semi-rural areas of the Outer Metropolitan Area are prosperous and have populations with good health. Most of the analyses reported in this chapter refer to the Greater London Authority area. For the World Cities project, the most appropriate area for comparisons with the City of Paris, Manhattan, and the urban core of Tokyo will be Inner London . Accordingly, several tables present information for Inner London, Outer London, and the Greater London Authority.

Profiles of London's Older People

Population. Greater London has over the last two decades become the English metropolitan area with the lowest share of its population in the older age groups. In 2002, 15.8 percent of its population was aged sixty years or more, compared to 20.7 percent in the rest of the United Kingdom. The older population of 1.17 million was 23.5 percent less (or 357,000 fewer) than the national age structure would imply. Taking the population in the officially recognized pensionable age (sixty or more years for women, and sixty-five or more for men), the "deficit" of older people in 2002 reached 24 percent, or 325,000 (Table 8.1). The shortfall is mainly of people in their midsixties to midseventies and, in comparison to the rest of England, there are relatively large shares in the youngest and the oldest age groups of older people. In 1995, the average age of both men and women aged sixty-five years or more in London was higher than in England—and the differential had widened during the early 1990s. At least four reasons can be identified for the rapid change and rejuvenation of the inner city. First, London's strong employment growth has strengthened its half-millennium-long attraction to young migrants, and during recent decades there has been an increase in the in-flow of economic migrants, particularly from Pakistan and Bangladesh, who tend to be young and to have high birth rates. Second, a large area of inner East London, formerly the London docks, has been redeveloped with housing, much of it attractive to young professionals, which has led to local population increases, reversing a long-established trend. Third, much of the housing stock that formerly provided affordable rental apartments to older people has been converted and rehabilitated as apartments for sale. This trend has particularly affected the middle- and upper-income residential areas of inner west and north London, and has probably increased the tendency for the older age groups to move away from the city. Fourth, London's property prices are exceptionally high and have been increasing at above-national rates for most of the last twenty-five years; this again provides a strong incentive for people to leave when they retire.

The age structures of the officially defined subregions of the GLA show only minor variations (Table 8.1). In 2002, northeast London was exceptional in having a higher representation of children than did England as a whole, and correspondingly a relatively low excess of those in the "adult midyears" (a term that is beginning to replace "working ages," which will soon become archaic). All parts of the GLA had, however, a substantial deficit of older people. The age structure of the Outer Metropolitan Area or Home Counties almost exactly reproduced that of England as a whole, but its different parts showed more variation than within the GLA. The coasts and adjacent semi-rural areas of Essex, Kent, and Sussex, to the east and south of London, had strong overrepresentations of older people, while regions to the north and west of London (as around Heathrow airport) had strong underrepresentations of older people and high child shares.

London's pensionable-age population has been falling, but during the second

Table 8.1. Broad Age Structure: English Subregions, 2002 (midyear population estimates)

	Total (millions)	0–15 years		16–60/65 years		60/65+ years	
		%	Ratio[a]	%	Ratio	%	Ratio
London	7,356	19.6	0.99	66.4	**1.07**	14.0	0.76
North Central London	1,215	19.0	0.96	67.3	**1.09**	13.7	0.74
North East London	1,538	21.8	**1.10**	64.5	1.04	13.7	0.74
North West London	1,785	18.1	0.91	67.9	**1.10**	14.0	0.76
South East London	1,514	19.9	1.01	65.7	**1.06**	14.4	0.78
South West London	1,304	19.0	0.96	66.6	**1.08**	14.4	0.78
England	49,537	19.8	1.00	61.8	1.00	18.4	1.00
Bedfordshire and Hertfordshire	1,607	21.0	**1.06**	62.1	1.00	16.9	0.92
Essex	1,622	20.0	1.01	60.6	0.98	19.3	**1.05**
Hampshire and Isle of Wight	1,788	19.4	0.98	61.7	1.00	18.9	1.03
Kent and Medway	1,589	20.6	1.04	60.3	0.98	19.1	1.04
Surrey and Sussex	2,560	18.9	0.95	59.8	0.97	21.3	**1.16**
Thames Valley	2,100	20.4	1.03	63.8	1.03	15.7	0.85
Home Counties	9,478	20.1	1.01	61.3	0.99	18.6	1.01
London and Home Counties	16,834	19.9	1.00	63.5	1.03	16.6	0.90

Source: ONS, 2003.

Note: Ratios of 1.05 or above (bold type) and 0.95 or less (italic type) denote the highest and lowest child, working-age, and retired age group values.

[a] Ratio of subregional percentage to percentage for all England

half of this decade a slight recovery is projected to 1,003,000 in 2011. The number aged eighty-five years and over increased during the 1990s from 101,000 to around 119,000 but is likely to fall during this decade by 5,000. Inner London's age structure has changed markedly in the last two decades, and its population is increasingly dominated by working-aged people. Twenty years ago, Outer London's population had a high share of people aged sixty years or more, but the excess has declined quickly (Table 8.2). It still has an overrepresentation of people aged seventy-five years and more. The characteristics of London's population, including the relative shares in different age groups, and several socioeconomic attributes such as income, proximity to relatives, and housing quality, are greatly influenced by the substantial in- and out-migration flows. London attracts young adults as students, trainees, and job entrants. It has been described as a "socio-economic escalator," raising the income and occupational status of many who begin their careers in the city.[3]

Migration. London attracts migrants from all continents but is a substantial exporter of its population to the rest of England and Wales. There is a strong age pattern to the migration movements, with only very young adults having a net in-flow to the city (Figure 8.1). In 2002, 15,200 people aged fifty-five to sixty-four years left the city, and only 3,600 entered. Even among those aged seventy-five or more years, there is a strong net outflow, with 8,100 leaving and 2,400 entering. Around 20–25 percent of the people approaching and passing through the age of retirement in London leave the city when they stop working (or shortly before or after), a much higher rate of retirement exodus than from any other region of the country.[4] The highest retirement-age out-migration rates have been from a contiguous belt of districts in the GLA and the Home Counties of Surrey, Berkshire, Hertfordshire, and Buckinghamshire. Rates of out-migration of older men from several districts in this core approach 5 percent each year. This export area consolidated and deepened from the late 1970s to the late 1980s. Female retirement out-migration rates have been lower and more variable by area of the city. Neither the extensive reach of the area around London that exports a high proportion of its retiring population, nor the fact that it includes districts of the highest-quality residential environments, are widely appreciated. The migration is selective of owner-occupiers, middle- and higher-income groups, and the white population. The net effect is to lower the average socioeconomic profile of those who remain. The exodus may also lower the average health status of the very old population of the city.

Minority ethnic populations. Greater London has the highest proportion of minority ethnic older people of any region of the United Kingdom (in 2002–2003, 29.9 percent compared to 8.1 percent for Great Britain) (Table 8.3). London has the highest proportion of people from minority ethnic groups apart from those who identified themselves in the 2001 census as of Pakistani origin, of whom there is a higher proportion in Yorkshire and the Humber (2.9 percent) and the West Mid-

Table 8.2. Changing Distribution of Pensioners: London Metropolitan Area, 1971–1991

	Pensioners (thousands)			Share of Total Population (%)			Location Quotients		
	1971	1981	1991	1971	1981	1991	1971	1981	1991
Inner London	375	335	273	16.1	17.5	15.4	1.05	1.04	0.91
Outer London	849	866	801	16.5	18.0	17.3	1.07	1.07	1.03
Outer Metro. Area	720	836	922	14.0	15.5	16.9	0.91	0.92	1.00
London Metro. Area	1,944	2,036	1,996	15.4	16.8	16.9	1.00	1.00	1.00

Source: ONS, 2001.

Figure 8.1. Net Out-Migration by Age Group: Greater London, 2002

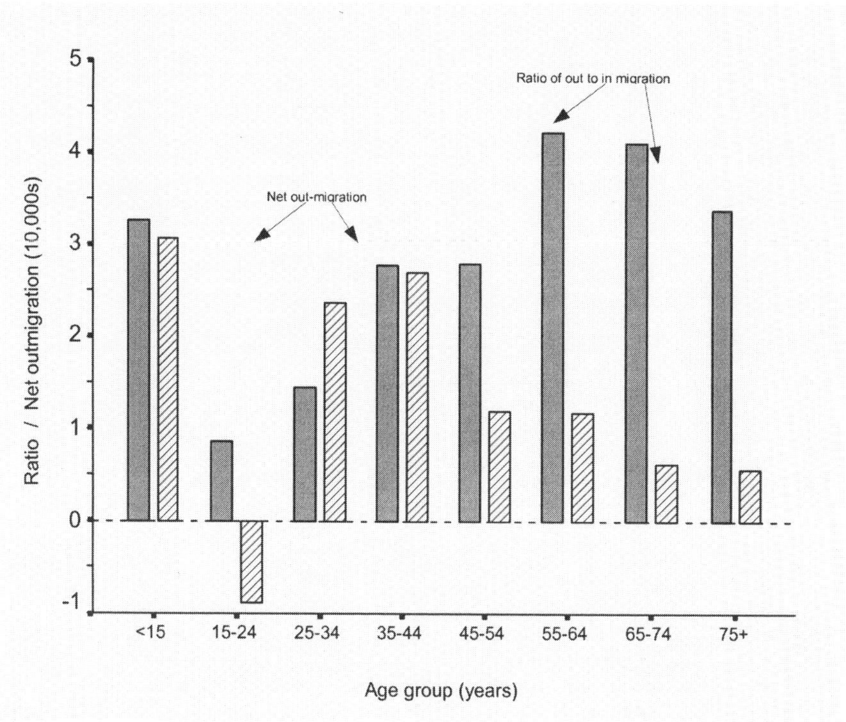

Source: ONS, 2003.

lands (2.9 percent). While Bangladeshis form only 0.5 percent of the population of England and Wales, no less than 33.4 percent of them are in the London borough of Tower Hamlets. Black Caribbeans form more than 10 percent of the population of the London boroughs of Lewisham, Lambeth, Brent, and Hackney. Over 10 percent of the populations of Southwark, Newham, Lambeth, and Hackney are black African. More than 2 percent of people describe themselves as "other black" in Hackney, Lambeth, and Lewisham. Chinese people form more than 2 percent of the population in Westminster, the City of London, and Barnet.

Rapid increases in the number of older people in the black Caribbean and Indian communities are now occurring (reflecting the high rates of immigration among young adults in the 1950s and 1960s) . There is a bold contrast between Inner and Outer London. In Inner London in 1991, there were approximately 18,000 black Caribbeans aged sixty to seventy-four years, and 2,000 aged seventy-five years and over.[5] Alongside were 5,000 self-ascribed Indians aged sixty to seventy-four years and 1,000 aged at least seventy-five years. In Outer London, the most numerous groups were Indians, with 17,000 aged sixty to seventy-four years and 1,000 aged seventy-five years and over. In both Inner and Outer London, there were many

Table 8.3. Residents by Ethnic Group: London and Great Britain, 2002–2003

	% of ethnic minority population	
	London	**Great Britain**
Mixed	7.4	10.9
Asian or Asian British	42.0	49.5
Black or Black British	35.4	25.5
Chinese	3.3	4.2
Other ethnic group	11.9	9.8
Total as percent of total population	29.9	8.1
Nonwhite (thousands)	2,219	4,654
White (thousands)	5,207	52,964
Total	7,434	57,643

Source: Labour Force Survey, *National Statistics 2003*, Table 2.3.

fewer in all other ethnic groups. The number of black Caribbeans aged sixty to seventy-four years may have decreased in Inner London during the late 1990s, but the number increased in Outer London (Fig. 8.2). The rate of increase of people aged seventy-five years or more in the minority ethnic communities will be very high during the next few decades, but the total number, presently around 12,000, will not reach 20,000 for another decade.

The black Caribbean older population is heavily concentrated in Inner London boroughs, particularly Brent, Hackney, Haringey, Lambeth, Southwark, and Lewisham. On the other hand, the Indian population is strongly clustered in Outer London, and there are separate concentrations in the northwest (the boroughs of Brent and Harrow), the west (Ealing and Hounslow), and the east (Newham and Redbridge). The much smaller Bangladeshi population is exceptionally concentrated in Tower Hamlets (the borough immediately to the east of the financial district) and has high rates of deprivation and sickness.

The health of older Londoners. Broadly, the health status of older people in London is similar to their counterparts' in the rest of the United Kingdom. Mortality rates among older people are generally a little lower in Greater London than in England and Wales as a whole (Table 8.4). There is, however, a considerable differential between Inner and Outer London, with the Standardized Mortality Ratio for people aged less than seventy-five years in 1994 being 20 percent higher than the England and Wales figure, while that in Outer London was 7 percent lower.[6]

The majority of those in their sixties and seventies are healthy, active, and without disability. While levels of disability increase with age, they remain a minority

Figure 8.2. Minority Ethnic Groups: Inner London, Persons 75+, 1990s

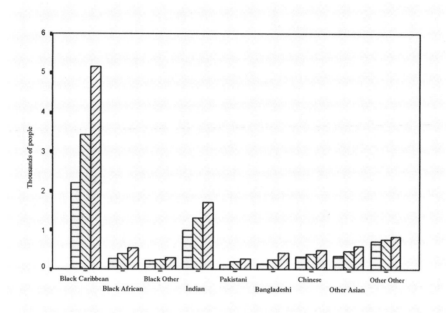

Source: ONS, 2001.

Note: Each group of three columns represents from left to right the populations for 1991, 1996, and 2001.

characteristic until around the late seventies. The incidence of acute clinical episodes increases with age from late middle age and rises sharply in the five years before death. Substantial improvements in late-life mortality have been achieved in London (and the rest of England and Wales) in recent years, but the United Kingdom has done far less well than several neighboring European countries. Comparisons with France, Switzerland, Spain, or Japan indicate that there is much premature morbidity and mortality in this country. Between 1960 and 1990 in sixteen western European countries, the prospects of an older person dying during any one year fell by 23–41 percent, depending on age and sex.[7] In the United Kingdom, the rate of improvement for older men broadly matched those figures but did not reduce a substantial disadvantage. For the United Kingdom's older women, however, the chances of dying in any one year changed from being roughly the same as in Europe in 1960 to being substantially higher in 1990. The differentials between the most and the least deprived areas of London have also increased during the 1990s for the all-age population.

On many standard measures of morbidity, perceived health, and functional abilities, London's older population appears marginally better off than its counterpart in the rest of England (and therefore in the rest of the United Kingdom). Late-age mortality rates from stroke and several cardiac disorders have been lower in London

Table 8.4. Deaths of Persons 55+ by Age Group: Greater London and England and Wales, 1992

	Males			
	55–64	**65–74**	**75–84**	**85+**
Greater London	13.3	37.6	87.3	187.4
England and Wales	13.4	37.3	90.1	193.9
Ratio	0.99	1.01	0.97	0.97
	Females			
	55–64	**65–74**	**75–84**	**85+**
Greater London	7.5	21.2	53.9	140.2
England and Wales	7.9	21.5	56.9	148.8
Ratio	0.95	0.99	0.95	0.94

Source: Office of Population Censuses and Surveys 1994, *Mortality Statistics 1992: Area, England and Wales.* OPCS Series DH5 No. 11, Table 2.

than elsewhere, but the differentials are narrowing in middle age. Remarkably, this advantage appears to extend to inner deprived areas, where the reported female rates are lower than in high-status areas. Inaccurate estimates of the "usually resident" population, particularly for the oldest ages and women, may distort the figures.[8] The poorest health conditions among older people are found in the inner deprived areas and among the more recently established minority ethnic groups, notably the Pakistanis and the Bangladeshis.[9] There is an overrepresentation of men in the young elderly age groups of the black Caribbean and the Bangladeshi populations, and both have relatively high rates of morbidity and mortality, as from coronary heart disease.[10]

Service Provision and Utilization

Hospital services for older people. London's hospitals provide above-national levels of service for the older residents of London, mainly through a relatively high rate of hospitalization for those aged less than seventy-five years who live in the intermediate and outer areas of the city. When the large proportion of the major London hospitals' episodes of acute treatment delivered to people from outside the city are subtracted, it is found that the hospitalization rate for the older population of Inner London is exceptionally low. This deficit is found in all five-year age groups of later life. The shortfalls in some age groups exceed 15 percent. Similarly, occupied-hospital-bed days per capita are at approximately national levels in London as a whole (except among women aged eighty years and over, for whom they are high), but the older residents of inner deprived London occupied around one-fifth *fewer* bed days than their equivalents in provincial urban areas (Table 8.5). Overestimates of the residential population (as noted earlier) may account for a proportion of the deficits, but Sir Leslie Turnberg has attributed the differentials to "shorter lengths of stay and more day-case treatment" in London compared to provincial cities.[11]

Geriatric beds are unevenly provided across London, with relatively high provision in scattered suburbs of north London. Shortfalls occur in several inner deprived areas, although this pattern is not consistently reflected in hospital episodes; the provision in some districts is at twice the rate of others. London's low provision of independent and voluntary sector nursing homes, particularly in its inner areas, combines with delays in completing "care assessments" by the borough social service departments, the high proportion of one-person households, and the prevalence of flats in multistory buildings to multiply the difficulties of discharge following acute hospital admissions. The issue of the blocking of acute beds by dependent older people who cannot look after themselves and have no informal caregivers, but for whom no place in a residential care or nursing home is available, has greatly exercised the Department of Health in recent years. A plethora of intermediate care schemes were introduced from the late 1990s, and most recently the government has introduced fines for borough social services that do not promptly find such patients a care-home bed and remove them from the hospital.

Psychogeriatric services have been developing quickly from a low base over the last decade, but their provision is very uneven across London. There is a low rate of hospital episodes throughout London for senile and presenile organic psychotic conditions (roughly equivalent to the most prevalent dementias), in strong contrast to large provincial cities. All parts of London are underprovided with psychogeriatric facilities, with the 60 percent shortfall in Inner London being the greatest deviation.

Community-health services. There are no comprehensive data on the community-health services, and contact data by age are particularly scarce. The available evidence suggests that rates of provision in London are equivalent to national levels but with considerable variability. As in the rest of the country, there is considerable diversity in the organization and profile of the services delivered by National Health Service (NHS) Care Trusts to older people. Superficial accounts suggest that the unit costs of these services are unusually high in London because of the city's high premises and wage costs but also related to the intensity of patients' needs. Some Care Trusts report a very rapid increase in the last few years in the number of older patients requiring intensive services. The male population aged eighty-five years or more increased unusually quickly during the 1990s (an echo of the recovery of the adolescent and young adult male population after World War I). The work of the

Table 8.5. Completed Hospital-Consultant Episodes for Persons 65+ by Age Group: England, 1994–1995 (per 1,000 residents)

Age Group	Inner/Deprived			Total		
	London	Non-London	London as % of non-London	London	Non-London	London as % of non-London
Men						
65–69	378	424	89	374	344	109
70–74	453	521	87	453	425	107
75–79	575	636	90	560	531	105
80–84	641	746	86	647	626	103
85+	725	825	88	743	716	104
Total 65+	489	552	89	492	461	107
Women						
65–69	271	308	88	267	248	108
70–74	310	363	85	306	297	103
75–79	370	447	83	373	371	101
80–84	447	528	85	454	451	101
85+	557	604	92	541	509	106
Total 65+	369	422	87	368	352	105

community-health services in London is especially hampered by its large scale and the multiplicity of acute hospitals. They may be most helped by radical innovations in information handling and exchange.

General practice (or primary care). The deficiencies of London's general practice services have been well recognized for two decades and have attracted not only a sequence of detailed analyses but also major investment programs. Until recently, the proportion of "single-handed" (one physician) practices and of substandard premises remained high in London, particularly in the inner deprived areas and in the eastern sector, and there were fewer practice nurses and support staff. The impact of the national and the London-specific reforms of general practice during the 1990s and of the reorganization of the services into Primary Care Trusts is unclear. Little evidence of the levels of patient satisfaction is available, but focus-group research has revealed a worrying frequency of complaints about the maladministration of appointments systems and about ageist and racist attitudes.

Around a quarter of a million of London's older people consult their general practitioners every two weeks. The consultation rate is higher than for most adult age groups but not markedly so. As in the rest of the country, patients at the oldest ages receive a high share of physicians' and practice nurses' home visits. The 2001–2002 *General Household Survey* found a substantially lower rate of consultation among people aged sixty-five or more years during the previous two weeks in London (15 percent) as compared to the United Kingdom (19 percent).[12] The annual health check for those seventy-five and older is not highly regarded by general practitioners, and many local initiatives for fulfilling the contractual obligations are evident. No widely accepted view about the health benefits or outcomes of the check has become established.

Residential and nursing-home places and care. Local authority residential home places remain relatively plentiful in Inner London but under present legislation and funding have no long-term future. Private sector residential and nursing care is, however, scarce in Inner London; the provision in Outer London, although more plentiful, is also below national rates. London relies on the relatively abundant provision in the outer suburbs, beyond the Greater London Area, and in the rest of the Southeast (there are, for example, high concentrations in many of the coastal towns of southeast England). Many placements into the independent residential sectors involve a migration toward the periphery of the urban area, which may make it more difficult for relatives to keep in touch with an older person admitted to a nursing home. The main impediments to the provision of independent and voluntary sector residential and nursing-home care in London are the high costs of land, property, and staff. By the *Care Standards Act 2000,* a new inspection and regulation system and higher minimum standards (particularly concerning the qualifications of the staff) have been introduced.

Personal social services—community care and multiagency delivery. As in the rest of the country, the implementation of the 1993 community-care provisions of the 1990 NHS reforms has been uneven. Fewer care assessments have been completed by the social services than are required, and the rate of completion varies considerably among the boroughs. There are many local initiatives for joint efforts between primary care and the community-health services, and between these and social services. These demonstrate the need for interagency and intersector arrangements but rely on goodwill and are vulnerable to changes in personnel. The frequent need among older patients and clients for interagency and intersectoral care of long duration meets with a systemic weakness: both the management of older patients' acute episodes of long duration, and multiagency care to moderately and severely disabled older patients, raise demands for levels of communication and patient-centered care that often are not met.

The Social Service Departments' Community Care Plans reveal many problems in implementing a consistent approach to care assessment and care plans for the most dependent people able to live in their own homes. Shortages of funds are usual, but no template for interagency cooperation and responsibility has been available and the success of joint efforts is a function of local circumstances and goodwill. Older people with complex needs are falling through the cracks between agencies. Services are fragmented, and there are problems with funding, a lack of proper assessment and reassessment, inequity, and inadequate communication.

The absence of any means to monitor the quality and effectiveness of multi-provider care is a serious impediment to the diagnosis of weaknesses in health and social services for older people and for their correction. The present blindness to system performance is lamentable. There is a strong case for a fresh start to the implementation of care management. The ambition to provide seamless care should, however, extend beyond the services for the most frail and dependent older people. The further challenge is to establish effective mechanisms for monitoring, evaluating, and managing the complex treatment pathways of acute episodes. There should be effective audit of multiprovider and intersectoral care. The powers and duty to correct suboptimal treatment and care should be clearly defined and allocated to a responsible body.

One of the most frequently identified problems of providing health and social services to older people in London is the sheer number and fragmentation of providers. To provide both local government and National Health services, the city has been divided among a great number of purchasing and providing bodies. While it is true in any part of Great Britain that a dependent older man or woman who is eligible for domiciliary social services may be cared for by three health sectors, as well as district social care staff, in London, more than elsewhere, they are likely to be served by agencies that do not have coterminous boundaries and have no more intensive a mutual working relationship than with several other similar bodies. This is particularly true of liaison between the acute Trusts in Inner London, which serve such a wide area, and the community-health and social services. London's great size also implies that on average a hospital consultant there will need to exchange information with many more general practitioners than elsewhere. The scope for communication gaps and administrative delays is great.

Recent developments in London's government and administration. There have been two important developments in London's governance in the last five years. As mentioned earlier, a single local government body, the Greater London Authority, has been restored, but by and large the boroughs have retained their powers and independence. In the mid-1990s, health services in London were administered by four separate NHS regions. These were first reduced to two, north and south of the river Thames, and in 1999 a single NHS Executive Region for London was created. This was partly in anticipation of the creation of the GLA, and partly a response to the many reports that had criticized the fragmentation of health administration. Then a further reorganization transferred much of the commissioning and planning functions to the new Primary Care Trusts, with some strategic and financial functions placed with very large Strategic Health Authorities.

In 1997, the government commissioned a report on the future of health services in London. Directly as a consequence, a single region of the NHS Executive was created to administer and develop London's health services. In March 1999, a modernization plan for the National Health Service in London for the following three years was published.[13] Among the proposals distinctive to London were:

- Increase community and hospital provision for severely mentally ill people, with an investment of at least £6m in staffed beds and community teams
- Improve London's thirty-two accident and emergency hospital departments
- Improve at least fifty general practice (family doctor) premises each year
- Implement the largest-ever hospital building and rebuilding plan in London, totaling over £1.2 billion, with major work underway at six acute hospitals in 1999–2000, and ten other major developments planned to start during 1999–2002.[14]

In addition to the initiatives specific to London, two policy developments in the United Kingdom are relevant to the situation of older people in the city. First, the Labour government elected in 1997 has made modernization of the National Health Service a key priority. Very many reforms, too numerous to summarize here, are being introduced to raise the quality and effectiveness of health care, and to make the service more responsive to the public's and the patients' concerns.[15] Among the quality measures, a *National Service Framework for the Care of Older People* was developed "to produce a high and nationally uniform standard of care, to eliminate unacceptable practice, to reduce local variations and to drive up the quality of care."[16] Considerable attention is also focused on the interface between health and social care, not least as a contribution to releasing acute hospital beds and reducing waiting lists for elective procedures.

Issues concerning the quality of life and participation in society of older people have risen much higher in the policy and research agendas over the last few years. As in other countries, this trend has been driven first by concerns over the adverse trends in the ratio of the working to the retired (or Social Security–dependent older) population. Another innovative exercise was launched by the government early in its administration, the *Better Government for Older People* program. This has involved twenty-eight local authorities throughout the country, in which extensive participation exercises between the statutory services and a wide range of community-based older people's organizations have been supported.[17]

Crude national accounting reactions to population aging have been greatly moderated in the United Kingdom by the effective national organizations that express the older person's perspective, among which Age Concern England and Help the Aged have been most active in raising the sophistication and information content of the debates. The "Debate of the Age" coordinated by Age Concern England during 1998–2000, the largest consultation exercise ever mounted in the country, utilized many innovative techniques for involving and giving voice to all age groups. From the vast collection of opinion, a summary, *Agenda for the Age*, has been published.[18]

Conclusion

This chapter has brought together extracts from completed research and archives, but is no more than an initial review of relevant issues. A priority task is now to contribute to the development of a database of standard indicators for the four world cities. The chapter concludes, however, by highlighting five issues that are of particular concern and interest concerning the situation of older people in world cities or the ways in which those cities must adjust to an increasingly aged society.

The advantages and disadvantages of being old in a world city. World cities are different from the generality of urban settlements. They have specialized national and international functions, more cosmopolitan and migratory populations, and unusually diverse amenities. But they also have high living densities; exceptional problems of congestion and pollution; high housing, living, and labor costs (making, for example, personal care services expensive); and greater income, educational, and occupational status inequalities than elsewhere. These distinctive attributes are bound to be expressed in the activities and quality of life of older people. There will be positive and negative effects. Among the negatives may be an exceptional level of dispersion and separation of families, which in turn may generate above-average levels of social isolation and anonymity. On the positive side, a world city is likely to have good local public transport, excellent national and international transport connections, wide choice and competition among retail services, and lavish leisure and cultural opportunities.

In London, it appears that the exceptional concentration of first-rate teaching and research hospitals in the inner city may be responsible for the perverse result of relatively poor hospital service to the local older population—despite the above-national volume of treatment. This is because a high proportion of hospital episodes are elective procedures to patients from outside the city. It would be valuable to examine the proportion of treatments to residents and to outsiders in Paris, New York, and Tokyo. Is there a conflict between being a center of medical excellence and the quality of "general" or "mundane" care in all countries? Another important factor in the quality of health and social care to older people in large cities is their great size and the large number of providing organizations. The coordination of care among multiple providers is inevitably more complex in a very large than in a small town.

Identifying and acting upon older people's views and preferences. The primacy given by world cities to commerce, government, and the production of economic wealth may reinforce the common neglect and demotion of the concerns of older people. Many of the facilities and customs of a large city are organized for the needs of the employed and trainees. The very sense that the city, even its own government agencies, is involved in vital economic and political developments may marginalize the domestic and welfare concerns of retired people. There is much evidence of increasing social inequalities and polarity in world cities: how can the opinions, preferences, and needs of relatively powerless and economically weak older people be heard and acted upon?

Raising the quality of services to the "elderly" in large cities. While the majority of the health care received by older people in world cities as elsewhere is provided by general physician and hospital services (ranging from immunization to elective surgery and emergency services), those who are chronically sick and functionally dependent are served by specialist elderly people's services, most obviously in diverse categories of long-term care. These services commonly have low prestige and are poorly funded. The quality of care in such services is commonly variable and sometimes low. The problems in very large cities may be especially severe, as a result of high property and labor costs and the fragmentation of commissioning and quality-control responsibilities. It would be valuable to assess the quality of elderly people's services in all four study cities relative to the standards achieved in the four nations.

Making services more responsive to ethnic and cultural differences. Reflecting the globalization of information transfer and the steep decrease in the cost of international air travel, New York, Paris, and London have exceptionally diverse ethnic populations. Technological, economic, and social forces may yet result in a similar trend in Tokyo. The great majority of economic migrants, refugees, and asylum seekers are young adults, and for two decades after an influx there are usually few older people in the immigrant populations. Among the Hispanic and Caribbean-born populations of New York City, the South Indian and Afro-Caribbean populations of London, and the North African, African, and Caribbean-born populations of Paris, however, the number of elderly people is now growing quickly. The diversification of the cultural and ethnic mix of the older population raises considerable problems in older people's services, especially in residential and nursing-home care. Making personal social services, community-health services, and residential and nursing-home care more sensitive to ethnic variations is clearly of growing importance and it is believed should be a priority for the World Cities project.[19]

Housing, the physical environment, and older people's health. In Britain, public health specialists have a long tradition of concern with insanitary and poor living environments in large cities. In recent decades, there has been much interest in the associations between health and overcrowding (living at high room densities), poor heating, dampness, and poor ventilation in homes. For older people with compromised mobility, there are also particularly difficulties associated with living in high buildings with poor access. The United Kingdom has an exceptional problem (as compared to other European countries) of "excess winter mortality" associated with cold room temperatures and a high vulnerability to respiratory diseases and cold-related cardiovascular problems. The above-average shares of renters and of subdivided apartment accommodation suggest that the problems of deficient home heating, cold-related disorders, and excess winter mortality are unusually high in London. Are these problems shared in deprived neighborhoods of all the world cities?

Notes

1. The creation of the GLA reflects the current administration's policy of devolving central government strategic planning and administrative functions to the regions (as with the reestablishment of the Scottish Parliament, the creation of a Welsh Assembly, and the unsuccessful referendum in late 2004 on an elected regional assembly in the northern region). The GLA is controlled by a directly elected executive mayor, who is subject to scrutiny from a twenty-five-member London Assembly, in part elected from constituencies, and in part on a proportional representation list system.
2. Hall, P. G. 1989. *London 2001*. London: Unwin Hyman.
3. Bruegel, I. 2000. The Restructuring of London's Labour Force: Migration and Shifting Opportunities, 1971–91. *Area* 32(1): 79–90.
4. Warnes, A. 1992. Temporal and Spatial Patterns of Elderly Migration. In J. Stillwell,

P. Rees, and P. Boden, eds. *Migration Processes and Patterns: Volume II, Population Redistribution in the 1980s*, 246–270. London: Belhaven. This estimate is based on the rates of net out-migration from the London Metropolitan Area for single years of age between fifty-five to sixty-nine years. Both the UK population census, which asks a "one-year" migration question—that is, the address one year before the census night—and the National Health Service patient re-registration data show the phenomenon clearly.

5. OPCS 1993. *Great Britain 1991 Census: Ethnic Group and Country of Birth*. London: Her Majesty's Stationery Office.

6. Health of Londoners' Project. 1998. *The Health of Londoners: A Public Health Report for London*. London: King's Fund, fig. 2.7; Griffiths, C., and J. Fitzpatrick, eds. 2001. *Geographic Variations in Health*. London: Stationery Office.

7. Warnes, A. M. 1999. UK and Western European Late-Age Mortality Rates: Trends in Cause-Specific Death Rates, 1960–1990. *Health and Place* 5(1): 111–118.

8. It is believed that many couples or families own (or rent) a home both in London and outside London. There are tax advantages in arranging affairs so that one property is owned by one person, and the other by that person's wife, husband, or partner. When completing the ten-yearly census forms, it would be logical for the married or partnered couple to report a single person living at each address. Detailed analysis has shown that there is a net movement of higher professionals and managers in their fifties and early sixties into Inner London; it seems likely that a high proportion would acquire a second home, a pied-à-terre, and not sell their principal home. Furthermore, it is probable that people in advanced old age who become very frail move out of London, often to live with or near a child or into a nursing home, but that there is a delay before their London property is sold or their lease expires. This would inflate (or exaggerate) the apparent residential population, particularly in the oldest age groups.

9. Qureshi, T. 1998. *Living in Britain, Growing Old in Britain: A Study of Bangladeshi Elders in London*. London: Centre for Policy on Aging.

10. Curtis, S., and K. Lawson. 2000. Gender, Ethnicity, and Self-Reported Health: The Case of African-Caribbean Populations in London. *Social Science and Medicine* 50(3): 365–386.

11. Department of Health [DH]. 1998. *Health Services in London: A Strategic Review*. London: DH, 6. Sir Leslie Turnberg, president of the Royal College of Physicians (1992–1997), chaired the review.

12. UK National Statistics 2003. *General Household Survey, 2001/02*. London: Stationery Office, table 7.15.

13. Department of Health. 1999. *The Modernisation Plan for the NHS in London, 1999–2002*. London: DH.

14. Ibid., 6.

15. Among the key policy documents are: Department of Health. 1997. *The New NHS: Modern, Dependable*. Cmnd 3807. London: Stationery Office; Department of Health. 1998. *A First Class Service: Quality in the New NHS*. London: DH; Department of Health. 1998. *Our Healthier Nation: A Contract for Health*. Cmnd 3852. London: Stationery Office; Department of Health. 1998. *Modernising Social Services:*

Promoting Independence, Improving Protection, Raising Standards. Cmnd 4169. London: Stationery Office. More information is available on www.doh.gov.uk/nsf/nsfhome.htm. Several of the key documents can be downloaded from the Internet.

16.   Department of Health. 2001. *National Service Framework for Older People*. London: DH, p. 3.

17.   Better Government for Older People. 2000. *All Our Futures*. Wolverhampton, West Midlands: BGOP. For further information, see *www.bettergovernmentforolderpeople.gov.uk*.

18.   Age Concern England. 2000. *The Debate of the Age: The Agenda for the Age*. London: ACE. For other *Debate of the Age* papers and further information, visit www.ace.org.uk.

19.   There is increasing research on the situation of older migrants and members of ethnic minority populations: Bhopal, K. 2000. South Asian Women in East London: The Impact of Education. *European Journal of Women's Studies* 7:35–52; Phillipson, C., E. Alhaq, S. Ullah, and J. Ogg. 2000. Bangladeshi Families in Bethnal Green, London: Older People, Ethnicity, and Social Exclusion. In A. M. Warnes, L. Warren, and M. Nolan, eds. *Care Services for Later Life: Transformations and Critiques,* 273–290. London: Jessica Kingsley; Phillipson, C., N. Ahmed, and J. Latimer. 2003. *Women in Transition: A Study of the Experiences of Bangladeshi Women Living in Tower Hamlets*. Bristol, Avon: Policy; Rehman, H. 1999. *Inequalities in the Health of Black and Minority Ethnic Groups*. London: Health Education Authority; Silveira, E. R. T., and S. Ebrahim. 1998. A Comparison of Mental Health among Minority Ethnic Elders and Whites in East and North London. *Age and Ageing* 27(3): 375–383; Warnes, A. M., K. Friedrich, L. Kellaher, and S. Torres. 2004. The Diversity and Welfare of Older Migrants in Europe. *Ageing & Society* 24(3), 307–326.

9. Inequalities among Older People in London: The Challenge of Diversity

Maria Evandrou

Introduction

Tackling inequality and reducing poverty are high on the British government's policy agenda. In 1999, the government published *Opportunity for All,* outlining its strategy to "eradicate child poverty, provide employment opportunities for all who can work and ensure that older people live secure, active and fulfilling lives."[1] A central part of that strategy is reduction of income inequality and inequalities in health. The 1999 policy document entitled *Saving Lives: Our Healthier Nation* aimed to improve the health of the nation and in particular that of the most disadvantaged. Targets for reducing inequalities at the national level were announced in February 2001.[2] An integral part of the strategy to achieve this goal has been the setting of local targets for reducing health inequalities by the Department of Health.[3] Thus, nationally set targets are to be achieved by improvements at the local level. The setting of targets has focused attention on the data needs of measuring and monitoring progress toward achieving these targets, with a concomitant increase in the quantity and quality of data being produced at the local level.

This chapter maps inequalities in the socioeconomic circumstances, health status, and access to health and social care services among older people in London. The discussion of inequality among London's older persons is located within the broader context of inequalities in later life in Britain as a whole. London is younger than Britain as a whole. In 2001, older people constituted just 10 percent of Inner London's population and 14 percent of Outer London's population, compared to one in six (17 percent) nationally.[4] This reflects both the high concentration of universities and other further education establishments in Inner London and the fact that many older people, particularly from the higher-income groups, choose to move out of London's urban core upon retirement. Of those who remain in Inner London, many move when they require care. Significant numbers of people aged seventy-five and over leave Inner London to be closer to relatives or move into residential or nursing homes in Outer London and other areas.[5] Despite London's being younger overall, there is a slightly higher proportion of older men and women in the oldest age groups, aged eighty-five and over, in Outer London compared with the national average (13 vs. 12 percent).[6] Although London is on average a young city, it is home to more than one million people aged sixty-five and over. Thus, aging in London remains a critical issue.

As seen in Chapter 8, older people in Inner London are more likely to be living alone than are their counterparts in Outer London or nationally. In 2001, 36 percent of men aged sixty-five and over in Inner London were living alone, compared to just 23 percent in Outer London and 22 percent in England and Wales a whole.[7] Family members, both within and outside the household, are a key source of practical and social support. That a higher proportion of London's older persons live alone may reflect the success of social services within the capital in terms of promoting older people's independence. However, it may also pose a continuing challenge to local authorities and policy makers in meeting the needs of older people in providing appropriate services and tackling social isolation.

London is one of the most diverse capital cities in the world and has the highest concentration of older people from minority ethnic groups in the country.[8] It is estimated that more than one hundred languages are spoken in London, and its residents include people from all the countries in the world and from all religious beliefs. London's distinctive demographic and socioeconomic profile presents both challenges and opportunities to policy makers and for the delivery of health and social care services to older people. For example, London includes neighborhoods that are among both the richest and the most deprived in Britain. It is home to the country's leading teaching hospitals, yet there is a shortage of general practitioners (GPs) in inner-city areas.

Socioeconomic Inequalities in London

London contains some of the most affluent and impoverished areas in the country; however, deprivation is concentrated in Inner London. According to an index of income deprivation constructed by the Department for Transport and the Regions, out of 354 local government administrations in England, London contains the 7th and 16th most deprived areas (Newham and Tower Hamlets, both in Inner London) and the 214th most deprived (Kingston upon Thames in Outer London).[9] Not surprisingly, the City of London ranks 353rd out of 354.

Differences in social deprivation between the urban core and periphery are also evident from the 2001 census data. A higher proportion of older people in Inner London than in Outer London live in overcrowded conditions and do not have access to central heating (Table 9.1). Furthermore, the likelihood of living in poor housing conditions increases with age.[10] The housing conditions in which people live reflect their economic resources and can also affect health and relations among household members; for example, households without central heating have a greater likelihood of suffering from dampness and condensation than other homes.[11] Overcrowding is associated with a higher rate of accidents in the home among the young and old, and may have a negative impact on health.[12]

Housing tenure is a powerful indicator of socioeconomic circumstances. A greater proportion of older people live in social housing in Inner London (46 percent) than in Outer London (19 percent) (Table 9.1). This figure reflects both the supply of social housing and differences in income, as most people's preferred tenure is the owner-occupied sector. The higher proportion living in accommodations on the fifth floor or higher is also a reflection of the housing stock, with more high-rise flats in Inner than in Outer London. This has implications for older people's physical access to shops and services.

Access to a convenient means of transport is an important determinant of an individual's ability to carry out aspects of daily living (such as going to the shops, banking, and attending hospital appointments), as well as to participate in social activities. Older people living in households without access to a car and dependent on public transport may have reduced opportunities for social contact and social participation. Car ownership, or lack thereof, is an important indicator of both economic deprivation and greater risk of social exclusion. The evidence illustrates that older people in Inner London are much less likely to live in a household with at least one car or van (39 percent) than those in Outer London (60 percent) or the population as a whole (63 percent) (Table 9.1). Lack of access to a car increases with age.[13] London's residents aged sixty and over qualify for a Freedom Pass, which provides free travel on London's public transport. Although this goes some way to improving mobility and access to services, it lacks the flexibility of private transport and poses difficulties for older people with disabilities or in wheelchairs.

On all indicators, a higher proportion of older people living in Inner London are disadvantaged, with implications for their health and their demand for and ac-

Table 9.1. Persons 65+ in Disadvantaged Circumstances: Inner and Outer London and England and Wales, 2001 (as a percent of all persons 65+)

	Inner London	Outer London	England and Wales
In overcrowded accommodation	14	6	4
Without central heating	14	11	14
Without sole use of bath/shower and toilet	1	1	<1
In local authority or other social housing	46	19	20
In private rental	10	5	6
On 5th floor or higher	5	1	1
With no car or van in household	61	41	38

Source: U.K. Census 2001.

Note: Number of rooms occupied is less than the number of rooms required by household members, based on their ages and relationship.

cess to health and social care services. Particular challenges are presented by some of Inner London's housing stock, where high-density terraced housing damaged during World War II was replaced with high-rise flats. Many of these were erected during the 1960s and their tenants have aged with them. Flats that were suitable for people earlier in their life course are no longer suitable for them in later life. Poor communal infrastructure, with lifts that frequently break down, entry phones subject to vandalism, and graffiti-ridden communal landings, all serve to heighten older people's sense of social isolation and exclusion. London has the highest rate of recorded crime per capita in England.[14] Although older people are less likely to be victims of a household or personal crime than are other age groups, they are more likely to worry about crime. Fear of crime is highest among older people living in Inner London, particularly those with poor health, with low income, living in social housing, and from Asian communities.[15] A third of all women over sixty in England report feeling unsafe when walking alone after dark. This problem is exacerbated in Inner London by lack of private transport, with many older persons dependent on public transport and effectively confined to their homes after sunset.

Inequalities in Health across the Capital

Life expectancy. The health status of London's older population varies significantly, both within and between Inner and Outer London. In 1999–2001, men aged sixty-five in Outer London could expect to live on average 0.8 years longer than men in Inner London. Similarly, women aged sixty-five in Outer London could on average expect to live 0.4 years longer than their counterparts in Inner London. However, these averages mask significant inequalities across London in life expectancy. Within Inner London, male life expectancy at age sixty-five varied from 14.4 years in Newham to 18.1 years in Kensington and Chelsea, a difference of 4.3 years. Only two of the fourteen Inner London boroughs report male life expectancies higher than the average for England (Kensington and Chelsea and the City of Westminster). There is a similar picture for women, with the above-average boroughs also including Hammersmith and Fulham. The picture is much more mixed in Outer London, with nine boroughs reporting life expectancies above the English average and ten below average.

Although women may expect to live longer than men in every borough, the differences are most marked in areas of high deprivation. For example, as we saw earlier, Hackney, Tower Hamlets, and Newham are the most deprived areas in London, and in these areas women outlive men at age sixty-five by 4.1, 3.6, and 3.5 years respectively. This contrasts with the least-deprived areas in Greater London of Kensington and Chelsea and Richmond upon Thames, where excess female life expectancy at age sixty-five is 3.0 and 3.2 years respectively. These results are confirmed by similar findings in other studies.[16] The differences in life expectancy by London borough have increased throughout the 1990s, and if current trends continue, this gap is expected to increase.[17]

These inequalities in life expectancy may reflect differences in the age structure of the population. Looking at the Standardized Mortality Ratios for Inner and Outer London in 2001, the split between the inner core and the outer periphery is clear, with most of Inner London experiencing excess mortality, along with Waltham Forest, Barking and Dagenham, and Greenwich in Outer London (Figure 9.1).[18] The concentration of boroughs with excess mortality in Inner London suggests a greater need for health and social care services in the inner core, despite its relatively younger age structure.

Self-reported health status. In addition to health status as measured by mortality, it is possible to examine inequalities in health using measures of self-reported morbidity collected in the 2001 census. Information was obtained on two measures: general health status over the past year, and the presence of a long-term illness, health problem, or disability that limits daily activities or work, including problems due to old age.

Fifty-two percent of persons aged sixty-five and over in Inner London reported a limiting long-term illness (LLTI), compared with 49 percent in Outer London, and 52 percent in England and Wales. However, three-quarters of older people reported their general health over the previous year as "good" or "fairly good." This suggests either that many chronic conditions do not affect health, or that perceptions of general health may change with increasing age so that long-standing illnesses, such as arthritis, are more likely to be accepted by the respondent as part of everyday living.

Figure 9.1. Standardized Mortality Rates, Inner and Outer London, 2001

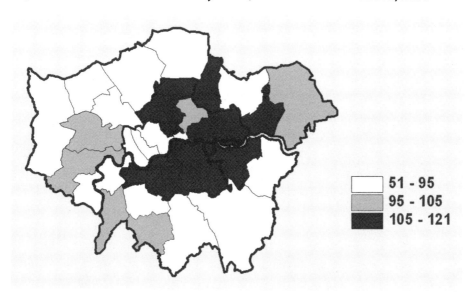

51 - 95
95 - 105
105 - 121

Source: ONS, 2002.

A higher proportion of older men and women in Inner London than in Outer London report being in poor health, but this is lower than for England and Wales as a whole (Table 9.2). This variation is in part due to the differences in age structure, with the older population in Inner London being relatively younger. However, higher levels of self-reported poor health in Inner London compared to Outer London remain once age is controlled for. Within age groups, self-reported morbidity in Outer London is actually lower than in England and Wales as a whole (as shown by the figures indicating the relative position of London to England and Wales, Tables 9.2 and 9.3). Thus, the health divide highlighted earlier with respect to life expectancy and mortality is mirrored in inequalities in self-reported health between Inner and Outer London.

The proportion of people age sixty-five and over reporting an LLTI varies across London boroughs, with the highest proportion of older men reporting ill health according to this measure being found in Newham (59 percent), Tower Hamlets (56 percent), and Hackney (56 percent)—again, the most-deprived boroughs. Among older women, the highest proportion reporting an LLTI live in Hackney (62 percent), Newham (62 percent), and Barking and Dagenham (59 percent). These are among the poorest boroughs in London, again highlighting the relationship between deprivation and health. This income effect is compounded by the out-migration of better-off (and healthier) older people from Inner London at retirement.

Health status by socioeconomic position. Empirical evidence clearly indicates a relationship between deprivation and ill health at the spatial level. Health status is also related to older people's individual socioeconomic characteristics. Older people living in social housing are much more likely than those living in owner-occupied housing to report ill health in terms of having both an LLTI and poor general health over the last year (Table 9.4). This is especially marked among those aged sixty-five to seventy-four. The decreasing differential with age reflects both differential mortality rates between tenures and the propensity for survivors to move into communal establishments.

Interestingly, the health gap between those in social housing and owner occupiers is greatest in Outer London, where people aged sixty-five to seventy-four living in social housing are almost twice as likely to report ill health as those in owner-occupied housing (25 vs. 13 percent). This may reflect the greater relative disadvantage of those living in social housing in better-off areas. Living in social housing is more a minority experience in Outer London than in Inner London (see Table 9.1).

Further light may be shed on socioeconomic differentials in health status among older people in London using data from the General Household Survey (GHS).[19] There is a clear negative relationship between LLTI and income, with a higher proportion of older people in Greater London reporting an LLTI among those living in households in the poorest fifth of the income distribution compared to those

Table 9.2. Self-Reported Health Status over the Last Year of Persons 65+, by Age and Sex: Inner and Outer London and England and Wales, 2001 (as a percent of all persons in age and sex category)

	Men				Women			
	65–74	75–84	85+	All 65+	65–74	75–84	85+	All 65+
Inner London								
Good health	37	32	26	35	35	30	24	32
Fairly good health	39	40	39	39	41	41	41	41
Not good health	24	28	35	26	24	29	35	27
Outer London								
Good health	44	34	27	39	41	31	23	34
Fairly good health	39	43	42	40	41	43	42	42
Not good health	18	24	31	21	18	26	35	24
England & Wales (E&W)								
Good health	42	32	26	37	39	29	22	33
Fairly good health	39	43	42	40	42	43	42	42
Not good health	19	25	32	22	19	28	36	25
Inner London relative position to E&W								
Not good health	1.26	1.12	1.07	1.18	1.25	1.05	0.98	1.10
Outer London relative position to E&W								
Not good health	0.92	0.94	0.96	0.94	0.94	0.93	0.97	0.95

Source: U.K. Census 2001.

Table 9.3. Persons 65+ Reporting a Limiting Long-Term Illness, by Age and Sex: Inner and Outer London and England and Wales, 2001 (as a percent of all persons in age and sex category)

	Men				Women			
	65–74	75–84	85+	All 65+	65–74	75–84	85+	All 65+
Inner London	45	56	68	50	45	58	74	54
Outer London	39	53	68	46	38	56	76	51
England & Wales (E&W)	43	56	70	50	41	59	78	53
Inner London cf. E&W	1.04	0.99	0.97	1.01	1.09	0.99	0.94	1.01
Outer London cf. E&W	0.91	0.95	0.97	0.94	0.94	0.95	0.97	0.96

Source: U.K. Census 2001

Note: The census question refers to limiting long-term illness, health problem, or disability that limits daily activities, including problems due to old age.

Table 9.4. Persons 65+ Reporting a Limiting Long-term Illness and "Not Good" Health over the Past Year, by Housing Tenure: Inner and Outer London, 2001 (as a percent of all persons in age category)

	Inner London			Outer London		
	65–74	75–84	85+	65–74	75–84	85+
Owned	15.7	23.1	31.4	13.4	20.6	30.1
Rented from council	27.3	29.6	34.6	25.4	28.3	35.4
Other social rented	25.2	27.0	33.5	24.1	27.7	33.2
Private rented & other	19.8	25.0	29.9	20.7	25.6	31.8
All in private households	21.2	26.2	32.5	15.7	22.6	31.4
Relative position renting from council v. owner	1.74	1.29	1.10	1.89	1.37	1.18

Source: U.K. Census 2001.

living in households in the richest fifth (42 vs. 22 percent) (Table 9.5). This gradient remains after controlling for differences in age structure, although the GHS sample sizes are low within London.

Health status and ethnicity. As has been found in other studies, there is a clear relationship between ethnicity and self-reported morbidity (Table 9.6), with older people from Asian ethnic groups reporting significantly higher levels of morbidity, and older people from Chinese communities reporting lower levels of morbidity, than white older persons.[20] (Given that white older persons are on average older than their counterparts from minority ethnic groups, it is likely that the differences in health status between Asian and white older persons are even more marked.) A number of factors may be associated with ethnic inequalities in health: first, differences between groups in health-related behavior (such as diet, smoking, drinking, propensity to exercise, etc.); second, attributes which relate to particular population subgroups or individuals (for example, the genetic inheritance of sickle-cell anemia among some of the black Caribbean population); third, differences in the material environment and resources enjoyed by different groups, including living arrangements, financial resources, and other indicators of standard of living; and fourth, differences associated with the consequences of direct and indirect racism.

Older people from ethnic minority groups, in particular Pakistani and Bangladeshi, are more likely to be among the poorest in terms of family income and to live in poor-quality housing (i.e., without central heating, overcrowded, and with lower access to consumer durables).[21] This finding has implications for their quality of

Table 9.5. Persons 65+ Reporting a Limiting Long-term Illness, by Income Quintile: Greater London and Great Britain, 1998–2001

	Poorest 20%	2d Quintile	3d Quintile	4th Quintile	Richest 20%
Greater London	41.9	43.7	41.2	26.7	22.4
(n)	(198)	(229)	(119)	(90)	(76)
Great Britain	46.2	44.9	41.0	31.6	24.9
(n)	(2090)	(3202)	(1736)	(838)	(558)

Source: Author's analysis General Household Survey, 2001.
Note: Differences in LLTI by income quintile are significant at p<0.01 in Greater London and p<0.001 in Great Britain. Income quintile is based on the distribution of equivalized gross household income of the population.

Table 9.6. Persons 65+ Reporting "Not Good" Health, by Ethnicity: Inner and Outer London, 2001 (as a percent of all persons 65+ in age and sex category)

	Inner London			Outer London		
	All	Men	Women	All	Men	Women
Limiting long-term illness						
All 65+	52.2	50.1	53.8	49.0	46.3	50.9
White	51.5	49.3	53.0	48.4	46.0	50.1
Mixed	50.4	48.5	52.1	46.8	44.6	48.7
Asian or Asian British	61.8	60.5	63.6	57.3	51.4	63.4
Black or black British	54.0	50.0	58.0	49.1	43.7	54.3
Chinese or other ethnic group	49.3	45.6	52.5	46.6	41.6	50.7
"Not good" health over the last year						
All 65+		26.2	27.5		20.8	23.5
White		25.3	26.3		20.4	22.5
Mixed		25.8	28.7		19.3	23.8
Asian or Asian British		33.4	37.8		24.7	36.1
Black or black British		29.3	35.0		24.1	31.0
Chinese or other ethnic group		23.6	28.3		18.7	25.6

Source: U.K. Census 2001.

life, as well as their ability to contribute financially to their packages of care in frail old age.

Material deprivation is one of the main drivers in health differences. Thus, policies that attempt to tackle and reduce deprivation may also contribute to the reduction in health inequalities. The 1998 Acheson Report, *Health Inequalities,* suggests that policies to reduce social and economic inequalities should be a key part of any strategy to reduce inequalities in health.[22] However, multivariate analysis has shown that even after controlling for deprivation, ethnic differences in the propensity to report ill health remain significant.[23] This finding highlights that indicators of socioeconomic position only partly account for the social disadvantage faced by ethnic minority groups and that other factors may also play an important role in contributing to ethnic inequalities in health.

In particular, other forms of disadvantage, such as the experience of racism, may also affect the health of older persons among ethnic minorities. A study on the health and health-care use among older persons from ethnic minorities in London found that minority ethnic older persons, with the exception of the Chinese, were at least as likely as white older persons to consult a GP.[24] High frequency of use may indicate an ineffective consultation, thus requiring further visits, or low patient satisfaction with the consultation outcome (e.g., no prescription, referral, or certificate). The higher relative use of GP services by Pakistani and Bangladeshi elderly people does not translate into higher outpatient attendance, suggesting a lower referral rate from primary to secondary care. Low referral rates by GPs were found to be one of the main factors related to low use of district nursing services by disabled people from ethnic minority communities.[25]

The Acheson Report stressed the importance of policies that specifically take into account the needs of ethnic minority groups with regard to health promotion and education, needs assessment, resource allocation, and health-care planning and provision. The National Health Service (NHS) and social services are undergoing modernization, with new policies and new service frameworks. The challenge is ensuring that health education is meaningful to minority ethnic communities, that goals and targets are clearly defined, and that services are culturally competent and acceptable to different groups.

To summarize, there are clear inequalities in health within London's older population when measured across a range of different dimensions: spatial, socioeconomic, and ethnic. Inequalities at the individual level are compounded by inequalities across neighborhoods.

Inequalities in Health and Social Care

Inequalities in the supply of health-care services. In response to the NHS Performance Assessment Framework (April 1999), the Department of Health has published a series of performance indicators for the NHS on a variety of domains, including access to health care. These indicators are designed to help managers and clinicians improve standards within health care to meet national and local targets. The data for February 2002 indicate that the supply of health-care services is unevenly distributed across the capital.[26]

London has often been viewed as having poor primary health care. The 1997 Turnberg Report highlighted that primary health-care services in London were lagging behind those in the rest of the country.[27] The report identified a number of difficulties, including recruitment and retention of GPs, a fall in the total number of GPs in London against a rise in the total number in England as a whole, a high proportion of single-person practices in London, and many premises of poor quality. Since then, a number of initiatives, such as the London Initiative Zone, have helped improve supply. In 2002, the supply of GPs in many parts of London exceeded the average for England (5.74 per 10,000).[28] However, the provision of GPs per ten thousand population remains particularly low in the eastern parts of Outer London (5.3/10,000 in Barking and Havering Health Authority), despite an increase of 5.5 percent since 2000. Although there have been improvements, it is clear that not all health authorities have benefited equally. There have been falls in provision since 2000 in south London. Between 2000 and 2002, provision in Bexley, Greenwich, and Bromley dropped by 2.2 percent to 5.5/10,000, and Richmond Health Authority fell by 4.1 percent to 6.6/10,000.

As of January 2004, all GPs in England are members of primary care trusts, which will commission and provide health care, as well as monitor the quality of health care. For older people, the GP is the key gatekeeper and provides the route to many health- and community-care services. The doctor's surgery is often viewed as the first point of contact for older people seeking advice concerning their health and social care concerns. Inequality in the distribution of GPs across London means that in some areas GPs may be unable to meet the demand for consultations, with the outcome that older patients in some areas experience long waiting times. Evidence from the *National Survey of NHS Patients* indicated that the wait to see a GP is longer in London than elsewhere in England. To see a GP, 36 percent of Londoners had to wait at least a day longer than they desired, compared to 29 percent nationally. This wait time means that some people may present with more severe symptoms than would otherwise have been the case, a possibility likely to be exacerbated among older patients with multiple pathology. Delays in accessing advice and services also cause older patients additional anxiety and stress. Londoners also spent longer, on average, waiting in the GP surgery than did patients from other regions, where waiting times were broadly similar.[29]

Interestingly, the boroughs with the lowest levels of service provision in terms of GPs per hundred thousand population are not necessarily those with the highest levels of patient dissatisfaction with that service. Nevertheless, the proportion of patients who complained or felt like complaining about GP surgery staff in the previous twelve months was significantly higher in London than in the country as a whole. For example, 19 percent of patients in Camden and Islington Health Authority were dissatisfied on this measure, compared to 12 percent for England as a whole.[30]

In terms of inpatient care, London is generally better provided for than is the rest of the country. Inpatient waiting lists are generally shorter than in England as a whole, where the average is twenty-one per thousand population.[31] Once again, the position is worst in the northern and eastern parts of Outer London. In Barking and Havering Health Authority, inpatient waiting lists in 2000 were twenty-seven per thousand. This indicator is useful in that it reflects general access to health services; however, it does not tell us anything about use of inpatient services by older people per se.

The number of finished consultant episodes for those aged sixty and over per thousand population of the same age reflects variations in both the supply of and demand for services. In 1999–2000, there was little variation between Inner London (423/1,000) and Outer London (419/1,000). However, the indicator varies significantly across the capital. Interestingly, for 1999–2000 it was highest in Newham and Tower Hamlets (493 and 494, respectively), both areas characterized by poor health and high deprivation and thus high demand. However, it was also high in Barnet, Brent and Hammersmith, and Fulham Health Authorities, areas that did not exhibit particularly high levels of ill health (see Figure 9.1). The lowest levels of finished consultant episodes were reported in Lambeth (356). Lambeth, in Inner London, is also an area of high deprivation and poor health, with a relatively high ethnic minority population, and so might be expected to have a high level of need. Thus, there appears to be no consistent pattern across the capital.

One indicator of the effective delivery of appropriate health care to older people is the percentage of patients aged sixty-five and over discharged home within twenty-eight days of emergency admission to a hospital with a hip fracture. This indicator acts as a proxy for successful outcome of rehabilitation. Rates in England as a whole fell slightly between 2000 and 2002, from 47 to 46 percent. Again, the picture is very mixed across the London health authorities, with no clear pattern of the urban core versus the periphery. The percentage of older people discharged within twenty-eight days was lowest in Ealing, Hammersmith, and Hounslow at just 38 percent. This compares to 64 percent in the best-performing health authority, Hillingdon, which is also in west Outer London. Of course, the proportion of older people able to return home depends partly on the availability of support at home and the quality of community services, as well as appropriate health-care services.

Patterns of social care provision. The provision of social care is pivotal in enabling older people to live independently in the community. Since 1998, the Department of Health has published data on various indicators of performance for Personal Social Services (PSS). The policy document *Modernising Social Services* sets out new arrangements to assess the performance of each local authority with social services responsibilities.[32] The PSS Performance Assessment Framework provides a statistical overview of the performance of each local council over the year.[33] Evidence for a range of indicators that have direct relevance for the quality of life of older people in London and elsewhere are presented here. In particular, there is a focus on evidence regarding progress in promoting older people's independence and ensuring standards are met and maintained in residential care.

Levels of provision. Social services are accessed through assessments, and the number of assessments per thousand older people (sixty-five plus) in each local council provides a useful indication of the distribution across London. Very low figures would suggest problems with either the referral system or the assessment process itself. In England in 2001–2002, an average of 113 assessments of older people were carried out for every thousand older people in the country. The level for Inner London was above the national average at 118, although the level of assessments in Outer London was below, at 111. The levels had fallen from 125 and 122, respectively, in 2000–2001. The figures for individual councils within London ranged from 64 (Ealing) to 111 (Kensington and Chelsea) to 213 (Southwark), demonstrating wide variability across the capital. However, once again, there was no distinct patterning between the urban core and the first ring in terms of high or low levels of assessments.

Promoting older people's independence. It has been an explicit aim of government policy since the early 1990s to reduce the number of older people living in residential and nursing homes and to promote and support older people to live independently in the community. The policy document *Modernising Social Services* outlines the government's aims to promote the independence and social participation of social service users.

There have been falls in the rate of older people admitted to supported residential and nursing care in both Inner and Outer London since 1997–1998.[34] The decline has been particularly marked in Inner London, falling from 186 admissions per ten thousand older people sixty-five and over in 1997–1998 to 109 in 2001–2002, reflecting the implementation of the independent-living policy agenda (Table 9.7). However, this drop needs to be examined alongside the provision of intensive home care for older people. As more people are helped to live at home and provided with rehabilitative care, a smaller proportion of people needs to be admitted permanently to institutions. Thus, a high figure for admissions may be explained in part by a low figure in the provision of home-care services that help people remain at home.

In general, provision of intensive home care for older people is higher in urban areas than rural areas, and provision is significantly higher in Inner London than elsewhere in England (Table 9.8). This may in part reflect the higher proportion of older men and women in Inner London than elsewhere who live alone. There is, however, significant variation across boroughs in both indicators. Supported

Table 9.7. Supported Admissions of Older People to Permanent Residential and Nursing Care per 10,000 Population 65+: Inner and Outer London and England, 1997–2002

	1997–1998	1998–1999	1999–2000	2000–2001	2001–2002
Inner London	186	127	126	108	109
Outer London	97	102	101	94	95
England	139	128	124	109	109

Source: Department of Health 2003, Social Services Performance Assessment Framework Indicators 2001–2002 (London: DOH).

admissions are lowest in Outer London (with the exception of Barnet and Barking and Dagenham). Interestingly, receipt of intensive home care is also lowest in these Outer London areas, suggesting that some people in need of care may not be receiving it (although most boroughs are above the national average of ten per thousand people aged sixty-five and over). Conversely, provision of intensive home care *and* supported admissions are both highest in Inner London. The picture is somewhat complex. Supported admissions may be higher in inner-city deprived areas because of higher physical need (as discussed earlier, health is worse in these areas) but also because of greater financial need. Support for residential care is means tested, so support admissions are likely to be higher in poorer neighborhoods. There is also a wide range of systems for charging for domiciliary services and in the maximum and minimum charges.[35]

Looking at the number of older people helped to live at home (by receipt of any

Table 9.8. Households Receiving Intensive Home Care per 1,000 Population 65+: Inner and Outer London and England, 1998–2002

	1998–1999	1999–2000	2000–2001	2001–2002
Inner London	16.7	21.8	23.7	23.8
Outer London	10.6	12.3	13.1	13.5
England	7.8	8.8	9.3	9.9

Source: Department of Health 2003, *Social Services Performance Assessment Framework Indicators 2001–2002* (London: DOH).
Note: Intensive home care is defined as more than ten contact hours and six or more visits per week.

social care services, including equipment and adaptations) provides an indication of how much low-level social care is being provided. The figures in Table 9.9 confirm the earlier picture of higher levels of support in London than in England in general, and the highest levels of support in Inner London. Furthermore, Outer London recorded a significant fall in social care services per thousand older people between 1999 and 2000 and between 2000 and 2001, then no change for 2001–2002—despite the fact that the age structure of Outer London, in terms of the percentage of people aged eighty-five and over, is older than for Inner London. Levels of provision are particularly low in Hounslow, where just 61 households per thousand older population received support, compared to a high of 154 in Tower Hamlets. This variation may reflect differences in need not captured by simple demographic indicators, with levels of deprivation being much higher in Tower Hamlets and with a significantly more diverse population.[36] As was discussed earlier, compared to Outer London, Inner London is more ethnically diverse and records higher levels of deprivation and poor health status (in terms of standardized mortality ratios, lower life expectancy, and higher proportions reporting an LLTI).

A final indicator of how well London's councils are performing in helping people live independently at home is provided by the number of hospital admissions of people aged seventy-five and over due to hypothermia or injury caused by a fall per thousand population of the same age cohort. This measure captures the extreme outcomes which social services can play a part in preventing. Given that there are comparatively few admissions for hypothermia, the indicator largely reflects admissions because of falls and includes falls that occurred in the person's home or in a residential care home. Rates of admission varied significantly across the capital from just two per thousand in Harrow to twenty-eight per thousand in the City of London and twenty-seven per thousand in Islington. Overall, hospital-admission rates are lower in Inner and Outer London than the average for England.

Table 9.9. Number of Older Persons Helped to Live at Home per 1,000 Population 65+: Inner and Outer London and England, 1998–2002

	1998–1999	1999–2000	2000–2001	2001–2002
Inner London	130	115	111	115
Outer London	98	101	89	89
England	82	85	83	83

Source: Department of Health, 2003, *Social Services Performance Assessment Framework Indicators 2001–2002* (London: DOH).

Note: Includes all recipients of any social care services following assessment, including the issuing of equipment and adaptations.

Table 9.10. Hospital Admissions due to Falls or Hypothermia, Persons 75+ per 1,000 population 75+: Inner and Outer London and England, 1997–2002

	1997–1998	1998–1999	1999–2000	2000–2001	2001–2002
Inner London	22	17	18	18	17
Outer London	22	18	20	18	17
England	24	21	23	21	21

Source: Department of Health 2003, *Social Services Performance Assessment Framework Indicators 2001–2002* (London: DOH).

Note: The numerator includes all admissions during the year to NHS hospitals where the primary diagnosis was injury caused by a fall (ICD codes are injuries S00-T98 caused by falls W00-W19) or any diagnosis of hypothermia (ICD code T68).

Furthermore, they have declined over time—reflecting an improvement in services in this area (Table 9.10).

Reducing mortality from accidents by 20 percent and serious injuries by 10 percent is one of the targets outlined in *Our Healthier Nation.* Around a third of all accidental deaths result from falls to people aged over sixty-five, so this area has been the focus of considerable attention in the last five years. Reducing falls among older people is one of the standards in the *National Service Framework for Older People.*[37] The Health Education Authority in collaboration with the Department for Trade and Industry produced a resource pack, *Avoiding Slips, Trips, and Broken Hips*, to improve awareness among health professionals of accident-prevention strategies for older people.

Quality of services provided. As well as targets in terms of the provision of social care services, the Department of Health has published standards regarding the quality of those services. Service users and their caregivers should be able to expect practical help and support to arrive in a timely fashion soon after their needs have been referred to Social Services. In 2002–2003, 33 percent of all new clients in Inner London waited more than six weeks from first contact by Social Services until they received their first service.[38] This contrasts with 34 percent in Outer London and 29 percent for England as a whole. Thus, older people in both Inner and Outer London face a longer wait between referral and receipt of services than is the case nationally. However, there has been some improvement since 2001–2002, when 38 percent of service users in Inner London waited for more than six weeks.

The Department of Health published in 2003–2004 a new target of a maximum four-week wait from completion of assessment to delivery of service. Meeting this requirement will require substantial improvements by those councils not yet meeting the former six-week target. The worst offenders include the two Inner London boroughs of Hackney and Tower Hamlets, where over half of all new clients waited more than six weeks. These boroughs are among the most deprived and also have a high concentration of minority ethnic older persons.

User perceptions of how they have been treated are also very important. Social Service Departments need to be responsive to racial, cultural, and religious needs, of particular relevance in London, where the population is so ethnically diverse. Table 9.11 shows percentage of survey respondents who answered in the affirmative when asked whether social services staff took note of important matters relating to their race, culture, or religion. In 2001–2002, 39 percent of users in England as a whole said that issues relating to race, culture, or religion had been taken into account, but this figure was slightly lower in Inner London (37 percent). Again, there are significant variations across the boroughs, with the lowest rates recorded in Lambeth (just 21 percent) and Lewisham (25 percent) and the highest in the City of London (78 percent). The low rates in Lambeth and Lewisham are cause for concern, given that these Inner London boroughs have higher-than-average concentrations of ethnic older persons.

Inequalities in the use of health and social care services—evidence from the General Household Survey. The previous section highlighted the experience of aging in a world city and the relationships between need and provision at the spatial level. The inner core of London has higher levels of deprivation and a more diverse population than the periphery, but also records higher levels of provision of health and social care services. However, older people in some Inner London boroughs have to wait longer for community services, and more work remains to be done to

Table 9.11. Yes Answers to Survey Question on Needs Assessment: London and England, 2000–2002

	2000–2001 %	2001–2002 %
Inner London	35	37
Outer London	36	39
All Metropolitan Districts	40	41
England	37	39

Source: Department of Health, 2003, *Social Services Performance Assessment Framework Indicators 2001–2002* (London: DOH).

Note: Respondents replied to survey question asking: "Did social services staff take note of any important matters relating to your race, culture, or religion?"

improve responsiveness to the needs of particular ethnic communities. To supplement this analysis, we now look in depth at the service utilization according to the characteristics of older persons in Greater London and Britain. (The constraints of the GHS data we use make it impossible to disaggregate the analysis of health and social care service use into Inner and Outer London, and thus we compare Greater London and Great Britain.)

Health care services. Just over one in five people aged sixty-five and over in Greater London consulted a doctor in the previous two weeks (21 percent), which was much the same as that for Britain as a whole (Table 9.12). The difference between men and women was marked, with 26 percent of men and 18 percent of women consulting a GP. Looking at hospital outpatient attendance, 28 percent of older Londoners reported that they had attended a hospital outpatient department in the previous three months, slightly higher than in Great Britain. Once again, utilization rates were higher among men than women (32 vs. 25 percent). Of all older Londoners, 10 percent reported that they had attended a hospital as a day patient in the last year, although there were no significant gender differences in London; 14 percent reported a hospital inpatient stay during the last year.

There are clear differences in patterns in health-care use once health status is taken into account, with those reporting a limiting long-term illness (LLTI) or reporting "not poor" general health status over the last year being significantly more likely to consult a GP or use hospital outpatient, day-patient, and inpatient services. Looking at differences in utilization rates between London and Britain after controlling for health, there is greater use of day-patient services among those with an LLTI in London than in Britain. Among those without an LLTI, there is higher use of outpatient services in London but lower use of inpatient services than in Britain as a whole (Table 9.13). A similar health-care-use pattern obtains when the analysis uses general health status over the last year as the control variable (Table 9.14). There are also differences in service utilization by socioeconomic status (Table 9.15)

The evidence shows that health varies by socioeconomic status, and we have seen that health-care use varies by health status. The key question is whether there are socioeconomic differentials in health-care use once health status has been taken into account. Multivariate analysis shows that older people from the top four income quintiles are more likely to consult a GP than are those from the poorest quintile, taking health status into account (Table 9.16). Among those with an LLTI, 32 percent of better-off London's older persons consulted a GP compared to just 19 percent of their poorer counterparts. Inequalities in health-care use by income are more marked in London than in Britain as a whole. Reducing inequalities in service utilization in London, as elsewhere in the country, will require tackling inequalities in health as well as in deprivation.

Table 9.12. Men and Women 65+ Using Health Services: Greater London and Great Britain, 1998–2001 (as a percent of all persons 65+ in age and sex category)

	Greater London			Great Britain		
	All	Men	Women	All	Men	Women
Consulted GP/doctor (last 2 weeks)	21.3	25.8[a]	17.8[a]	21.2	21.0	21.4
Hospital outpatient (last 3 months)	28.0	31.8[b]	24.9[b]	23.9	25.7[c]	22.5[c]
Hospital day patient (last year)	10.1	8.3	11.6	8.5	8.7	8.4
Hospital inpatient (last year)	14.2	15.7	12.9	14.4	15.7[a]	13.4[a]
Total (n)	(820)	(363)	(457)	(9588)	(4232)	(5356)

Source: Author's analysis using pooled General Household Survey 1998, 2000, 2001.
[a] Difference between men and women significant at p<0.01
[b] Difference between men and women significant at p<0.05
[c] Difference between men and women significant at p<0.001.

Table 9.13. Persons 65+ Using Health Services Who Reported a Limiting Long-Term Illness (LLTI): Greater London and Great Britain, 1998–2001

	Greater London %		Great Britain %	
	With LLTI	Without LLTI	With LLTI	Without LLTI
Consulted GP/doctor (last 2 wks)	27.8	16.8	27.9	16.4
Hospital outpatient (last 3 months)	37.4	22.0	33.0	17.4
Hospital day patient (last year)	16.0	6.4	11.4	6.4
Hospital inpatient (last year)	26.5	6.4	22.5	8.7
Total (n)	(313)	(499)	(3,968)	(5,608)

Source: Author's analysis using pooled General Household Survey 1998, 2000, 2001.
Note: The difference in health-care use between those reporting a LLTI and those without is significant at p<0.001 within London and Britain. The difference in use rates between London and Britain within health groups was significant at p<0.01 for day patients among those with LLTI, p<0.01 for hospital outpatients for those without LLTI, and p<0.05 for hospital inpatient stays for those without LLTI.

Table 9.14. Persons 65+ Using Health Services, by General Health Status over the Last Year: Greater London and Great Britain, 1998–2001

	Greater London %		Great Britain %	
	Good/ Fair Health	Not Good Health	Good/ Fair Health	Not Good Health
Consulted GP/doctor (last 2 wks)	18.3	29.7	16.9	34.6
Hospital outpatient (last 3 months)	22.3	46.3	18.5	41.3
Hospital day patient (last year)	7.4	18.3	7.0	13.2
Hospital inpatient (last year)	7.3	33.1	8.4	31.0
Total (n)	(605)	(175)	(7017)	(2178)

Source: Author's analysis using pooled General Hospital Survey 1998, 2000, 2001.
Note: Difference in health-care use between those reporting good/fair health or not good health is significant at p<0.01 within Greater London and at p<0.001 within Britain. The difference in use rates between London and Britain within health groups was significant at p<0.01 for day patients among those with not good health and p<0.01 for hospital outpatients for those with good/fair health.

Table 9.15. Persons 65+ Using Health Services, by Poverty Status: Greater London and Great Britain, 1998–2001

	Greater London %		Great Britain %	
	Poorest 20%	Richest 80%	Poorest 20%	Richest 80%
Consulted GP/doctor (last 2 wks)	15.1[a]	23.6[a]	21.5	21.0
Hospital outpatient (last 3 months)	20.1[b]	30.2[b]	20.7[c]	25.0[c]
Hospital day patient (last year)	13.1	9.1	8.2	8.7
Hospital inpatient (last year)	17.6[a]	12.0[a]	14.5	14.1
Total (n)	(199)	(517)	(2091)	(6340)

Source: Author's analysis using pooled General Household Survey 1998, 2000, 2001.

Note: Poverty is defined as the individual residing in a household where the equivalized gross household income is in the bottom 20% of the income distribution for the whole population.

[a] Difference in health-care use between poor and not poor respondents significant at p<0.05

[b] Difference in health-care use between poor and not poor respondents significant at p<0.01

[c] Difference in health-care use between poor and not poor respondents significant at p<0.001

Community health and social services. Use of community-care services is known to be related to age, disability, and household composition (i.e., the availability of coresidential informal care). Levels of service use within age groups in Greater London are similar to those in Britain as a whole, with the exception of use of lunch clubs among people aged seventy-five and over, which is higher in London (9 percent vs. 5 percent). Private domestic help and use of Meals-on-Wheels among those aged seventy-five and over is also higher in London than in Britain, although the differences are less marked. As expected, older people living alone are more likely than those living with others to make use of community-care services. Comparing older people living alone in London and Great Britain, a slightly higher proportion of solo older Londoners use local authority home helps (11 vs. 9 percent) and lunch clubs (8 vs. 6 percent).

Discussion

Although London is younger than the United Kingdom, the sheer number of older people living in the capital and their diverse needs and characteristics ensure that aging in the city remains high on the policy agenda. Average figures across the capital mask important differences between Inner and Outer London, between the constituent boroughs within the urban core and the first ring, and between subgroups of the older population. It should not be overlooked that the variation within the inner core and the periphery is often as great as the variation between them.

Table 9.16. Persons 65+ Using Health Services, by General Health and Poverty Status: Greater London and Great Britain, 1998–2001

| | Greater London | | Great Britain | |
| | % | | % | |
	Poorest 20%	Richest 80%	Poorest 20%	Richest 80%
Among those reporting limiting long-term illness:				
Consulted GP/doctor (last 2 wks)	19.3[a]	31.6[a]	26.5	28.0
Hospital outpatient (last 3 months)	26.5[a]	41.1[a]	27.9[c]	34.7[c]
Hospital day patient (last year)	18.1	15.8	10.4	11.8
Hospital inpatient (last year)	26.5	23.7	20.4	22.5
Total (n)	(83)	(190)	(963)	(2554)
Among those reporting not good general health over the last year:				
Consulted GP/doctor (last 2 wks)	18.2[a]	36.3[a]	31.1	35.2
Hospital outpatient (last 3 months)	30.9[b]	53.9[b]	31.9[c]	45.0[c]
Hospital day patient (last year)	16.4	18.6	12.5	13.9
Hospital inpatient (last year)	25.5	35.3	26.0[b]	33.9[b]
Total (n)	(55)	(102)	(560)	(1384)

Source: Author's analysis using pooled General Household Survey 1998, 2000, 2001.
Note: Poverty is defined as the individual residing in a household where the equivalized gross household income is in the bottom 20% of the income distribution for the whole population.
[a] Difference in health-care use between poor and not poor respondents after controlling for health status significant at $p<0.05$
[b] Difference in health-care use between poor and not poor respondents after controlling for health status significant at $p<0.01$
[c] Difference in health-care use between poor and not poor respondents after controlling for health status significant at $p<.001$

In terms of the key drivers of the need for health and social care within London, a higher proportion of older people are living alone and a greater proportion are from ethnic minority groups in Inner London than in Outer London. Furthermore, deprivation is concentrated in Inner London in terms of both low income and poor housing quality. Life expectancy is lower and Standardized Mortality Rates are higher in Inner London. Thus, given the differentials in demographic, socioeconomic, and health drivers, one would expect a greater need for health and social care services in the inner core, despite a relatively younger age structure. That older people from ethnic minority groups generally report worse health, with the exception of the Chinese, highlights the need for these services to be culturally competent.

The evidence examined in this chapter indicates that provision of health and social care services is greater in Inner London than in Outer London. There are more GPs per hundred thousand population, higher completed hospital episodes per ten thousand population aged sixty and over, higher supported admissions to residential care, *and* higher levels of provision of intensive home care. However, indicators of the quality of services show a somewhat different picture. In particular, waiting time to see a GP and waiting time between referral and receipt of community services are both longer in Inner London than in Outer London and in England as a whole. Despite Inner London's having the most ethnically diverse population in Britain, fewer older people report that matters relating to their race, culture, or religion were taken into account by social services staff, presenting a challenge for social service managers. If waiting times are an indication of the mismatch between supply and demand, then the greater provision of health and social care services within Inner London still falls short of that required to meet its higher demand.

Moving away from analysis based on geographic units and looking at patterns of utilization at the individual level, the evidence shows that inequalities in health-care use remain after taking health status into account. Inequalities between subgroups of individuals are compounded by inequalities across boroughs. This emphasizes the need for integrated policy programs to tackle inequalities in later life at the individual level, as well as at the level of the neighborhood. It highlights the need for a range of interventions, at both the national and regional levels, targeted at local communities with particular needs. Diversity and aging in the city present both challenges and opportunities to policy makers and providers and for the delivery of appropriate health and social care services to older people. Tackling poverty, deprivation, and social exclusion of older people, as well as the dynamic nature of their health and social care needs, is critical. Improved service provision and delivery goes hand-in-hand with finding innovative ways of working with professionals from different backgrounds.

The modernizing of health and social services in the United Kingdom will go some way toward improving the quality of life of older people, in London and nationwide. The *National Service Framework for Older People* (NSFOP) sets out a program of action and reform for older people's services. It specifies eight national standards aimed at modernizing NHS and social services, and promoting innovative ways of working. These standards are: combating age discrimination; focusing on person-centered care; improving access to a new range of intermediate care services at home or in care settings; providing appropriate hospital care delivered by specialist multidisciplinary teams; delivering improved treatment and rehabilitation to stroke patients; reducing the risk of falls; providing integrated mental health services; and promoting an active healthy life in older age. As part of the NSFOP, each local heath authority has developed a local action plan. A key tool in implementing the framework in London has been the London Older People's Service Development Program. This has been successful in bringing together a variety of stakeholders, including patients, hospitals, GPs, and leisure and other local services, to work in partnership to improve primary health and social care services. In particular, the program has found that targeted preventative work can be successful in reducing the number of accident and emergency attendances, as well as the length of hospital-bed stays.

The new publicly available data facilitate further monitoring and accountability of provision and quality, both from within local government and from outside. As part of ensuring progress and meeting targets, NHS regional offices plan to use the *NHS Performance Framework* data to assess performance locally. Some improvements have already been achieved in health and social care, as evidenced by the analysis of the NHS and PSS Performance Framework data presented in this chapter. However, there is much more work to be done in improving the quality of life of older people. Strengthening multidisciplinary work involving older people is key, particularly the partnerships between general practice–based staff and other health and social care providers. Improving coordination between health-service providers, particularly between GPs, community nurses, occupational therapists, social care services, housing, and transport, has been recommended by various voluntary organizations working with older people.[39] The real challenge is ensuring that the implementation of the new reforms and interventions makes a difference in terms of older people's health and well-being today.

Notes

I am grateful to the Office for National Statistics, in particular Barbara Toson, Health Statistics, for providing unpublished data on life expectancy. I am also grateful to the ESRC (Economic and Social Research Council) Data Archive for access to the GHS data for 1998–2001, which has been used by permission. The analysis and interpretation of the data are the responsibility of the author alone.

1.   Department for Work and Pensions. 1999. *Opportunities for All*. London: Stationery Office.

2.   Department of Health. 2001. *Tackling Health Inequalities: Consultation on a Plan for Delivery*. London: Stationery Office.

3.   Ibid. 2002. *Tackling Health Inequalities: Cross Cutting Review 2002*. London: DOH. November 20; Department of Health. 2002. Improvement, Expansion, and Reform: The Next Three Years. *Priorities and Planning Framework, 2003–2006*. London: Stationery Office.

4.   Office of National Statistics. 2003 (www.statistics.gov.uk/census2001); see also Chapter 8 by Tony Warnes.

5.   London Research Centre [LRC]. 1999. *Social Care in London: Trends in Social Services Activity, 1993–1997*. London: LRC.

6. Evandrou, M. 2004. *Growing Old in London: Social and Economic Inequalities*. ESRC SAGE Research Group Discussion Paper No. 16. London: London School of Economics.

7. Ibid.

8. Lowdell, C., M. Evandrou, M. Bardsley, D. Morgan, and M. Soljak. 2000. *Health of Ethnic Minority Elders in London*. London: Health of Londoners Project.

9. Department of the Environment, Transport, and the Regions. 2000. *Indices of Deprivation, 2000*. London: DETR.

10. Evandrou, *Growing Old in London*.

11. Howarth, C, P. Kenway, G. Palmer, and C. Street. 1998. *Monitoring Poverty and Social Exclusion—Labour's Inheritance*. York: Joseph Rowntree Foundation.

12. Home Office. 1997. *Fires in the Home, 1995*. London: Stationery Office.

13. Evandrou, *Growing Old in London*.

14. Aitchison, A., and J. Hodgkinson. 2003. *Crime in England and Wales, 2002/2003: London Region*. London: Home Office.

15. Home Office. 2000. *The 2000 British Crime Survey*. Home Office Statistical Bulletin 18/00. London: Home Office.

16. Greater London Authority [GLA]. 2002. *Health in London: 2002 Review of the London Health Strategy High-Level Indicators*. London: GLA/London Health Observatory.

17. Fitzpatrick, J., and B. Jacobson. 2001. *Mapping Health Inequalities across London*. London: London Health Observatory.

18. Such rates control for differences in age structure between subgroups of the population by applying the age-specific death rates of a standard population (in this case England and Wales) to the age structure of the boroughs. Observed and expected deaths are then compared. A value above one hundred means that mortality is higher than would be expected if the borough had the average mortality of England and Wales, and a value of less than one hundred means that it is lower than expected.

19. The General Household Survey is a multipurpose cross-sectional survey carried out annually in Britain. The survey collects detailed information on a range of topics, including health and socioeconomic position, from around twenty thousand adults aged sixteen and over living in private and sheltered accommodation. The analysis in this chapter uses data pooled across three years (1998–99, 2000–2001, 2001–2) to provide a sufficiently large sample of older people living in Greater London.

20. Evandrou, *Growing Old in London*; Lowdell et al., *Health of Ethnic Minority Elders*; Nazroo, J. 1997. *The Health of Britain's Ethnic Minorities*. London: Policy Studies Institute; Balarajan, R., and V. S. Raleigh. 1995. *Ethnicity and Health in England*. London: Stationery Office.

21. Evandrou, M. 2000. "Ethnic Inequalities in Health in Later Life." *Health Statistics Quarterly* 8:20–28.

22. Acheson, D. 1998. *Report of The Independent Inquiry into Inequalities in Health*. London: Stationery Office.

23. Ibid. .

24. Lowdell et al., *Health of Ethnic Minority Elders*.

25. Evers, H., F. Badger, E. Cameron, and K. Atkin. 1988. *Community Care Project Working Papers*. Birmingham: Department of Social Medicine, University of Birmingham.

26. Department of Health. 2002. *NHS Performance Indicators, February 2002*. London: DOH.

27. London Strategic Review Independent Advisory Panel. 1997. Health Services in London: A Strategic Review (the Turnberg Report). London: Department of Health.

28. The indicator is the number of full-time-equivalent GPs per ten thousand weighted population, where the population is adjusted for cross-boundary flows and temporary residents and weighted for age and need.

29. Department of Health. 1999. *National Survey of NHS Patients: General Practice, 1998*. London: NHS Executive.

30. Department of Health. 2000. *NHS Performance Indicators, July 2000*. London: DOH.

31. Waiting list is expressed as per one thousand population, weighted to take account of differences between populations that affect the need for NHS care, including age.

32. Department of Health. 1998. *Modernising Social Services: Promoting Independence, Improving Protection, and Raising Standards*. London: Stationery Office.

33. Department of Health. 2003. *Social Services Performance Assessment Framework Indicators, 2001–2002*. London: DOH.

34. Supported residential and nursing care is care provided either directly in a local authority–run home or in a private or voluntary home where the local authority pays part or all of the costs.

35. LRC, *Social Care in London*.

36. Of the population in Tower Hamlets, 97 percent live in wards ranked in the bottom decile, compared to none in Hounslow; of the older population in Tower Hamlets, 22 percent are from nonwhite minority ethnic groups, compared to 17 percent in Hounslow.

37. Department of Health. 2001. *National Service Frameworks for Older People*. London: Stationery Office.

38. Department of Health. 2004. *Social Services Performance Assessment Framework Indicators, 2002–2003*. London: DOH.

39. Age Concern London. 2002. *Access to Primary Care*. Age Concern London Policy Briefing. April.

10. Long-Term Care Facilities in London

Inge Strüder and Tony Warnes

Introduction

Few aspects of Britain's welfare services have changed as much over recent decades as has residential and nursing-home care. Up to the late 1970s, there were many long-stay geriatric nursing homes and wards (and even hospitals) run by the National Health Service (NHS), and local authorities had built up a considerable number of their own residential care homes. But from the early 1980s, successive governments have promoted the involvement of independent (or private sector) proprietors, social housing providers, and voluntary organizations, and discouraged direct NHS and local authority provision. Under the community-care provisions of the 1990 National Health Service and Community Care Act, the new mixed economy of residential care has been consolidated. NHS, and therefore "free," long-term care provision has been curtailed, extending the range of disabilities and care needs that are provided for through means-tested social care. The results have confused and dismayed many older people with chronic impairments and their caregivers. How to pay for long-term care became a juridical and politically contentious issue.

The new Labour administration of 1997 fully appreciated the complexities and sensitivity of the issue and appointed a Royal Commission on the Financing of Long Term Care (1997–1999) to appraise options and make recommendations. After thorough consultation and research, the majority report made the radical proposal that both the "nursing" and "social care" elements of residential care should be free at the point of delivery and financed through general taxation. A dissenting report, heavily influenced by alarmist (and dubious) projections of the likely increase in the prevalence of disability, took the view that the costs would be "insupportable" and should in large part be passed to the residents or users. The government's response was distinctly cool and evasive. It has accepted that nursing care should be free, and accepted the procedural recommendations designed to improve the technical qualities of care. These are being implemented through the Care Standards Act 2000 and the establishment in April 2002 of a more centralized system of quality regulation through a new independent body, the Commission for Social Care Inspection. Interestingly, the newly devolved Scottish Parliament has more fully implemented the royal commission's proposals; in Scotland, personal care in residential homes is free.

Meanwhile, the government is giving high priority to its modernization plans for the NHS.[1] These include the implementation of National Service Frameworks (NSF), one of which concerns older people's services.[2] The NSFs are wide-ranging statements of principles, objectives, and good practice. They have been accompanied by a wide range of "intermediate care" initiatives, designed inter alia to develop support for frail older people in their own homes. These initiatives have affected all sectors of the statutory health and social care services for older people, and have meant that despite a high rate of closure of independent and voluntary homes, the issue has claimed relatively little attention and the government is not responding urgently or with additional funds to maintain the existing level of provision. This chapter takes stock of the changes in residential and nursing-home care provision in London over the last two decades by examining the volume, nature, and locations of current provision and the characteristics of the residents.

Provision in London

The national transformations have been repeated in London and confounded by its high property prices and staff costs. The 1991 census established that London had many fewer nursing-home places per capita than had either large provincial cities or the country as a whole (Table 10.1). As measured by the percentage of persons eight-five and over in such homes, there was a particularly large shortfall in Inner London, where only 6.3 percent were accommodated. The underprovision was slightly compensated by above national rates of those eighty-five and over living in other types of communal establishments—including almshouses and specialized dwellings for independent older people managed by religious organizations and the boroughs.

A King's Fund London Commission study, *The Health Economy of London,* provided additional evidence of trends in residential places between 1985 and 1995 using an analysis by "inner-deprived," "mixed-status," and "high-status" boroughs.[3] The number of places in local authority homes for older people in London's inner-deprived areas decreased by 54 percent over the decade (the fall in the equivalent zones of provincial cities was similar). In London's "mixed-status areas," the number fell by 21 percent, compared to a 33 percent increase in provincial cities; while the available places in London's "high-status areas" hardly changed, compared to an increase of 31 percent in provincial cities.[4] Turning to independent residential care homes, during the decade the available places for older people in England increased by 95 percent. In inner-deprived London, however, the growth was only 10 percent, compared to 136 percent in the equivalent areas of provincial cities. There was a 25 percent increase in London's mixed-status areas and a 38 percent increase in high-status areas, compared to 209 percent and 104 percent respectively in the

Table 10.1. Residence of Persons 65+ in Local Authority Residential Homes and in Nursing Homes, by Age Group and Urban-Area Settlement Type: Great Britain, 1991

	85+ in Nursing Homes		85+ in Other Communal Establishments		75+ in Local Authority Res. Homes	
	%	Ratio	%	Ratio	%	Ratio
Inner London	6.3	0.40	5.9	1.05	2.5	1.09
Outer London	9.3	0.59	5.3	0.93	2.1	0.92
Principal cities[a]	10.6	0.67	6.6	1.16	1.1	0.49
Other metropolitan areas[b]	15.6	0.98	6.7	1.19	3.6	1.55
Great Britain	15.3	1.00	5.7	1.00	2.3	1.00

Source: Lewis, J. and H. Glennerster, 1996. *Implementing the New Community Care*. London: Open University Press, 25.

Notes: Ratio = the percentage in the area to the percentage in Great Britain.

[a] Core authorities of Birmingham, Glasgow, Leeds, Liverpool, Manchester, Newcastle, and Sheffield.

[b] Suburbs of the principal cities and Aberdeen, Bristol, Cardiff, Derby, Edinburgh, Dundee, Hull, Leicester, Nottingham, Plymouth, Portsmouth, South.

provincial cities. Clearly, London's provision has become relatively more deficient over the decade.[5]

Further detail is provided in Lewis and Glennerster's evaluation of the 1993 community-care procedures in four anonymous London boroughs and an adjacent suburban county. The boroughs were chosen "to reflect a cross-section of authorities politically—some strongly supportive of the government's changes, others more traditional, and some marginal politically and in terms of their adherence to the mixed-economy model at the outset."[6] They contain around one-eighth of London's population. The changing balance of the sectors of residential home provision from 1988 to 1993 is tabulated, and a selection of the figures has been entered in Figure 10.1. The columns represent the rate of provision per thousand residents aged sixty-five and over, and show that the overall level of provision remained around eighty-three places per thousand throughout the period. But the composition has changed quickly, with places in the local authority homes decreasing from 59 percent in 1988 to 49 percent in 1993, and the private sector's contribution increasing from 11 percent to 25 percent. Voluntary sector provision was relatively stable at around 30–33 percent.

The changing pattern of ownership and the expansion of provision continued

Figure 10.1. The Changing Composition of Residential Home Places, by Sectors: Four London Boroughs, 1988–1993

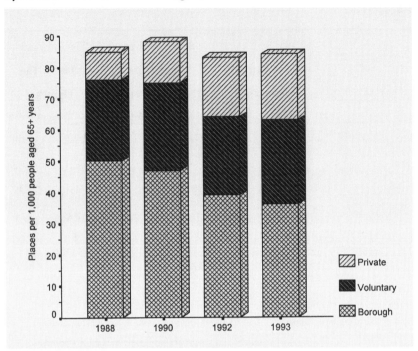

Notes: Residents aged 65+ in homes for elderly and younger physically disabled perople per 1,000 pupulation aged 65+ years as of 31 March in the given years.
Source: Lewis, J. and H. Glennerster. 1996. Implementing the New Community Care. London: Open University Press, 25.

nationally until 1998, but for the next two years there was retrenchment. The annual survey of care provision by the industry market-research group Laing and Buisson found that during 2000, nearly 10,000 places in homes for the elderly and physically disabled were lost, 7,300 in the private and voluntary sector, and 2,500 in local authority–run homes.[7] With other changes in the types and number of residents, there was a net decline of 7,267 places. In the local authority sector, forty-eight homes closed, with a loss of 2,481 places, making a fall of 9,748 for the year.

According to the long-term care providers' associations, the immediate prospect in England and Wales is of increasing costs to meet the raised minimum wage, higher nurse salaries, and staffing and room-standards requirements of the Care Standards Act 2000. In April 2001, the government announced above-inflation increases to meet the fees of residents in homes since before 1993 (they for legal reasons have "preserved rights"). This has been described "as a political gesture and a sign of the government's frustration with the way that local authorities, who are responsible for funding the majority of care-homes residents, distribute cash to care home operators." LCS International Consulting has noted that in the early months of the year, "local authorities across the country set their fee levels for 2001–2002. On an average weighted basis, the increase is hardly 3 percent, or £10–11 per bed per week, insufficient to meet the costs of running a care home or to stem the wave of receiverships [bankruptcies] affecting the sector."[8]

Enumerating Current Provision

Nursing and residential homes have been required by law to be registered and inspected by the health authorities and the local authorities respectively (although residential care homes with three or fewer residents have been subject to less-stringent registration requirements and have not been routinely inspected). To determine the numbers of home and beds within each borough, all thirty-two borough and seventeen health-authority registration authorities in Greater London were contacted.[9] The reference dates vary considerably, from September 2000 to July 2001, for some boroughs update their lists annually and others monthly.

Although the lists identify the homes that care for older people and those that offer convalescent, elderly mentally ill, and elderly mentally handicapped beds, not all homes are exclusively for one age group and a minority operate flexible admissions policies. Age limits varied across the lists. Some of the borough registration units explicitly limit the age of "older" clients to under sixty-five or sixty years and indicate which homes accept people beyond that age. Others use forty-plus years as a client category; all such beds have been included in the count. Some dual-registered homes provide both nursing-home and residential home care, and the relative number of residents in each grade can change from week to week. Consequently, for a minority of homes it is not straightforward to identify the number of places intended for, or occupied by, older people. The number of places for mentally ill or handicapped older people is higher than presented in the table, as some dual-registered homes are dedicated to mentally frail people but not exclusively older people, and others have places for mentally ill residents in generalist homes. Some home descriptions name the categories of clients who are admitted but do not specify the number of places. Another complication arises from the poor descriptions and incomplete registration of very small residential care homes—some are less a business venture than a spontaneous result of the occupier caring first for an elderly relative and then taking in other frail people. The exact addresses on the lists have enabled all the homes to be allocated to the boroughs. Given all these complexities, the estimates of the numbers of homes and beds in various categories are clearly approximations.

Homes and Places in 2001

Throughout Greater London in 2001, there were 749 registered care homes, 288 nursing homes, and 76 dual-registered homes (Table 10.2). The 1,101 homes in all categories provided 32,218 beds, with approximately half in residential care homes. The City of London had no provision, and there was very low provision in the inner boroughs of Hackney, Westminster, Kensington and Chelsea, and Hammersmith and Fulham. The greatest provision was by far in Barnet in northwest Outer London. There were no registered nursing homes in Kensington and Chelsea or Westminster, and three or fewer in Camden, Hammersmith and Fulham, Hackney, Tower Hamlets, Merton, and Richmond upon Thames. Barnet and Croydon had the greatest provision. Most boroughs have only a handful of dual-registered homes, but Croydon had six and Redbridge eight unusually large establishments that provided over 1,400 places. Official statistics presently use five subdivisions of Greater London. They show that there are many more homes and beds in Outer than in Inner London, and that provision is particularly low in the inner west, the area with the highest land and property prices, and that it is highest in the outer northern boroughs.

The variation in provision across London can be further assessed by examining the rates of provision in relation to the local older population. The average age of admission to long-term care has characteristically been around seventy-five to seventy-nine years. Estimates in 1998 of the eighty-year population are available and rates of provision per hundred thousand of the local resident population in this age group are presented in Table 10.3. The boroughs are ranked for each category of provision in this table, and the standard deviations are shown. One should note, however, that rigid catchment areas do not apply, particularly for places in private sector and voluntary organization homes. Some residents of London's institutional homes will have moved from outside the capital and even the country.

For each thousand people aged eighty years or more in Greater London, there were in 2001 64 residential care beds and 41 nursing-home beds. With dual-registered homes, the total was 126. The variation among the thirty-three boroughs was greater for nursing than for residential care homes, although the latter produced the most extreme values, with Barnet and Waltham Forest having very high provision, and Hackney very low. The boroughs with rates of provision that were ±0.5 standard deviations from the borough average have been shaded on Table 10.3. For residential care provision, all the "high-rate" authorities are outer boroughs, and all the "low rate" providers except Hillingdon and Brent are inner boroughs. The inner-outer dichotomy breaks down for nursing homes, with low rates of provision in the outer boroughs of Merton, Richmond upon Thames, Waltham Forest, and Bexley. When all provision including that in dual-registered homes is aggregated, less variation by borough is found. Two boroughs have exceptionally high provision—Barnet with 232 places per thousand, 2.2 times the average, and Redbridge with 274 (sd=3.0). In other words, the long-term residential population in Redbridge equals more than one-quarter of its noninstitutional population eighty years and over.

Implications and Issues

A persistently low rate of provision of nursing homes in the inner areas of London is now being exacerbated by the progressive reduction in the real value of government support (through subsidized fees) for residential care and nursing-home places. The money paid by central government to local authorities as a contribution to the funding of care homes has not been "ring-fenced," leaving local authorities open to the claim of diverting the funds. A representative of the *Coalition for Quality in Care* claimed that "local authorities have been raiding the long-term care budget. The provision of an important service is being very badly mismanaged, bringing hardship to old people and bad value to the taxpayer."[10] The crisis engulfing the care-homes sector intensified during the following months, partly because of the uncertainty caused by a raft of new legislation. Most importantly, the rise in the minimum wage from £3.70 to £4.10 per hour in October 2004, increases in nurses' pay, and adaptations and increased staffing levels to meet the forthcoming standards are expected to add substantially to operators' costs.

A severe shortage of institutional accommodation implies that residential places that do become available are allocated to those with the severest needs, and that many admissions are made under "crisis" circumstances. The cumulative effect is to alter the ambience and functions of the homes. The situation is inimical to achieving a good match between the resident's care needs and the home's services and staff skills. It also militates against informed choice in the selection of an institution that becomes a person's home, and probably increases the average distance between the institutional home and the resident's address of origin (and that of their caregivers and family). No recent studies are known of the experience of those who are unable to be admitted to homes.

The ownership and management of homes has become dominantly "nonstate." The homes now offering care vary immensely in size, location, ambience, and—it has to be said—quality of care. A persistent problem for the potential residents and their families is the difficulty of obtaining consistent, systematized information about the services that these diverse homes offer. As a study of thirty recent placements in Sheffield discovered, "the complexity of UK funding arrangements produces high levels of anxiety for older people and their families about whether they will be able to afford to move into their home of choice." The authors concluded that "there is an urgent need to examine the ways in which health and social care staff can better support relatives when they are helping an older person to relocate."[11]

The severe shortage of residential and nursing-home accommodation may also be harming the efficiency of acute services by delaying discharge. In response to a 2001 Audit Commission report on lengthening waiting times for treatment in accident and emergency departments (emergency rooms)—in which London's hospitals performed far worse than those in the rest of the country—Dr. Liam Fox, the opposition health secretary, said that "the loss of 50,000 beds in the care home

Table 10.2. Residential Care and Nursing-Home Provision: London, March 2001

Borough	Residential Homes		Nursing Homes		Dual-Registered		Total	
	Homes	Beds	Homes	Beds	Homes	Beds	Homes	Beds
Camden	17	349	3	78	1	61	21	488
Hammer' & Fulham	6	160	2	140	0	0	8	300
Kensington & Chelsea	7	265	3	110	1	82	8	347
Wandsworth	18	311	6	315	5	307	29	933
Westminster	5	204	1	39	1	110	6	314
Hackney	4	50	3	126	2	108	9	284
Haringey	20	553	6	202	0	0	26	755
Islington	10	198	4	151	1	60	15	409
Lambeth	20	323	11	403	3	85	34	811
Lewisham	44	434	19	570	4	170	67	1163
Newham	11	281	6	334	1	21	15	543
Southwark	12	308	10	356	1	81	23	745
Tower Hamlets	7	206	1	27	1	51	10	284
Barking & Dagenham	12	451	4	186	2	191	18	828
Bexley	11	388	4	141	4	377	19	906
Enfield	35	806	14	641	1	32	50	1479
Greenwich	15	461	9	498	2	170	26	1129
Havering	34	947	14	539	2	83	50	1569
Redbridge	27	640	8	389	8	1441	43	2470

Waltham Forest	34	956	12	37	1	25	36	1018
Bromley	48	1067	16	592	2	134	66	1793
Croydon	45	945	26	832	6	269	77	2046
Kingston/Thames	34	450	9	369	1	39	44	848
Merton	31	433	3	133	5	181	49	749
Sutton	30	565	10	300	4	141	44	1006
Barnet	60	1868	24	820	5	378	89	3066
Brent	23	283	11	389	4	270	38	942
Ealing	45	687	12	453	1	6	58	1146
Harrow	33	529	19	509	2	131	45	1169
Hillingdon	17	430	13	440	2	106	32	976
Hounslow	13	380	7	385	0	0	20	765
Richmond/Thames	21	606	2	114	3	217	26	937
Inner London	181	3642	75	2851	21	1136	275	7525
Inner West	53	1289	15	682	8	560	76	2531
Inner East	128	2353	60	2169	13	576	199	4994
Outer London	568	12892	217	7767	55	4191	830	24842
Outer East & Northeast	168	4649	65	2431	20	2319	242	9399
Outer South	188	3460	64	2226	18	764	280	6442
Outer West & Northwest	212	4783	88	3110	17	1108	308	9001
Greater London	749	16534	292	10618	76	5327	1105	32367

Table 10.3. Rates of Long-Term Care Provision for Persons 80+ (per 1,000): London Boroughs, 1998

Residential Homes	Beds		Nursing Homes	Beds		Total (Including Dual)	Beds	
	Rate	sd		Rate	sd		Rate	sd
Barnet	**141.5**	**2.8**	**Croydon**	**78.5**	**1.7**	**Redbridge**	**274.4**	**3.1**
Waltham Forest	**124.2**	**2.2**	**Lewisham**	**73.1**	**1.4**	**Barnet**	**232.3**	**2.2**
Havering	**110.1**	**1.6**	**Greenwich**	**67.3**	**1.2**	**Croydon**	**193.0**	**1.4**
Haringey	**97.0**	**1.2**	**Kingston/Thames**	**64.7**	**1.1**	**Havering**	**182.4**	**1.2**
Croydon	**89.2**	**0.9**	**Brent**	**63.8**	**1.0**	**Brent**	**154.4**	**0.6**
Bromley	**82.7**	**0.7**	**Havering**	**62.7**	**1.0**	Greenwich	152.6	0.5
Kingston/Thames	78.9	0.5	**Barnet**	**62.1**	**0.9**	Kingston/Thames	150.5	0.5
Barking & Dagenham	77.8	0.5	**Newham**	**60.7**	**0.9**	Lewisham	150.5	0.5
Sutton	77.4	0.5	**Enfield**	**59.9**	**0.8**	Barking & Dagenham	142.8	0.3
Ealing	77.2	0.5	**Harrow**	**59.9**	**0.8**	Bromley	139.0	0.3
Richmond/Thames	75.8	0.4	**Lambeth**	**58.4**	**0.8**	Enfield	138.2	0.2
Enfield	75.3	0.4	**Hounslow**	**56.6**	**0.7**	Sutton	137.8	0.2
Redbridge	71.1	0.2	**Southwark**	**54.8**	**0.6**	Harrow	137.5	0.2
Merton	64.6	0.0	Ealing	50.9	0.4	Haringey	132.5	0.1
Greenwich	62.3	-0.1	Hillingdon	47.8	0.3	Waltham Forest	132.2	0.1
Harrow	62.2	-0.1	Bromley	45.9	0.2	Ealing	128.8	0.0
Hounslow	55.9	-0.3	Redbridge	43.2	0.1	Lambeth	117.5	-0.2
Lewisham	55.6	-0.3	Sutton	41.1	0.0	Richmond/Thames	117.1	-0.2
Camden	52.1	-0.4	Wandsworth	36.2	-0.3	Newham	115.6	-0.2
Newham	51.1	-0.5	Haringey	35.4	-0.3	Southwark	114.6	-0.3

Area		sd
Kensington & Chelsea	**48.2**	**-0.6**
Southwark	**47.4**	**-0.6**
Tower Hamlets	**46.8**	**-0.6**
Lambeth	**46.8**	**-0.6**
Hillingdon	**46.7**	**-0.6**
Brent	**46.4**	**-0.6**
Bexley	**46.2**	**-0.7**
Islington	**39.6**	**-0.9**
Wandsworth	**35.7**	**-1.0**
Hamm & Fulham	**35.6**	**-1.0**
Westminster	**27.6**	**-1.3**
Hackney	**9.6**	**-2.0**
Inner W	**39.3**	**-0.9**
Inner E	50.1	-0.5
Outer E & NE	**80.7**	**0.6**
Outer S	**80.1**	**0.6**
Outer W & NW	78.8	0.5
Inner London	**45.5**	**-0.7**
Outer London	**79.8**	**0.6**
Greater London	**68.5**	

Area		sd
Barking & Dagenham	32.1	-0.5
Hamm & Fulham	31.1	-0.5
Islington	30.2	-0.5
Hackney	**24.2**	**-0.8**
Kensington & Chelsea	**20.0**	**-1.0**
Merton	**19.9**	**-1.0**
Bexley	**16.8**	**-1.2**
Richmond/Thames	**14.3**	**-1.3**
Camden	**11.6**	**-1.4**
Tower Hamlets	**6.1**	**-1.6**
Westminster	**5.3**	**-1.7**
Waltham Forest	**4.8**	**-1.7**
Inner W	**20.8**	**-1.0**
Inner E	46.1	0.2
Outer E & NE	42.2	0.0
Outer S	51.5	0.4
Outer W & NW	51.2	0.4
Inner London	**35.7**	**-0.3**
Outer London	**48.1**	**0.3**
Greater London	**44.0**	

Area		sd
Hounslow	112.5	-0.3
Merton	111.5	-0.3
Bexley	107.9	-0.4
Wandsworth	107.2	-0.4
Hillingdon	106.1	-0.4
Kensington & Chelsea	**83.1**	**-0.9**
Islington	**81.8**	**-0.9**
Camden	**72.8**	**-1.1**
Hamm & Fulham	**66.7**	**-1.3**
Tower Hamlets	**64.5**	**-1.3**
Hackney	**54.6**	**-1.5**
Westminster	**47.7**	**-1.6**
Inner W	**77.2**	**-1.0**
Inner E	108.5	-0.4
Outer E & NE	**163.2**	**0.8**
Outer S	149.3	0.5
Outer W & NW	148.3	0.4
Inner London	**95.6**	**-0.7**
Outer London	**153.9**	**0.6**
Greater London	**134.6**	

Note: sd = standard deviation of the borough from the average for Greater London. Bold type indicates those areas where the sd is greater than 0.5.

sector has made it more difficult to discharge patients into the community" and implied that this contributed to the delays in admitting patients from accident and emergency departments.[12]

These increases have been sanctioned by the government, but additional funds are not made available for care-home operators. While currently there are numerous "intermediate care" innovations to increase the support of sick and vulnerable older people in their own homes, their scale is unlikely to compensate for recent reductions in both residential provision and "low-intensity" social service support. The implications of the rapid reduction in provision and of continuation of the trend for both the welfare of frail older people and the good functioning of the social and health-care delivery system require urgent examination. Circumstances have conspired during the last five years to discourage the government, the Department of Health, and regional and local health-service planners to give much attention to residential and nursing-home care. There is perhaps a widespread view that these services are no longer the responsibility of the public health and social service agencies. The absence of coordinated planning gives signs of producing mounting adverse effects on frail and dependent older people, and on other sectors of the health-service system.

Notes

1. Department of Health. 1999. The Modernisation Plan for the NHS in London, 1999–2002. London: DOH.
2. Department of Health. 2001. National Service Framework for Older People. London: Stationery Office.
3. London's social geography does not follow a simple pattern. The innermost boroughs include both wealthy and low-income boroughs (e.g., respectively, Westminster and Tower Hamlets). Similarly the southwestern and northwestern sectors of Outer London are relatively affluent, but the eastern and southern are (largely) not; Boyle, Sean, and Richard Hamblin. 1997. The Health Economy of London. A report to the King's Fund London Commission. London: King's Fund, 237–242.
4. Ibid., Table 2, 238.
5. Ibid., Table 3, 239.
6. Lewis, Jane, and Howard Glennerster. 1996. Implementing the New Community Care. London: Open University Press, 25.
7. Hawkes, N. 2001. Care Home Places Lost. The Times, April 19; Laing and Buisson. 2001. Community Care Market News. London: Laing and Buisson.
8. Court, M. 2001. Care Home Crisis Hit Young and Old Alike. The Times, April 6.
9. Their cooperation in sending lists of registered homes is acknowledged. The Department of Health collates the numbers of establishments and beds each year; the figures for March 31, 2000, were published in Community Care Statistics 2000 in February 2001 for the registration-authority areas (see www.doh.gov.uk/public/sb0028.htm). To establish figures of the two types of homes for the boroughs, an independent tabulation

for the local authorities has been carried out. The provisional tables were sent to the various registration authorities for verification. The presented figures are, however, entirely the authors' responsibility.

10. Court, Care Home Crisis.

11. Davies, S., J. Sandberg, and U. Lundh. 2000. The Entry to a Nursing Home: Residents' and Relatives' Experiences. In A. M. Warnes, L. Warren, and M. Nolan, eds. Care Services for Later Life: Tramsformations and Critiques, 152–170. London: Jessica Kingsley. Quote, p. 168.

12. BBC Radio 4. 2001. Today. October 25.

11. Living Arrangements and Housing among Older People in London

Tony Warnes and Inge Strüder

Introduction

"When a man is tired of London he is tired of life; for there is in London all that life can afford." Samuel Johnson's familiar quotation of 1777 aptly poses an issue about the relation between contemporary cities and the older population, men and women. On ceasing formal employment, do retired people find capital or world cities inimical to or supportive of the lifestyles and activities that they wish to pursue? They spend more time at home than people who work and may feel keenly the restricted space of the city's housing. Do the high rates of crime, population and traffic densities, and levels of noise and atmospheric pollution outweigh the advantages of plentiful retail and transport services, commercial entertainments, cultural institutions, and voluntary associations? In particular, do the exceptional housing costs and the scarcity of houses with gardens (as opposed to apartments) persuade older and retired people to shun world cities? Empirical evidence from London and Paris suggests that for large numbers they do, for as many as one-quarter of those passing through retirement have been leaving Greater London over at least the last thirty years.[1]

This chapter examines the household and housing characteristics of older people in London. It is based on evidence from the *Census of Population* for 1991 and 2001, which enables variation by electoral wards to be examined. Data from the 1998–1999 *General Household Survey* (GHS) are also examined to establish trends during the 1990s; while its sample size of 301 pensioner households in London is too small to examine the variation by borough, analyses by ethnic group, deprivation, and health measures are possible.

Some explanation of special features of British housing markets and data will be helpful. Many UK official statistics on older people tabulate data for the "pensioner population," which for many decades has been and until 2010 is statutorily defined as women aged sixty years and more, and men aged sixty-five years and more.[2] As in all countries, "public" and "social" housing have specific features. Between the 1890s and the 1970s, the United Kingdom built more public housing than did any other western European country, and some London boroughs were in the lead. During the last twenty-five years, however, new building has ceased and many properties have been sold to their occupiers through a "right-to-buy" principle. The remaining public housing is owned by local government authorities—in London, the boroughs and the City of London—but increasingly managed by commercial companies.[3] Since the 1970s, other types of non-profit-making "social housing" providers have been stimulated by the Housing Corporation, a government funding agency, mostly through nonprofit "housing associations" that provide dwellings for rental and partial equity sale. As in all countries, private landlords range from large property-management companies to individuals who rent single properties or rooms. A small fraction of dwellings is provided by employers to employees (as for caretakers and in hotels) and is often described as "tied" accommodation. Another important characteristic of London's housing is its high cost. In 2002, the average price of a dwelling in Greater London was £241k, compared to £148k throughout England.[4] The average price had risen by 19 percent during the previous year.

The Changing Urban Distribution of the Population

Greater London's population decreased from 1920 to 1980, and the rates of decline after 1940 were high.[5] During the 1980s, however, the all-age population stabilized, and during the 1990s it grew through an increase in the population of working age.[6] The growth has continued, from 6.8 million in 1991 to 7.3 million in 2001. The pensionable population continued to fall, from 1.22 million in 1971 to 1.07 million in 1991 (by 1.1 percent a year during the 1990s) and 1.03 million in 2001. The total doubles if the outer suburbs (Outer Metropolitan Area) are incorporated (Table 11.1). From 1991 to 2001, there was a marked reversal of the decline in Inner London, but despite the increase of around 56,000, the pensionable share declined from 15.4 to 11.5 percent because younger age groups grew even faster.

As recently as 1981, a larger percentage of London's (17.9) than of Great Britain's (17.7) population was of pensionable age, but in the last two decades the positions have reversed. The 2001 census showed that London's pensioner population had fallen to 1.03 million, just 14.2 per cent of the total, only 0.78 of the national percentage. And although during the first decade of this century there will be slight growth (a result of the high birth rates in the 1940s), the older population will continue to fall as a share of the total (Table 11.2). Only during the 2010s will the "elderly share" in London return to the level of the 1970s. By 2021, 16.0 per cent of the city's population will be in the (soon to be revised) pensionable age groups, 0.70 of the national percentage. The relative rejuvenation of London's population has come about through the high fertility of its recent in-migrants and its attraction for young adult national and international migrants, but the out-migration of the later working-aged and older people themselves makes a substantial contribution. It is estimated that during 1999, 12,600 (9,600 net) people aged fifty-five to sixty-four years left the city, and 15,400 (11,000 net) aged sixty-five years or more.[7] If the 1.2 percent annual *net* rate for the older population applied from fifty-five to seventy-four years, more than a quarter (26.9 percent) of the survivors through these ages would leave the city.

Table 11.1. Distribution of Pensioners: Greater London Region, 1971–2001

	Number (thousands)				Share of Total Population (%)				Location Quotients[a]			
	1971	1981	1991	2001	1971	1981	1991	2001	1971	1981	1991	2001
Inner London[b]	375	335	273	329	16.1	17.5	15.4	11.5	1.05	1.04	0.91	0.82
Outer London[c]	849	866	801	702	16.5	18.0	17.3	15.7	1.07	1.07	1.03	1.12
Greater London	1,224	1,201	1,074	1,032	16.4	17.9	16.8	14.0	1.07	1.06	1.00	1.00
Outer Metro Area[d]	720	836	922		14.0	15.5	16.9		0.91	0.92	1.00	
London Metro Area	944	2,036	1,996		15.4	16.8	16.9		1.00	1.00	1.00	

Source: Population Censuses of England and Wales (because there was significant underenumeration in the 1991 census, especially of adolescents and minority ethnic groups, the 1991 figures have been revised) for 2001, *Region in Figures: London*, Table 2.12 (available online from Office for National Statistics Web site).

[a] Ratio of the zone percentage to the percentage for the entire Metropolitan Area; in 2001, for the GLA only

[b] Approximates to the area of the London County Council (1889–1965) and extends approximately 10 km from the center over the 1914 built-up area

[c] Remainder of the former Greater London Council (1965–86), now the Greater London Authority (2000–) area, extends to about 25 km from the center, approximately the 1939 built-up area

[d] A statistical entity only, includes London's greenbelt and the commuter towns and suburbs beyond, to about 65 km from the center

Table 11.2. Estimates and Projections for Men 65+ and Women 60+: Greater London, 1999–2021

	Number (thousands)			Share of Total Population (%)			Location Quotients[a]		
	1999	2011	2021	1999	2011	2021	1999	2011	2021
Inner London	360			12.8			0.71		
Outer London	703			15.7			0.87		
Greater London	1,063	1,068	1,021	14.6	14.3	16.0	0.81	0.73	0.72

Source: ONS (2001). *Region in Figures: London.* London, HMSO. Table 6.4.

[a] Ratio of the zone percentage to the percentage for the entire Metropolitan Area

Pensioner Household Trends during the 1990s

In 1991 in Greater London, 833,138 households contained at least one pensioner, 30.2 percent of all households in the city. The variation by borough was from 24 percent in high-status, inner-west Kensington and Chelsea, to 38 percent in low-status Barking and Dagenham (the most easterly Thames north-bank borough). More generally, the percentage was low in many inner boroughs and high in most of the outer boroughs (Table 11.3).

Table 11.3. Distance of Pensioner Households from Center: London Boroughs and Greater London, 1991

| | | | % of Pensioner Households | |
	Distance from Center (km)	% of All Households	Owner-Occupied	Public Housing
Highest percentages				
Barking and Dagenham	18.5	37.7	43.3	51.8
Havering	25.8	34.2	71.9	21.0
Bromley	20.1	34.2	73.6	14.8
Barnet	13.1	33.6	68.9	16.8
Redbridge	16.4	33.6	74.8	15.9
Harrow	17.4	33.3	75.6	13.0
Lowest percentages				
Islington	4.0	26.9	18.1	62.5
City of London	2.5	26.7	37.4	41.0
Hackney	6.0	26.3	18.3	59.7
Hammersmith and Fulham	6.4	25.7	31.4	34.7
Lambeth	6.0	25.5	30.5	43.6
Haringey	8.5	24.8	45.6	33.4
Kensington and Chelsea	4.4	24.2	38.1	19.5
Greater London	N/A	30.2	53.0	29.8

Source: Census of Population of England and Wales 1991, accessed through University of Manchester national online data depository.

Household Size and Type

Nearly one-half (47.7 percent) of London's pensioner households in 1991 were people living alone: 308,000 were women, three and one-half times the number of men (Table 11.4). Although this percentage is higher than the national average, it is matched by the shares in both remote rural districts (as in most of Wales and southwest England) and in coastal retirement areas.[8] The higher the age, the greater the imbalance, so the 40,000 women aged eighty-five or more years who lived alone was five times the number of men. A quarter (24.8 percent) of all pensioner households comprised exclusively two or more pensioners, and 27.5 percent also contained younger people (in many cases, of course, a spouse).

Older people's household types vary markedly in different parts of the city, the strongest feature being the high prevalence of relatively young (sixty/sixty-five to seventy-four years) older people living alone in the central boroughs, especially of men in the City of London (Table 11.4), and of women in the City of Westminster and Camden (the borough to the north of Westminster, which extends into the center in Bloomsbury). In the City of London, these households accounted for a quarter of older people's households (and 8.7 percent of all households). The occupiers include service staff (caretakers, security personnel, and caterers), senior company managers working beyond the statutory retirement age (many of whom will have other homes, the address being a pied à terre), widows, and widowers.

The single-person percentage of all pensioner households declines regularly with distance from the center of the city, and linear relationships are found for both men (r_{xy} = 0.87) and women (r_{xy} = –0.63), the only aberrant value being the exceptionally high percentage of single male pensioner households in the City of London (Figure 11.1).[9] The other clear geographical variation is in the proportion of pensioner households of two or more without younger people, which is low in Inner London and high in the outer zone.

The exceptionally high number of households with *both* pensioners and non-pensioners in Brent, a northwestern borough that straddles the inner and outer city, suggests a high relative frequency of two-generation households. The borough has late-nineteenth-century housing areas, as in Willesden and Harlesden, and 1930s speculatively built housing estates, as in Wembley, as well as high representations of residents from Ireland, the Caribbean, and India. By the 1970s, many of the oc-cupiers of the 1930s housing were in the older age groups (many having been the first occupiers), and a wholesale turnover of the population had begun, as many young immigrant families moved in.[10]

The high ratios of households of two or more pensioner *without younger people* in the outer boroughs of Barnet, Harrow, Bromley, and Havering can be associated with their high socioeconomic status and extensive low-density residential areas of high environmental quality. Not only do they have many detached and semi-detached (duplex) houses, but also the favorable survival rates of upper-income groups keep

Table 11.4. Household Status of Pensioners, by Age Group and Gender: London Boroughs, 1991 (in percents)

	km[a]	1 Man			1 Woman			2+ pensioners		Others
		<75	75–84	85+	<75	75–84	85+	all <75	any 75+	any 75+
Greater London		5.6	4.1	1.0	17.6	14.7	4.7	13.4	11.4	27.5
Inner London[b]		1.33	1.12	1.00	1.10	1.02	1.03	0.82	0.85	0.98
Outer London[b]		0.81	0.93	1.00	0.94	0.99	0.98	1.10	1.08	1.01
Borough[c]										
Westminster	2.4	1.58	1.21	1.13	**1.22**	**1.13**	1.16	0.66	0.86	0.84
City of London	2.5	**2.29**	**1.30**	**2.37**	1.13	***0.86***	***0.76***	0.98	0.96	***0.71***
Camden	3.9	1.44	1.21	1.06	**1.22**	1.10	**1.23**	0.71	0.85	0.85
Islington	4.0	1.44	1.09	1.17	1.15	0.97	0.94	0.82	1.00	1.00
Kensington & Chelsea	4.4	1.45	1.10	1.05	**1.38**	1.10	1.17	***0.64***	***0.77***	***0.84***
Tower Hamlets	6.5	1.58	1.14	0.88	1.05	0.92	0.93	0.91	***0.75***	1.04
Southwark	6.6	1.39	1.17	***0.82***	1.09	1.00	0.93	0.92	0.82	0.97
Brent	11.0	1.01	1.01	1.06	***0.86***	***0.87***	0.84	0.84	0.98	**1.26**
Waltham Forest	12.2	0.91	1.06	1.19	0.92	1.12	**1.22**	0.99	1.11	0.91
Barnet	13.1	0.73	0.95	1.06	0.92	1.02	1.00	1.01	**1.23**	1.00
Harrow	17.4	***0.66***	0.83	1.09	***0.80***	1.06	1.07	1.02	**1.25**	1.06
Bromley	20.1	***0.70***	0.83	0.89	0.98	0.98	0.99	1.29	1.09	0.93
Havering	25.8	0.74	***0.77***	0.85	0.95	***0.86***	***0.76***	**1.50**	0.96	1.02

Source: Census of Population of England and Wales 1991, accessed through University of Manchester national online data depository.

Note: Figures in bold type are the highest ratios for each tenure; figures in bold italic type are the lowest.

[a] Kilometers from city center (Trafalgar Square)

[b] Percent as ratio of Greater London figure

[c] Boroughs with highest and lowest ratios to Greater London

Figure 11.1. Single-Pensioner Households by Distance from City Center, London Boroughs, 1991

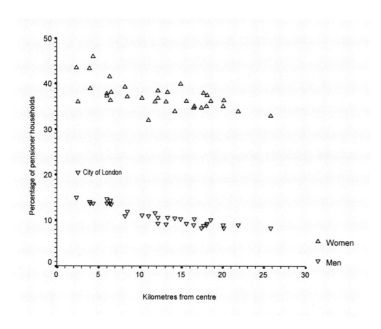

Source: Census of Population of England and Wales 1991.

married and partnered-couple households together to a greater age than in low-income areas. The inner-west boroughs also have high-income areas (as in Mayfair, Knightsbridge, and South Kensington), as we have seen with above-average shares of single-women pensioner households, but they have the lowest ratios of two-plus pensioner households. Low-status boroughs, like Tower Hamlets and Southwark, have overrepresentations of young pensioner households, and underrepresentations of the oldest households.

Pensioner Households in 2001

During the 1990s, the escalation of London's house prices and the conversion of its dwellings from privately rented to owner occupation continued (Figure 11.2). The trends during the 1990s in older people's households can be described from the 1998–1999 *General Household Survey.* It appears that the representation of single-person pensioner households fell during the decade, particularly those of people aged seventy-five or more years (Table 11.5). But one-person female households still formed a substantially higher percentage of all pensioner households in London than in Great Britain. Table 11.6 presents a tabulation of 2001 census data, which shows that 555,266 households, 18.2 percent of the total in Greater London, were comprised of pensioners only. Of these, 69.6 percent were of just one person. The relatively few older-people households in London is demonstrated by the fact that in England and Wales, 23.8 percent of all households were formed exclusively by pensioners. The "deficit" in London is greatest among pensioner households of two or more persons, for they formed 39.4 percent of all-pensioner households in England and Wales, compared to 30.4 percent in London.

Tenure

London's housing stock has relatively few (semi-) detached houses and owner-occupied properties and, the complement, many apartments and privately rented homes. The last forty years have seen radical changes in the tenure pattern (partly reversing the increase of public housing up to 1980).[11] In 1961, 63 percent of Inner London's households rented from a private landlord, but by 1991 the percentage had halved (Figure 11.2). In the Greater London Area (GLA), private rented dwellings formed 16 percent of all households in 1993, since when the figure has not changed. Turning to public housing, it peaked in Inner London around 1981 at 43 percent of all households, but had fallen to 16 percent throughout the GLA by 2003. It is owner occupation that has grown strongly, in Outer London to 70 percent of all households by 1991, and in the GLA to 59 percent of all dwellings in 2003 (Figure 11.2). "London is now characterised by a large and growing number of high income earners . . .who have substantial sums to put into the housing market [and their] purchasing power is able to outgun other groups, . . . leading to a growth of 'socio-tenurial polarisation.' The process involves the concentration of the less skilled, unemployed and low-paid workers . . . into what remains of the council [borough] rented sector."[12] Formerly, older people were to an extent protected from the full

Table 11.5. Pensioner Household Status, by Age and Gender: Greater London, Great Britain, 1991–1999 (in percents)

| | Male | | Female | | | Total in |
	65–74	75+	60–74	75+	Others	Thousands
Greater London, 1991	5.6	5.1	17.6	19.4	52.3	
Greater London, 1999	5.0	3.3	16.3	15.6	59.8	301
Great Britain, 1999	4.5	4.2	12.3	13.1	65.8	3,759
Ratio GL:GB, 1999	1.10	0.79	1.32	1.19	0.91	

Sources: Census of Population of England and Wales 1991; Office of National Statistics online Table KS20N Household composition (London); General Household Survey 1998/99.

rigors of London's competitive housing market by both "controlled rents" and a relatively abundant supply of public housing. Those on low incomes and without assets do qualify for housing benefit (a Social Security benefit), but some find it stigmatizing and the take-up rates are low.

Among pensioner households in 1991, just over one-half (53 percent) were in owner occupation, 30 percent in public housing, and 10 percent in rentals from private landlords (Figure 11.2). Public housing provision was generally highest toward the center, and the prevalence of owner occupation highest toward the periphery (Figure 11.3). Socioeconomic and cohort-succession influences can also be identified. The former were expressed through much of the twentieth century by the enthusiasm for public housing in working-class (Labour) boroughs and lack of investment by affluent (Conservative) boroughs. The result by 1991 was that public housing was most abundant in the inner eastern and southeastern boroughs of Hackney, Islington, Tower Hamlets, and Southwark, while in Kensington and Chelsea there was little provision (Figure 11.3). Similarly in Outer London, while public housing provision was generally low, the extensive estates built by the London County Council (LCC) disturbed the general pattern. The largest, Becontree in Barking and Dagenham, was begun in the 1920s and built for working-class East Enders.[13] It was extended after World War II, partly to replace the housing lost during the war (in some dockland areas, two-thirds of the housing had been blitzed). There were similar but smaller interwar LCC estates scattered across the outer boroughs, as at Bellingham and Downham (Lewisham), St. Mary Cray (Bromley), Morden (Merton), Roehampton

Figure 11.2. The Changing Tenure of Housing: Greater London, 1961–2003

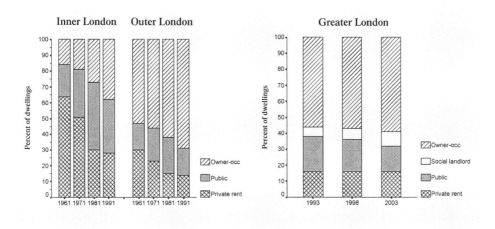

Source: Censuses of Population of England and Wales: 1961, 1971, 1981, and 1991; ONS. 2003. Region in Figures: London. Stationery Office, London, Table 6.4.

(Wandsworth), and Watling (Barnet). The cohort dimension is revealed in the areas that were first settled during the 1950s and 1960s, for by 1991 they had considerable overrepresentations of older households. In 1991, 37.7 percent of Barking and Dagenham's households included pensioners, a quarter above the Greater London percentage, and 52 percent of them were in public housing.

Privately rented, housing-association tenant, and "tied" pensioner households are much more concentrated in particular parts of the city than are either of the two predominant tenures, and in all three cases they are especially found in the inner city (Table 11.7). Tied accommodations are a special feature of the City of London (the majority are likely to be for porters and security staff, but beefeaters at the Tower of London add to the number). Privately rented accommodation is most concentrated in the high-status inner-west boroughs of the City of Westminster and Kensington and Chelsea. It is a surprising fact that housing-association pensioner households are relatively scarce in the low-income outer boroughs: as investment in public housing has declined in these areas, the provision of social housing through housing-association investment has not correspondingly grown. While the spatial association between public housing and this alternative social housing tenure is positive, the correlation is weak and insignificant (r=0.4). Housing-association properties are consistently low in the northeastern quadrant, from inner low-status Tower

Figure 11.3. Owner-Occupied and Public Housing Pensioner Households, London Boroughs, 1991

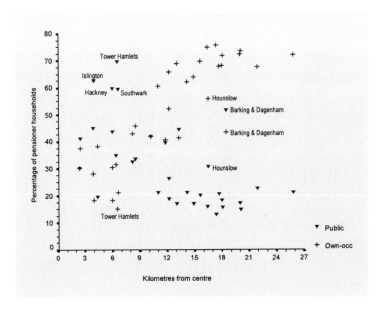

Source: Census of Population of England and Wales, 1991.

Table 11.6. Households with Pensioners:
Greater London, England and Wales, 2001 (in percents)

	Single Pensioner	One Family, All Pensioners	Others, All Pensioners	Others[a]	Total in Thousands
Greater London	12.7	5.4	0.4	81.6	3,016
England & Wales	14.4	9.0	0.4	76.2	21,660
Ratio: GL:E&W	0.88	0.60	0.91	1.07	

Sources: Census of Population of England and Wales 2001; Office of National Statistics online Table KS20N Household composition (London); *General Household Survey 1998/99.*
[a] Households with both pensioners and younger people

Hamlets to outer low-status Barking and Dagenham and mid/high-status Havering and Redbridge. The very high percentages of housing-association households in the high-status inner-west boroughs reflect a more general pattern across the city, of a positive correlation between the prevalence of these households and those that are in privately rented dwellings (Table 11.8).

Tenure by Household Size and Type

The evidence is therefore of several broad patterns in the tenures occupied by different types of pensioner households. Housing-association and privately rented properties largely accommodate single-person households, especially of the oldest age groups. The most overrepresented group in housing-association dwellings is lone women aged eighty-five or more years (with a ratio of 1.68 to their percentage in all tenures). By contrast, in privately rented tenancies, the greatest overrepresentation is of lone men aged eighty-five or more years (ratio 1.64 to all tenures) (Table 11.9). The orientation of public housing is also toward single-person households but less strongly, perhaps because of the lower socioeconomic status of its tenants, their lower life expectancy, and the alternative accommodation that the boroughs have until recently provided in residential care homes. The complement of the special role of social housing in providing accommodation for one-person pensioner households is that two-person-plus pensioner households are strongly overrepresented in owner-occupied housing, especially when the householder is less than seventy-five years of age.

Table 11.7. Tenure of Older People's Households: Greater London and Boroughs, 1991

	km[a]	Owner Occupied	Privately Rented	Tied[b]		Housing	
				Unfurnished	Furnished	Association	Borough
Greater London (%)		53.0	1.5	8.1	1.0	6.6	29.8
Inner London[c]		0.59	1.37	1.31	1.42	1.62	1.47
Outer London[c]		1.23	0.79	0.83	0.76	0.65	0.73
Boroughs[d]							
City of Westminster	2.4	0.57	2.69	2.19	2.37	2.36	1.01
City of London	2.5	0.71	1.61	1.30	5.57	0.45	1.38
Islington	4.0	0.34	0.89	0.76	1.26	1.61	2.10
Kensington and Chelsea	4.4	0.72	3.62	2.05	2.20	2.75	0.65
Hackney	6.0	0.35	1.04	0.90	1.54	1.76	2.00
Hammersmith and Fulham	6.4	0.59	1.78	2.10	1.08	1.98	1.17
Tower Hamlets	6.5	0.29	0.31	0.42	1.91	1.43	2.34
Southwark	6.6	0.40	0.52	0.88	1.36	1.56	1.99
Greenwich	13.3	0.78	0.41	0.76	1.03	0.97	1.50
Enfield	15.6	1.31	0.59	0.77	0.69	0.38	0.67
Redbridge	16.4	1.41	0.84	0.68	0.63	0.30	0.53
Harrow	17.4	1.43	0.84	0.80	0.67	0.45	0.44
Sutton	17.7	1.28	0.61	0.61	0.78	0.74	0.69
Kingston upon Thames	18.1	1.35	0.83	0.91	0.75	0.49	0.52
Barking and Dagenham	18.5	0.82	0.25	0.24	1.00	0.23	1.74
Bexley	20.0	1.36	0.41	0.68	0.45	0.64	0.57

Bromley	20.1	**1.39**	0.58	0.61	0.78	0.76	0.50
Havering	25.8	**1.36**	***0.40***	***0.44***	***0.57***	***0.36***	0.71

Source: Census of Population of England and Wales 1991, accessed through University of Manchester online national data depository.

Note: Figures in bold type are the highest ratios for each tenure; figures in bold italic type are the lowest.

[a] Kilometers from city center (Trafalgar Square)
[b] "Tied" housing is provided by employers to employees
[c] Percent as ratio of Greater London figure
[d] Boroughs with highest and lowest ratios to Greater London

Table 11.8. Associations between Tenure and Ownership Status of Older People's Households: London Boroughs, 1991

Tenure	Owner Occupied	Rented from			
		Tied	Housing Association	Borough	Private Owner
Owner-occupied	1.00	-	-	-	-
Tied	-0.49[a]	1.00	-	-	-
Rented from:					
Housing association	-0.73[b]	0.26	1.00	-	-
Borough	-0.90[b]	0.36	0.40	1.00	-
Private owner	-0.34	0.37	0.72[b]	-0.09	1.00

[a] Correlation significant at the 0.01 level (Pearson two-tailed correlation coefficient)
[b] Correlation significant at the 0.001 level (Pearson two-tailed correlation coefficient)

Living Densities and Amenities

Space standards, housing amenities, and the standards of maintenance of British housing have improved immensely in recent decades. Broadly, it is no longer the case that poor housing is associated with older occupants. London has shared in these national trends, but, of course, poor-quality housing has not been eliminated (it tends now to be associated with recent, low-income immigrant groups, as in Tower Hamlets). First, there is an unsurprising inner-outer dimension to the prevalence of *relatively* high densities of persons per room (ppr; this once closely monitored index does not count pantries, small kitchens, lavatories, or bathrooms as inhabited rooms). Figure 11.4 shows the clear association between distance from the center and the percentage of pensioner households living at densities of more than 0.5 ppr. Only the atypically high prevalence (38 percent) in the City of London departed from a remarkably regular linear trend. Up to eight kilometers from the center, over a quarter of pensioner households lived at these relatively high room densities.

Among the 783 electoral wards in Greater London in 1991, there was inevitably

Figure 11.4. Prevalence of High Living Densities and Poor Housing Amenities among Pensioner Households by Distance from Center: London Boroughs, 1991

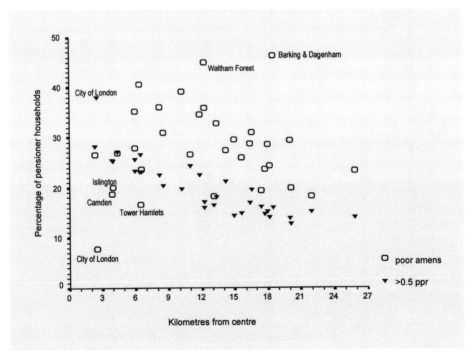

Source: Census of Population of England and Wales, 1991.

Note: >0.5 ppr – average room density more than 0.5 persons per inhabited room (excluding bathrooms and pantries). Poor housing amenities – Lack or shared use of bath/shower and/or inside lavatory (water closet) and/or central heating.

a great deal more variation in living densities and amenity standards than among the boroughs. Excluding the City of London's tiny wards that had none, the average number of pensioner households in a ward was 1,092 (N=764). In 19 wards, more than a third of the pensioner households were living at the relatively high room density (Table 11.10). They were scattered, although there were concentrations in low-income areas of the inner boroughs, notably north Kensington, and there were minor clusters farther out to the north and west in Ealing and Brent. The wards with the lowest shares of pensioner households living at a high room density were all in the outer boroughs, many of the names being well known as the highest-status suburbs.

The most useful single indicator of housing amenity in 1991 was whether the property had exclusive use of central heating *and* a bath or shower *and* a toilet. For the whole city, 28.1 percent of pensioner households came in this category. Figure 11.4 shows the relationship between distance from the center and the percentage of pensioner households living with substandard housing amenities. This shows that among the majority of the boroughs, a regular linear relationship applied, but six boroughs (including those mentioned) returned aberrant results. There was considerable variation among the boroughs, from 8 percent in the City of London (there is very little pre-1950 housing in this area), to 46 percent in Barking and Dagenham and 45 percent in Waltham Forest. As we have seen, the former has an unusually high proportion of public housing, but Waltham Forest, an outer-northeast borough, has extensive areas of high-density terraced housing built under late-nineteenth-century bylaws (that was of sufficient quality to escape comprehensive clearance during the 1950s and 1960s), and a large amount of privately rented unfurnished dwellings (14 percent of pensioner households). The electoral ward statistics give more detail (Table 11.11). In eight wards of these two boroughs, over 60 percent of pensioner households failed the amenity standard, the worst score being in Campbell Ward— Barking and Dagenham, with 78 percent (983 pensioner households). Campbell and Goresbrook are contiguous wards at the southern extremity of the LCC Becontree estate. The five wards of Waltham Forest listed in Table 11.11 are from the nineteenth-century suburbs of Leyton and Walthamstow, and form London's most extensive cluster of poor-quality housing.

The figures for these two boroughs are unusual and a cause for concern. Most postwar public housing has high standards of basic amenities, as in the inner boroughs of Camden, Islington, and Tower Hamlets, where there is a large stock of multistory council flats (Figure 11.4). The low-rise public housing estates developed in Barking and Dagenham during 1917–1939 and the 1950s, however, were built to lower specifications, before central heating was a standard installation. The subsequent programs of modernization and improvement have clearly been inadequate in these areas, and there are large numbers of older people living in substandard homes. Equally, the curtailment of the government's home-improvement financing

Table 11.9. Tenure of Pensioner Households by Size and Type: Greater London, 1991

| | All tenures | | % of Group in Tenure as Ratio of % for All Groups | | | |
| | | | | Rented from | Housing | |
	Thousands	%	Owner Occupied	Borough	Association	Private Owner
Lone male 65–74	46	5.6	0.70	**1.35**	**1.31**	**1.32**
Lone male 75–84	34	4.1	0.75	**1.21**	**1.31**	**1.47**
Lone male 85+	8	1.0	0.78	1.11	**1.32**	**1.64**
Lone female 60–74	146	17.6	0.86	1.16	**1.34**	1.05
Lone female 75–84	122	14.7	0.77	1.15	**1.59**	**1.43**
Lone female 85+	40	4.7	0.71	**1.20**	**1.68**	**1.54**
2+ pensioners, all <75	112	13.4	**1.20**	0.87	0.59	0.63
2+ pensioners, any 75+	95	11.4	1.10	0.84	0.78	1.13
Others containing pensioners	229	27.5	**1.23**	0.81	0.52	0.62
All containing pensioners	833	100.0	1.00	1.00	1.00	1.00
Percentage by tenure		100.0	53.0	29.8	6.6	9.6[a]

Source: Census of Population of England and Wales 1991, accessed through University of Manchester online national data depository.

Note: Figures in bold type indicate ratios of 1.2 and above.

[a] 1.0% lived in accommodation tied to employment.

Table 11.10. Pensioner Households Living at High Room Densities: Electoral Wards of Greater London, 1991

Highest % Wards and Boroughs		Lowest % Wards and Boroughs	
Northcote, Ealing	51.7	Bickley, Bromley	9.2
Glebe, Ealing	44.9	Cranham East, Havering	9.2
Chalk Farm, Camden	44.7	Danson, Bexley	9.1
Cripplegate, City of London	43.1	Spring Park, Croydon	9.1
Portsoken, City of London	41.4	Carshalton Beeches, Sutton	9.0
Avondale, Kensington and Chelsea	41.3	Coombe, Kingston upon Thames	8.7
Earls Court, Kensington and Chelsea	39.4	Cranham West, Havering	8.7
Golborne, Kensington and Chelsea	38.1	Purley, Croydon	8.6
Aldersgate, City of London	36.5	Ickenham, Hillingdon	8.6
Mount Pleasant, Ealing	35.6	West Wickham South, Bromley	8.6
Westbourne, City of Westminster	35.4	Emerson Park, Havering	8.3
Carlton, Brent	35.3	Kelsey Park, Bromley	8.2
Bayswater, City of Westminster	35.1	Selsdon, Croydon	8.2
Brunswick, Camden	34.8	Grange, Enfield	7.9
Colville, Kensington and Chelsea	34.7	Petts Wood and Knoll, Bromley	7.8
Spitalfields, Tower Hamlets	34.5	Upminster, Havering	7.4
Liddle, Southwark	34.0	Shortlands, Bromley	7.3
Millbank, City of Westminster	33.8	Deansfield, Greenwich	7.2
Pembridge, Kensington and Chelsea	33.6	Cheam South, Sutton	4.8
Upton, Newham	33.2	Woodcote, Sutton	4.1

and the inactivity of private landlords have combined to produce the concentration of poor housing standards in Waltham Forest.

Conclusions

As throughout the United Kingdom, housing space and amenity standards in London have improved vastly during the last sixty years. Population and living densities have increased; much of the worst nineteenth-century housing has been replaced; and kitchen, bathing, heating, and sanitation arrangements have been transformed. If during the 1950s and 1960s there was an association between the worst housing and the oldest households, this is no longer the case. By the early twenty-first century, the worst housing conditions are generally found in subdivided rental housing. The supply of low-cost rental housing has contracted, and it is predominantly occupied by recent migrants to the city, including students and young adult trainees. There are nonetheless remaining clusters of poor-quality housing, and they are not all in

Table 11.11. Poor Amenities and Renters of Nonpublic Housing among Pensioner Households: Electoral Wards of Greater London, 1991

Poor Amenities[a]		Renters of Nonpublic Housing	
Highest % Wards and Boroughs		**Highest % Wards and Boroughs**	
Cambell, Barking & Dagenham	77.5	Farringdon Without, City of London[b]	92.3
Goresbrook, Barking & Dagenham	71.6	Victoria, City of Westminster	68.1
Lloyd Park, Waltham Forest	70.4	St James, City of Westminster	66.4
High Street, Waltham Forest	66.1	Earls Court, Kensington & Chelsea	64.2
Thames, Barking & Dagenham	64.5	St. George's, City of Westminster	61.0
Grove Green, Waltham Forest	63.8	Brompton, Kensington & Chelsea	58.4
Higham Hill, Waltham Forest	63.4	West End, City of Westminster	57.7
Graveney, Wandsworth	61.0	Church, Kensington & Chelsea	57.5
Shaftesbury, Wandsworth	60.7	Baker Street, Wandsworth	54.2
Chapel End, Waltham Forest	60.2	Hamilton Terrace, City of Westminster	53.6
Lowest % Wards and Boroughs		**Lowest % Wards and Boroughs**	
Northwood, Hillingdon	3.1	Coldharbour, Greenwich	2.1
Portsoken, City of London[c]	2.3	Albion, Barking & Dagenham	2.1
Park, Tower Hamlets	1.9	Middle Park, Greenwich	2.0
Thamesmead Moorings, Greenwich	1.4	Cranham West, Havering	1.1
Cripplegate, City of London	0.9	Deansfield, Greenwich	0.7
Aldersgate, City of London	0.7	Woodcote, Sutton	0.5

Source: Census of Population of England and Wales 1991. Accessed through University of Manchester online national data depository.
[a] No or shared use of bath/shower and/or inside lavatory (wc) and/or central heating
[b] Ward had 65 pensioner households
[c] Ward had 133 pensioner households

the inner city. Almost all is rental housing, and it is found in both the private and public sectors.

The major housing problem facing London's older people is its high cost. It is true that most older people on low incomes who are social housing tenants (and not recent migrants) have the majority of their rental costs paid by Housing Benefit. Their choice of housing types and locations is then severely restricted. Not even those who own their housing outright (without a mortgage) are immune, for council tax (a local property tax) and maintenance charges are high. The combination of high costs, the ability to purchase equivalent housing at much lower prices outside the city, and environmental factors prompts a high proportion of London's people to move away when they retire or approach old age. No other region of the country, not even the industrial cities of the Midlands and North, drives so many older households away. It must therefore be concluded that the economic dynamism and governmental, financial, commercial, and creative media functions of London that make it a world city also create an environment that is on balance unsupportive and uncongenial for a large proportion of its older population.

Notes

1. Cribier, F., and A. Kych. 1993. A Comparison of Retirement Migration from Paris and London. *Environment and Planning A* 26:1399–1420; Warnes, A. M. 1994. Cities and Elderly People: Recent Population and Distributional Trends. *Urban Studies* 31:799–816.
2. To comply with European antidiscrimination legislation, from 2010 the female UK statutory pensionable age will be raised in steps to sixty-five years by 2020.
3. Note that the Greater London Authority is not a housing provider, unlike its predecessor until the late 1970s, the Greater London Council.
4. ONS. 2003. *Region in Figures: London*. Issue 7. London: Stationery Office, Table 7.11.
5. Hall, P. G. 1989. *London 2001*. London: Unwin Hyman.
6. Champion, A. G., and P. Congdon. 1988. Recent Trends in Greater London's Population. *Population Trends* 53:7–17.
7. ONS. 2001. *Region in Figures: London*. London: Stationery Office, Table 2.9.
8. Hall, R., P. E. Ogden, and C. Hill. 1997. The Pattern and Structure of One-Person Households in England and Wales and France. *International Journal of Population Geography* 3:161–181.
9. If the aberrant City of London is removed, the correlation coefficient is –0.92.
10. Stuart, A. 1987. Migration and Population Turnover in a London Borough: The Incidence and Implications of Retirement Out-Migration. *Espaces Populations Sociétés* 1:137–151.
11. Dennis, R. 1986. Housing Problems. In H. Clout and P. Wood, eds. *London: Problems of Change*, 83–91. Essex: Longman, Harlow.
12. Hamnett, C. R. 2001. London's Housing. *Area* 33(1): 82.
13. Young, T. 1934. *Becontree and Dagenham: The Growth of a Housing Estate*. London: Pilgrim Trust.

12. Growing Older in the City of Light

Victor G. Rodwin

Paris evokes many of the images of a world city. It is a center of political power and transnational corporations, a place for the pursuit of science and artistic creation, a hub for museums and libraries, a transmission belt for fashions and ideas, and so much more. In its heyday (1870–1910)—la belle époque–Paris radiated a sense of youth and boundless energy, since so many young artists were uniquely well anchored in this "capital of light."[1] Even at the time of Napoleon Bonaparte, most members of the French Academy were under forty years of age, in contrast to over seventy years today. And a century later, in the 1920s, when Ernest Hemingway recalled memories whose impact stays with you "wherever you go for the rest of your life," Paris also evoked images of youth.[2]

Today Paris remains a world city, even if it is often excluded from the big three—New York, London, and Tokyo—because of its smaller stock market and banking sector.[3] But more so, perhaps, than these big three, Paris will have to revise its image of itself, for it stands out now as having the highest share of persons eighty-five years and over—not just with respect to these world cities, but also in comparison to its greater metropolitan region and to France as a whole (Table 12.1). Despite its proportionally high cohort of students eighteen to twenty-four years old, a recent report from the Paris Planning Agency notes that there are over a hundred thousand older old (eighty years and over) in Paris.[4] Moreover, although over the past decade its age cohort sixty years and over declined slightly, still it represents one-fifth of the French capital's population.

Beyond the statistics, there is palpable evidence of population aging in Paris. One cannot walk through the streets and parks of the city without being struck by the number of older persons going about their daily routines. Whether one witnesses older persons taking their daily constitutionals, sitting on park benches or in neighborhood cafés, shopping in the open markets and small shops, or sitting on the metro, casual empiricism suggests that older persons abound. Some are well dressed and appear as distinguished as the personalities in Daumier's caricatures; others are distinctly less well groomed and less well dressed, particularly in the northeastern, North African parts of the city and in the Asian enclaves of the

Table 12.1. Persons 85+ as Percent of Total Population: Paris, France, and Urban Cores of New York, London, and Tokyo, 2000

	85+ as % of Total
Paris	2.4
First Ring	1.6
Second Ring	1.4
France	2.1
Manhattan	1.7
Inner London	1.6
Inner Tokyo	1.8

Sources: France: INSEE, local population estimates, January 2001; U.S.: U.S. Census 2000; U.K.: U.K. Census 2001; Japan: Japan Census 2000.

thirteenth arrondissement. There are, of course, many more nonwhite faces than in the past due to decades of immigration to Paris. And the combination of growth in numbers of older persons and greater diversity makes Paris an important place in which to study the consequences of human longevity and population aging for cities in the future.

The Paris city authorities are well aware of their aging population. Indeed, the new mayor has a special advisor for issues related to older persons. Even before the 1999 census revealed the presence of more than five hundred centenarians in Paris, the city government had decided to launch a small survey of these "city seniors" born before 1900, whose lives spanned three centuries. Based on interviews with forty Parisian centenarians, the city government decided to celebrate this outcome of the longevity revolution with the publication of a book, in 2002, prefaced by the new socialist mayor, Bertrand Delanoë.[5]

Neither the special advisor, however, nor the many generous programs for older persons, nor another publication could be expected to focus significant intellectual and financial resources on the myriad problems associated with the growing number of vulnerable older persons in Paris. It took the heat wave—*canicule*—of August 2003 to bring these issues into sharper focus and raise them a bit higher on the policy agenda. That is the only positive impact of the devastating heat that resulted in close to 5,000 "excess" deaths in Ile-de-France and 1,067 in Paris, alone.[6]

This chapter reviews the distribution of older persons in Paris and its surrounding region, examines their migration patterns and socioeconomic characteristics, and calls attention to the high rates of older persons, especially women, living at home alone. Finally, the chapter reviews the range of services available to them and speculates on the key issues that must now be confronted in the postcanicule period that lies ahead.

Overview of Older Persons in Paris and Its Surrounding Region

Among the arrondissements of Paris, there are significant variations in the distribution of older Parisians that reflect income disparities, differences in the quality of housing, and historic—as well as current—patterns in the level of neighborhood amenities. Most older Parisians live in the wealthier western areas of the city–the sixth, seventh, eighth, fifteenth, and sixteenth arrondissements; and this pattern is even more pronounced for those seventy-five years and over.[7] Overall, the geographic distribution of the older population coincides with that of the general population—the fifteenth arrondissement is the most highly populated, but with the exception of the fifteenth and sixteenth arrondissements, most people, including older people, live outside the center of Paris. An important challenge for the future is how to improve the quality of life of older persons living in the poorer northeastern part of the city and the thirteenth arrondissement.

The Paris metropolitan region—Ile-de-France—is made up of 1,300 local jurisdictions, or communes, of which 20 comprise the arrondissements of Paris. Together with the three *départements* of the first ring (Figure 2.1) and an additional four comprising the second ring around Paris, Ile-de-France is the most prosperous region in France. With a population of roughly eleven million (18.8 percent of the French population), it generates 28 percent of France's gross domestic product and includes 36 percent of households in which the head works in an executive or managerial position.[8]

The inhabitants of Ile-de-France—Franciliens—are young in comparison to their fellow citizens in the other twenty-one regions of France: in 2001, only 12.1 percent of the population was sixty-five years and over, in comparison to 16.1 percent in France and 23.1 percent in France's "oldest" region, Limousin. In contrast, within the context of the region, the Paris population is relatively old. There is a clear gradient in the distribution of older persons among Paris, its first ring (*proche couronne*), and the second ring, both of which make up what remains of Ile-de-France. Within the region, as distance from Paris increases, the share of older persons declines (Table 12.2).[9] During the entire post–World War II period, older persons in Ile-de-France have been concentrated in Paris. This reflects different rates of aging among these cohorts, as well as differential patterns of out-migration among age cohorts.

Over the next thirty years, differences in population aging between Paris and its surrounding region will gradually dwindle. Demographers project that in 2030, the number of people seventy-five years and over will increase by 23 percent in Paris, 63 percent in the first ring, and 169 percent in the second ring.[10] While Paris is older than its surrounding region, which is relatively young, over the next thirty years

**Table 12.2. Persons 65+ and 85+ as Percent
of Total Population: Paris and France, 2000**

	65+	85+
Paris	14.7	2.4
First Ring	12.4	1.6
Second Ring	10.8	1.4
Ile-de-France	12.1	1.7
France	16.1	2.1

Source: INSEE, local population estimates, January 2001.

these projections indicate that Ile-de-France will catch up with Paris. In 2000, 36.5 percent of Franciliens seventy-five years and over lived in the second ring around Paris; in 2030, INSEE demographers project, this share will reach 51 percent.

Projections through 2014 indicate that the population sixty years and over will remain lower in Paris than in France, and that the gap will increase: 19.4 percent versus 20.3 percent in 1998, 19.0 percent versus 20.9 percent in 2006, 20.4 percent versus 24.5 percent in 2014.[11] This trend, however, should be tempered by the fact that the average age of older persons remains higher in Paris than in the rest of the region and France. Not only is the share of persons eighty-five and over higher in Paris than in Ile-de-France and France as a whole (Table 12.2); the share of the older old (eighty-five plus), as a proportion of persons sixty-five and over, is also higher. It is 16 percent in Paris, 13.3 percent in the first ring, and 12.8 percent in France.

Several factors have contributed to the stabilization of the population sixty and over in Paris. Most important is the impact of changing migration patterns to and from the capital, since many students and young employees have traditionally come to Paris and significant cohorts of retirees have emigrated upon reaching the legal retirement age of sixty.

Migration. Since the post–World War II period, an average of 2 to 3 percent of the population sixty years and over has left Ile-de-France each year to retire to the provinces.[12] Like the migration of many older New Yorkers to Florida, many Franciliens head south to "retirement cities" such as Nice. Others have migrated to other coastal cities or simply returned to the regions where they were born. Over the last census period—between 1990 and 1999—approximately 26 percent of Franciliens between the ages of fifty-five and seventy-five left the region for the provinces to begin their retirement. Previously, this proportion reached 29 percent (1982–1990) and 33 percent (1975–1982).[13] The decrease may be explained by several factors—a reduction of the number of Franciliens who originally came from the provinces, an increase in new generations of children who have remained in Ile-de-France, and an increase in seasonal migration as opposed to more definitive departures from the region previously.

Data on migration patterns of Parisians only are more difficult obtain. Based on the 1990 census, it appears that there is very little migration of persons sixty years and over from the first and second rings of Ile-de-France to Paris.[14] But disentangling Parisians' migration patterns, by age cohort and time period, to capture the evolution of these trends since World War II is a complicated task. From what information is available at this level of disaggregation, it appears that retirement out-migration of persons sixty years and over from Paris has been lower than in the rest of the region in the most recent census period.[15] These different rates of out-migration probably reflect different patterns of labor-force participation between Paris and its surrounding region. For example, in 1999, for persons aged sixty to sixty-four the labor force participation rate was 36.1 in Paris, 23.1 percent in the first ring, and 14.9 percent in France.[16]

That a world city like Paris should differ from its surrounding region and the rest of the nation should not come as a surprise. It has, throughout French history, distinguished itself from the rest of the nation to such a degree that geographer Jean-François Gravier wrote a classic book entitled *Paris and the French Desert*.[17] And it is for this reason that the remainder of this chapter focuses on the distinctive characteristics of those Parisians who remain in Paris and grow older there.

Socioeconomic Characteristics of Older Parisians

One of the social characteristics of global cities is the growth of income inequality and the polarization among occupational groups.[18] A telling set of statistics that distinguishes Paris from its surrounding two rings and the rest of France would focus on indicators of gentrification.[19] For example, with 4 percent of the active population in France, Paris has 14 percent of all executives, managers, and CEOs. On average, there are as many people in these occupational groups in Paris as there are employees and blue-collar workers. In the rest of Ile-de-France, as well as in France as a whole, there are typically twice as many employees and blue-collar workers as executives, managers, and CEOs combined.[20]

In comparison to the Paris agglomeration (an area which concentrates 88 percent of the region's population), more Parisians have higher incomes and there is slightly more poverty when measured as the percentage of households whose income falls below half of the median.[21] If one compares Paris with the first ring only, the percentage of population with low-income levels is roughly the same.[22] This phenomenon results in greater income inequality within Paris than in the first and second rings surrounding it. Moreover, income inequality has increased significantly over the 1990s.[23] Poverty levels of older persons are similar to those of all ages: in 1996, 37 percent of older households (sixty-five and over) had incomes low enough to qualify for exemption from income taxation, only slightly more than the 35 percent of households for all ages.[24] Likewise, there is a higher proportion of older persons in lower income brackets in Paris than in the first ring.[25]

Despite the slightly higher level of poverty compared to the surrounding region, Paris remains an urban core with a higher-strata population. In terms of educational status, older persons (aged sixty plus) are more educated in Paris than in the first ring (Table 12.3). In 1999, 19.1 percent of older persons in Paris had a higher-education degree; in the first ring, 8.2 percent of older persons had such a degree. What is more, whereas this proportion went up only slightly between 1990 and 1999 in the first ring, in Paris it increased from 11.3 to 19.1 percent. Within Paris, of course, there are significant inequalities among arrondissements. For example, income inequalities among all households increase for older persons. The ratio of median income from the higher-income arrondissements to the lower-income arrondissements is 1.8 for all ages; for ages sixty to seventy-four and seventy-five and over, it is 2.3.[26]

Perhaps the most important change in the socioeconomic characteristics of older Parisians is the increase of older immigrants (Table 12.4). In Paris, where there have always been more immigrants than in the first ring, the share of immigrants in the total population did not increase between 1990 and 1999, but the share of im-

Table 12.3. Education Levels of Persons 60+: Paris and First Ring, 1990 and 1999

		BAC+2[a]	%	Higher Education Degree	%	Total
1990	**Paris**	18,964	4.3	50,229	11.3	69,193
	Hauts-de-Seine	8,612	3.5	21,788	8.8	30,400
	Seine-Saint-Denis	2,412	1.3	3,164	1.7	5,576
	Val-de-Marne	4,532	2.3	7,768	3.9	12,300
	First Ring	15,556	2.4	32,720	5.1	48,277
1999	**Paris**	25,242	6.1	79,610	19.1	104,852
	Hauts-de-Seine	13,114	5.1	35,693	13.8	48,807
	Seine-Saint-Denis	4,647	2.2	6,170	3.0	10,817
	Val-de-Marne	8,156	3.8	14,471	6.7	22,627
	First Ring	25,917	3.8	56,334	8.2	82,252

Source: INSEE, Census (25% sample), 1990, 1999

Notes: For location of First Ring departments surrounding Paris, see Figure 2.1.

[a] BAC+2 refers to high school and two years toward a college degree.

migrants over sixty years of age rose from 15.9 to 18.8 percent. In the department of Seine St. Denis (93), where the share of immigrants is even higher than in Paris and grew from 24.1 to 28 percent between the two census periods, the share of older immigrants grew as well (18.3 to 23.2 percent). Still, in comparison to the first ring, which has now caught up to Paris in its share of immigrants, Paris continues to have a slightly higher share of older immigrants.

There is relatively scant information for Paris, in comparison to New York and London, on the socioeconomic characteristics of the immigrant population—largely because census data are not collected by ethnicity under the laws of the French Republic. Nonetheless, there is increasing awareness among the Paris city authorities that aging immigrants represent a vulnerable population. Based on 1990 data, Marc Esponda of the Paris Planning Agency completed a careful analysis at the request of the mayor's office in which he compiled a portrait of aging immigrants over fifty years of age from outside Europe.[27] The rationale for using fifty as the cutoff was simply that unemployment rates were so high among these groups that this age seemed to be a kind of entry into early retirement for those who continued to stay on in Paris.

Based on his estimates of 45,800 older immigrants, Esponda notes that two-thirds were foreigners (62.9 percent), the rest having become naturalized French citizens. Two-thirds were also men, which reflects the economic nature of immigration, since men have been drawn to the work opportunities for manual laborers. After excluding all immigrants from Europe, three-quarters of older immigrants in Paris were from Northern Africa. The rest were from Southeast Asia (14 percent), sub-Saharan Africa (8 percent), Turkey (4 percent), and India (1 percent). After focusing only on the situation of isolated migrants either living alone or in various group quarters—a population that consists mostly of men (70 percent)—Esponda reveals their socioeconomic characteristics in comparison to a comparable age cohort of isolated, nonimmigrant Parisians: high rates of unemployment (15 vs. 3 percent), high proportions of manual laborers (63 vs. 17 percent), and deplorable housing conditions, as measured by the proportion living in units without toilets and bathrooms.

In all these respects—the convergence of wealthy and highly educated older persons with different groups of poor minorities—Paris is, indeed, a global city with the kinds of social polarization analyzed by Saskia Sassen.[28] But as Sophie Body-Gendrot argues, Paris is a "soft" global city because of the traditionally protective role of the state toward the less well-off.[29] This state role goes beyond the support of an incomes policy across occupational groups. It also tempers the tendency toward spatial segregation that is more pronounced in New York and London. Although there are increasingly small neighborhoods with concentrated ethnic minorities—for example, the Goutte-d'Or, Barbes, Belleville, Chateau Rouge, and parts of the thirteenth arrondissement—there are still no neighborhoods the size of an arrondissement that can claim a spatial division along ethnic lines. This outcome

Table 12.4. Immigrant Population:
Paris, Departments of First Ring, and First Ring, 1990 and 1999

	1990				
	Total	French	Naturalized	Foreign	% of Immigrants
Paris					
60+	445,892	414,768	39,725	31,124	15.9
Total pop.	2,151,245	1,810,755	126,152	340,490	21.7
Hauts de Seine					
60+	248,564	233,556	16,180	15,008	12.5
Total pop.	1,390,592	1,209,842	61,664	180,750	17.4
Seine Saint Denis					
60+	191,528	172,304	16,176	19,224	18.5
Total pop.	1,381,180	1,120,182	72,389	260,998	24.1
Val de Marne					
60+	198,665	186,249	17,768	12,416	15.2
Total pop.	1,215,143	1,059,957	59,188	155,186	17.6
First Ring					
60+	638,757	592,109	50,124	46,648	15.2
Total pop.	3,986,915	3,389,981	193,241	596,934	19.8
	1999				
Paris					
60+	417,182	378,526	39,899	38,656	18.8
Total pop.	2,125,017	1,819,233	155,607	305,784	21.7
Hauts de Seine					
60+	259,549	237,570	18,073	21,979	15.4
Total pop.	1,428,384	1,264,815	94,111	163,569	18.0
Seine Saint Denis					
60+	207,873	178,421	18,824	29,452	23.2
Total pop.	1,382,892	1,121,895	126,008	260,997	28.0
Val de Marne					
60+	215,801	196,465	17,054	19,336	16.9
Total pop.	1,225,594	1,081,126	93,627	144,468	19.4
First Ring					
60+	683,223	612,456	53,951	70,767	18.3
Total pop.	4,036,870	3,467,836	313,746	569,034	21.9

Source: INSEE Census, compiled for Paris by Atelier Parisien d'Urbanisme, 1990 and 1999.
Notes: Immigrants are defined as foreigners and French citizens, by naturalization. For location of First Ring departments surrounding Paris, see Figure 2.1.

is partly the result of the explicit attempt to support social heterogeneity across spatial units of Paris—the policy of *mixité social*.[30] As we shall see, the central state, as well as the Paris authorities, attempts to alleviate the harsher impacts of globalization and the general difficulties of growing older in a city characterized by increasing polarization.

Living Alone at Home

Whether one is an immigrant man or a third-generation Parisian woman, the problems that eventually emerge when one grows older are universal. What distinguishes Paris, however, from its surrounding region, the rest of France, and even our other world cities, is the unusually high number of persons eighty-five and over who avoid institutional long-term care and spend their final years living alone at home.

Marc Chagall once wrote: "Paris reflects my heart. I should like to dissolve in it, never to be alone with myself."[31] Yet in Paris, he would have been saddened to learn, 57 percent of the population eighty years and over lives alone, in contrast to 47.4 percent in the first ring. For women, the equivalent figures are 67 and 56 percent. Of course, these aggregate rates for all Parisians reflect important differences among arrondissements, which, in turn, reflect differences among ethnic groups. Nonetheless, these rates do distinguish Paris from the rest of France and from its first ring. For a French citizen living alone, the probability of ending up in a long-term care institution is more than twice as high in the first ring as in Paris.[32] This is as true for women as for men and for those eighty years and over, as well as for those ninety years and over. It also applies to foreigners living in Paris and in its first ring.

How might one explain these high rates of living alone at home in Paris? Do they reflect the fact that Parisians are generally in better health than their counterparts in the first and second rings and in the rest of the nation and live longer (see Chapter 13)? Alternatively, do these rates merely reflect the high land costs in Paris, which have led to a low level of retirement and nursing-home beds compared with the rest of Ile-de-France (Chapter 15)? Even if one counts long-term care beds outside Paris in which older frail Parisians are placed, as documented in Chapter 15, there are still significantly lower levels of nursing-home care. Or do high rates of living alone at home in Paris reflect the fact that Parisians have access to home-nursing services and a range of other home-help and amenities that accompany population density in the urban core?

For all age groups in Paris, living alone has become dominant among traditional living arrangements, such as in couples, families, and institutions. Of course, this household categorization does not automatically lead to loneliness. Nor does it specify anything about the material conditions of single households. Nevertheless, it is well known that many of the older old who live alone are indeed lonely and many—whether or not they live alone—have to put up with substandard housing conditions. As noted in Chapter 15, the 1999 census indicates that 7.1 percent of

Parisians sixty years and over had no toilet in their primary residence and 8.7 percent had neither a shower nor a bathtub. Fortunately for frail persons living alone, Paris offers a range of services aimed at delaying loss of autonomy and thereby avoiding institutionalization. These services did not prevent the unprecedented number of deaths during the canicule. But they are important for many of the older old, including centenarians who still remember the Paris flood of 1910 and share recollections of walking the *grands boulevards* only decades after they were laid down by Baron Haussmann.

When Mme. Yvonne Masse was interviewed for the city's book on centenarians, she summarized her life in the capital thus: "Paris—it was chic, it was gay, it was the city where one sings and cries softly." For frail older persons, the programs and services available in Paris have traditionally been considered generous in comparison to those in most other parts of France.[33] Together with their families, friends, and not least, as Marie-Ève Joël and Robert Haas argue in Chapter 14, the character of their local neighborhood community, such services can shape the quality of their lives.

The Role of Paris Authorities in Supporting Older Persons Living at Home

Paris has a unique administrative status in France. As a capital city, it has both a city government and mayor and at the same time functions as a département under the authority of the central government. The département implements government programs and regulations affecting health and social services through the Division of Health and Social Affairs (DASES). The city runs its specific Paris-initiated programs through its Center for Social Action (Centre d'Action Sociale de la Ville de Paris [CASVP]).[34]

Services operated by these entities, as well as those organized by the local Paris office of the National Pension Fund and a host of nonprofit organizations (*associations*) and health-care institutions, are guided by the *schéma directeur géron-tologique*—Long-Term Care Master Plan of 1999, an official document approved by the Paris City Council.[35] This document grew out of a collaborative planning process among different partners engaged in activities that serve older Parisians, and its aim is to improve coordination and integration of services by the multiple actors involved. Since its most important goal was to strengthen coordination among the many interventions in support of frail older persons, the city established Emerald Coordination Centers for all Paris neighborhoods.

These centers offer free call-in lines, as well as on-site counseling and information about the wide gamut of services available for older Parisians:

- A help line for victims of elder abuse, information on cultural and recreational activities, as well as intergenerational and continuing education programs. This includes free tickets or discounted prices to improve access to cultural activities, education, and travel.

- Emerald restaurants, where payment for meals is means-tested based on income
- Temporary housing and adult day care (less well developed than the senior centers in New York City)
- Temporary housing provided by the CASVP; this includes short-term-stay (maximum three months) residences with fully independent apartments; others offering independent living but with a variety of support services (food service, security, nurses on duty, social club, etc.); and others with nurses and other health professionals for older persons who cannot live on their own

Many older Parisians have meager resources and are eligible for supplemental retirement payments under French social security (the National Pension Fund). Eligibility for this benefit is determined on the basis of age and income. The average age of beneficiaries in France is 77.3, and 63.9 percent are women.[36] In Paris, twenty thousand persons sixty-five years and over (6.2 percent of older persons in contrast to 4.5 percent in the first ring) receive this benefit.[37] For those who are not eligible and still come under an income ceiling, the city runs a special program to cover unreimbursed health expenditures and social care.[38] Beyond this city-run income-supplement program, all older Parisians are entitled to special passes for free transportation and a range of services for home improvements to increase safety.

For persons sixty years and over with high levels of dependency, since 2002 the central government finances a universal program—*allocation personnalisée d'autonomie* (APA)—to cover payments for home help and assistance with the daily activities of living. This benefit is means tested, but even the wealthy receive a token payment. The determination of eligibility and administration of payment are managed at the local level, and there were seventeen thousand older Parisians receiving this benefit in 2003. Most of them were over eighty-five years old. Roughly half were using the benefit to support the room-and-board costs of nursing homes; the remainder were using it to support costs associated with home help. In this regard, three kinds of service covering all arrondissements are available:

- *Home Help:* This service provides home helpers (for a maximum of thirty hours a month) to assist older persons who are unable to perform household tasks (shopping, housecleaning, etc.) on their own.
- *Home Nursing Services:* These services, financed by the local health-insurance fund upon prescription by a physician and pending local availability of neighborhood nurses, provides assistance with personal hygiene and other activities of daily living.
- *Paris Home Care:* This program offers five kinds of service to support older persons living at home: installation of alarm systems for requesting rapid assistance; delivery of home meals; home hairdressing; pedicure; and home-assessment services.

For family caregivers there are also two noteworthy programs—a payment for those who choose to cease working to care for a parent who is ill, and a means-tested payment for families who take a parent over seventy-five years of age into their own home.

This catalogue of available services might appear to be a frail older person's dream come true. Many of these services, however, reach an exceedingly small share of older persons. For others, it is almost impossible to obtain data on the number of people served, let alone how well. What is more, in Paris, as elsewhere, home-help services are characterized by a lack of integration, since multiple institutions (social security pension funds, private insurance, local authorities) are in charge of different financing streams and no single authority is responsible for overseeing the social needs of specific groups of frail older persons. Consequently, for a given level of need, there exist wide disparities in the magnitude of resource and service provision to older persons, most often explained by their socioprofessional status and place of residence.[39]

Problems and Opportunities for Older Persons

The high percentage of older Parisians who leave the city on reaching retirement suggests that there are many characteristics of life in this world city that repel older persons. There is no compelling evidence on this score. But it is not difficult to speculate that congestion, pollution, weather, and high prices could be deterrents. On the other hand, as in New York, there is anecdotal evidence of a second wave of migration back to Paris when older persons grow older. Once again, one might imagine that high culture, teaching hospitals and specialist physicians, great educational institutions, many nonprofit organizations, and many more amenities would attract those who can afford it.

France, since World War II, has always engaged in a national planning process, even though critical decisions made were not necessarily direct outcomes of that process.[40] With respect to planning for population aging and longevity, there has been no exception to this rule. Numerous task forces have come and gone. White papers have been produced. Every local county (département) has even been required to produce a master plan to confront the challenge of population aging. Paris has been no exception, because so many of the complex policy issues must ultimately be solved at the local level. Thus, the Long-Term Care Master Plan of 1999.

The master plan succeeds in invoking just about every new idea in the field of gerontology and long-term-care services for an aging population. Also, it assembles much needed data, highlights some critical problems, and reviews what remains to be done. Without attempting to summarize its major findings and recommendations, and reading carefully between the lines, it seems appropriate to conclude by raising three themes that appear submerged in the first master plan and a final theme that will no doubt emerge out of current work on the next master plan:

1. The city as a center of medical care excellence versus a provider of medical care for the community

Since the end of the nineteenth century, Paris has been a center of medical excellence. Its public hospital system, Assistance Publique-Hôpitaux de Paris (AP-HP) was originally established to care for the poor.[41] Since the 1960s, however, it has become one of the great medical centers in France, including for specialty training and research in geriatrics. AP-HP beds are concentrated in Paris, but the system extends to the first and second rings around Paris. Moreover, AP-HP includes acute and long-term care beds, as well as entire nursing-home facilities. Since it is a public hospital system—and one with more power in many respects than the entire Ministry of Health has—AP-HP is torn between promoting the interests of its specialized physicians and meeting all its responsibilities to serve as a system of last resort for the poor and disenfranchised.

The mayor of Paris is president of the board of directors of AP-HP, which also includes local officials from Ile-de-France. In this capacity, the mayor has typically attempted to persuade the director of AP-HP (chosen by the president of the Republic and accountable to the board and powerful physician committees) to pressure AP-HP hospitals to improve services for the poorest segments of the Paris population so that the city does not have to bear the full burden in its social services and health-care centers. The mayor of Paris has also tried to persuade AP-HP to close some of its long-term care facilities outside Paris and to relocate them within the city. Since the canicule, however, there has been no constituency for closing down any of these facilities.

2. The city as a catalyst for coordinated strategies to assist frail older persons

In France, as in most OECD countries, there is a trend toward greater harmonization of diverse institutions caring for frail older persons. The idea behind proposed reforms is that institutions should be paid based on indicators of dependency and health status of their clientele, not specific institutional cost structures. In this respect, the trend in Paris is to design a "continuum" of services for frail older persons.[42] For example, the master plan recommended the expansion of:

- *Small temporary housing units.* The aim of small temporary housing units is to avert premature and useless institutionalization of frail older persons. These units function as a bridge between hospital and home to facilitate coming back home. They also can be a temporary solution to the absence of a regular helper. Although there are now only four such units in Paris (fifty-four beds), they are considered a "valuable link [in the] . . . continuum of care for older persons."

- *Day-care centers.* The goal of day-care centers is to prevent functional, psychological, and social dependencies, treat current dependencies, and "resocialize" isolated older persons. They can serve as an alternative to full housing and contribute to maintaining older persons with mobility limitations at home.[43]

3. The city as a vehicle for giving voice to older persons, particularly the frail

Older persons have been effective at forming organizations to defend their interests. They have also acted as a considerable political force in elections and interest-group lobbying. What is more, the economic power they exercise in the marketplace has had increasing influence. Parisians over sixty years old have household incomes that are 40 percent higher than the national average.[44]

As population aging has evolved, however, this constituency has revealed fractures due to its increasing heterogeneity. Also, frail older persons have always exercised a soft voice and depended on advocates. Buried in annex 11 of the Paris master plan is a bill of rights for older Parisians, which reveals the extent to which the city may already serve as a political amplifying device for its older, particularly frail citizens.

4. The city as the authority responsible for identifying where vulnerable older persons reside and developing an emergency preparedness strategy

Paris began the postcanicule era by establishing a new city agency charged with monitoring its population's health—the Paris Agency for Public Health. What is more, the Paris authorities have embarked on an unprecedented strategy to merge information files from the local health-insurance fund, the local pension fund, the CASVP, and the DASES so that these organizations, all of which serve older persons, will be able to locate those who seem most vulnerable, because of their economic or social circumstances, in the event of a crisis.

To suggest that the canicule had political implications and policy repercussions is no exaggeration. Whether or not such measures will save the most vulnerable older persons in a future heat wave, let alone improve their quality of life if crises are averted, remains to be seen. In the meantime, ideas about the value of clinical disease prevention and health-promotion programs for older Parisians will surely gain currency.[45] Concurrently, proposals to study and act upon the social determinants of health for older Parisians are likely to receive more searching examination.[46]

Notes

1. Peter Hall devotes Chapter 6 to Paris as the "Capital of Light" in his 1998 *Cities in Civilization* (New York: Pantheon).

2. Hemingway, Ernest. 1964. *A Moveable Feast.* New York: Charles Scribner's Sons. From a letter to a friend in 1950, inscribed on the title page of his book.

3. Sassen, Saskia. 2001. *The Global City: New York, London, Tokyo.* 2d ed. Princeton: Princeton University Press; Llewelyn-Davies. 1996. *Four World Cities: A Comparative Study of London, Paris, New York, and Tokyo.* London: Llewelyn-Davies, University College London Bartlett School of Planning, and Comedia.

4. Paris-Prôjet. 2003. *Paris 2020, Eléments pour un plan d'aménagement et de développement durable.* Collection Paris Prôjet, nos. 34–35. Paris: Atelier Parisien d'Urbanisme, 128.

5. *Hommage à nos ainés qui ont connu trois siècles.* 2002. Paris: Mairie de Paris.

6. *Conséquences sanitaires de la canicule d'août 2003 en* Ile-de-France-*Premier bilan.* 2003. Paris: Observatoire Régional de la Santé (ORS). October. www.ors-idf.org.

7. Esponda, M. 2002. *Les Personnes agées: Eléments de diagnostic.* Paris: Atelier Parisien d'Urbanisme. March.

8. INSEE, data cited in *Le Monde,* September 19, 2003.

9. There is one exception to this general pattern. Among the first and second rings around Paris, there are more than one hundred small *communes* in which over 20 percent of the population is over sixty years of age. These are the least urbanized areas of Ile-de-France, where farmers and agricultural workers still represent a significant share of the local population. See Louchard, P. 1999. An Overview of the Aging Population in Ile-de-France. *Le défi de l'âge. Les Cahiers de l'IAURF* 2(122 [March]).

10. INSEE. Departmental population projections 2000–2030 based on the following assumptions: maintenance of fertility rates for 1999—1.8 children per woman, the average rate observed over the past twenty-five years; decrease in mortality based on average rates observed over the past thirty years; and maintenance of existing migratory patterns observed over the period 1982–99.

11. Projections are from Department of Health and Social Affairs. 2000. *Premières rencontres de la vie sociale: Vivre à Paris après soixante ans.* Paris: Cahiers de Chaligny, Mairie de Paris.

12. Cribier, F., and A. Kych. 1992. La migration de retraite des parisiens, une analyse de la propension au départ. *Population* 47:677–717; and Cribier, F., and A. Kych. 1993. A Comparison of Retirement Migration from Paris and London. *Environment and Planning* 25:1399–1420.

13. *Population et modes de vie.* 2002. Vol. 3 of *Atlas des Franciliens.* Paris: Institut d'Aménagement Urbain de la Région Francilienne (IAURF)–INSEE Ile-de-France.

14. In 1990, 93 percent of persons aged sixty to seventy-four and 96 percent of persons aged seventy-five and over declared that they were residing in Paris nine years before, which indicates that only 7 percent of people aged sixty to seventy-four at that time and 4 percent of people aged seventy-five and over came from somewhere in France outside Paris. Even fewer people aged sixty to seventy-four (3 percent) and seventy-

five and over (1 percent) came to Paris from the rest of Ile-de-France (1990 census, INSEE).

15.   Lucas-Gabrielli, V., and F. Tonnellier. 2000. *Les personnes agées dans l'agglomération de Paris.* Paris: Centre de Recherche, d'Etude et de Documentation en Economie de la Santé (CREDES).

16.   For persons over sixty-five, the labor-force participation rate was 4.1 percent in Paris compared to 1.8 percent in the first ring and 1.2 percent in France as a whole (figures based on 1999 census, INSEE).

17.   Gravier, J. F. 1947. *Paris et le Désert Français.* Paris: Flammarion.

18.   Sassen, *The Global City.*

19.   See, e.g., the analyses of 1999 census data by Marc Esponda: "Profil socio-démographique des Parisiens." 2003. *Paris Prôjet* (34–35), 90–100.

20.   Ibid.

21.   The Paris agglomeration corresponds to Paris, the first ring, and only the most populated parts of the second ring. In 1996, average taxable income in Paris was $32,136 ($1=FF 6) versus $24,687 in the first ring (Direction Générale des Impôts [Division of Internal Revenue]). The income distribution is also more unequal in Paris than in the Paris agglomeration: in 1994, the Gini coefficient was .444 versus .325. (Chambaz, C. , F. Guillaumat-Tailliet, and J. M. Hourriez. 1999. Le revenu et le patrimoine des ménages. In *Données sociales.* .Paris: INSEE). Poverty is also higher in Paris than in the Paris agglomeration: 12.8% versus 10.2% percent of households had incomes that were less than one-half of the median household income in 1994 (ibid.).

22.   Debras, B., D. Chemineau, and A. Quiroga. 2001. Une approche de la pauvreté en Ile-de-France. *Ile-de-France à la page,* January.

23.   The Gini coefficient increased 30 percent from 1990 to 1994 (.341 to .444) (Chambaz, Guillaumat-Tailliet, and Hourriez, Le revenu).

24.   From 1990 to 1996, this figure declined from 39 to 37 percent (Direction Générale des Impôts).

25.   Of older persons aged sixty-five and over, 6 %, in Paris, have sufficiently low incomes to meet eligibility qualifications for a supplementary pension benefit versus 4.1 % in the first ring. Personal communication with Alain Rozenkier, National Pension Fund, Paris, July 2004.

26.   Based on data from the Direction Générale des Impôts, assembled by the Atelier Parisien d'Urbanisme [Division of Internal Revenue, Paris Planning Agency], 2001.

27.   Esponda, M. 2001. *Portrait socio-démographique des migrants agées—pour la création d'un café sociale.* Paris: APUR, May.

28.   Sassen, *The Global City*; Pinçon, M., and M. Pinçon-Charlot.2001. *Paris Mosaïque.* Paris, Calmann-Lévy.

29.   Body-Gendrot, S. 1996. Paris: A "Soft" Global City? *New Community* 22 (4 [October]): 595–605.

30.   Pinçon, M., and M. Pinçon-Charlot. Entre Soi ou Mixité Sociale? In Paris Prôjet, *Paris 2020.*

31.   Chagall, M. Cited by Julian Cain. 1960. *The Lithographs of Chagall.* New York: George Brazillier, 23.

32.   These probability analyses are based on 1999 French census data. See Gossiaux, S.,

M. Simon, and V. Rodwin. 2002. A Paris, plus de six femmes sur dix vivent seules après 80 ans. *INSEE Ile-de-France à la page,* no. 210 (May–June) (www.insee.fr/ile-de-france): fig. 5.

33.   Chesnais, Jean-Claude. 1988. Retirement Systems and Social Policy in Ageing Cities: The Case of Paris. In *Ageing and Urbanization: Proceedings of the United Nations Conference on Ageing Populations in the Context of Urbanization, Sendai, Japan, 12–16 September 1988.* 1991. New York: United Nations.

34.   See Web site of the City of Paris at www.paris.fr/FR/Solidarites/seniors.

35.   *Schéma Directeur Gérontologique du Département de Paris* (Health plan for older persons for the City of Paris). 1997. Paris: Division of Health and Social Affairs, October. Also see *Vieillir à Paris: Quels choix de vie à l'horizon 2010?* 1998. Vols. 1 and 2. Paris: Cahiers de Chaligny, Mairie de Paris.

36.   Chaput, H. 2002. *L'allocation supplémentaire du minimum vieillesse—Bénéficiaires au 31 décembre 2001.* Série statistiques n°45, Direction de la Recherche, des Etudes, de l'Evaluation et des Statistiques (DREES).

37.   In calculating these percentages, it was not possible to isolate those in Paris who were under sixty-five years of age. For all of France, 9 percent of the beneficiaries fall into this category.

38.   Thirteen thousand Parisians received benefits under this program in 2003. Many who are eligible, however, choose not to accept them because the full amount of benefits must be repaid from the beneficiary's estate.

39.   Huteau, Gilles, and Eric Le Bont. 1997. *Sécurité sociale et politiques sociales.* Paris. Armand Colin, 319.

40.   Cohen, S. 1975. *Modern Capitalist Planning: The French Model.* 2d ed.. Berkeley: University of California Press.

41.   Rodwin, V., with C. Brecher, D. Jolly, and R. Baxter, eds. 1991. *Pubic Hospitals in New York and Paris.* New York: New York University Press.

42.   See "*Offre de soins et problèmes de santé prioritaires en* Ile-de-France." 1992. Paris: ORS, July.

43.   *Schéma Directeur Gérontologique du Département de Paris. 1997.* Paris: Department of Social Affairs, Children's Services and Health. October. 45, 67.

44.   Study conducted in 1989–90 by the CERC (Centre d'Etudes sur les Revenus et les Capitaux. Cited in the *Schéma Directeur Gérontologique.*

45.   Forette, F. 1998. The Path toward the Prevention of Aging. *Le défi de l'âge. Les Cahiers de l'IAURF* 1(121).

46.   Henrard, J. C. 1998. The Health and Social Challenges of an Ageing Population in the European Union. *Le défi de l'âge. Les Cahiers de l'IAURF* 1(121).

13. The Health of Older Parisians

Véronique Lucas-Gabrielli, Philippe Pépin, and François Tonnellier

Introduction

The most striking aspect about the health of older Parisians is that their life expectancy, at sixty-five years, is among the highest not only in France but also in the world. In this chapter, we begin by examining the basis for this finding over the period from 1990 to 1999—before the heat wave of 2003. We also refine it by presenting a typology of health status for groups of arrondissements within Paris and groups of communes (jurisdictions) in the first ring. Next, we examine the results of a household survey in France, to see if individual-level data support the more general finding on the health of older Parisians. Finally, we examine patterns of medical care use among Parisians, as a prelude to our concluding interpretations.

Health Status by Geographic Units

The health status of the French population is characterized by an average life expectancy, at birth, comparable to other Western nations. This general measure, however, reveals some important contrasts. French men and women have the highest life expectancy after sixty-five years among the countries of the European Union. In contrast, however, premature mortality (before sixty-five years) is very high.[1] Paris reflected these distinctive characteristics in 1990, but by 1999, premature mortality had fallen, once again, to the average levels for France, due probably to the progress in treatments for HIV and AIDS.[2]

Life expectancy at sixty-five years is a good health-status indicator for older persons. In Paris, it is 18.2 for men and 22.1 for women, the highest among all ninety-five *départements* in France. The average figures for France were respectively 16.5 and 21.0. Differences in life expectancy at sixty or seventy-five years, among the départements, are similar to the differences in life expectancy at birth. Moving from west to east (Bretagne to Alsace), there is a rise in mortality. These geographic disparities have endured for half a century; the secular increase in life-expectancy trends has not modified these differences.

In 1999, the life expectancy of Parisians, at sixty, was higher than that of other départements in France. Even in 1990, Paris was well positioned and ahead of other départements (Table 13.1). Between Paris and the first ring, there was, on average, a one-year difference in life expectancy at sixty for men and for women.

Table 13.1. Life Expectancy for Persons 60+, by Gender: Paris, First Ring, Ile-de-France, and France, 1990 and 1999

	Males			Females	
	1990	**1999**		**1990**	**1999**
Paris	20.3	21.9		24.9	26.3
First Ring		21.0			25.7
Ile-de-France	19.5	21.0		24.5	25.7
France[a]	19.0	20.2		24.1	25.2
Départements					
Minimum	Pas de Calais 16.8	Pas de Calais 17.8	Moselle 22.6	Nord 23.7
Maximum	Deux Sèvres 20.4	Paris 21.9	Alpes Maritimes 25.1	Paris 26.3

Sources: 1990: INSEE; 1999: ORSIF.
[a] Includes overseas territories in 1990

In Paris proper, there are striking contrasts between the western and eastern parts of the city, which reflect the well-known differences between the wealthy neighborhoods of the west and the older working-class neighborhoods of the east. The lowest life-expectancy rates, at sixty, are in the northeast (in the départements of Seine Saint Denis). On the scale of France, Paris and the first ring appear more homogeneous: the large majority of communes are among those with the highest life-expectancy rates at sixty.

Life expectancy at birth. We performed simple correlation analysis among factors known to be related to life expectancy at birth across the 143 communes of Ile-de-France (Table 13.2). Not surprisingly, we found that life expectancy at birth is positively correlated with the characteristics of wealthier areas (e.g., percentage of professionals, mean taxable income, percentage of persons with higher levels of education) and negatively correlated with indicators of more disadvantaged areas (share of workers, unemployment rates, percentage of households exempt from tax payments). The magnitude of the correlation coefficients is often very high. For women, the correlations are significant and of the same order, but always weaker than those for men. Finally, we note that life expectancy at birth is also correlated with the percentage of persons seventy-five years and over. Evidently, the majority of the older old reside in areas where life expectancy is high.

Life expectancy at sixty and at seventy-five. For both sexes, life expectancy at different ages is correlated with life expectancy at birth. However, the magnitude of correlations with socioeconomic characteristics diminishes with age—for both men and women (Table 13.2). The local social environment, therefore, seems to have less impact after seventy-five years of age, a well-known finding in studies of life-course epidemiology.

Life expectancy and migration. Life expectancy is an index derived from mortality rates at a given time. Since it is based on cross-sectional rather than panel data, life expectancy cannot tell us anything about the possible effects of migration on this measure of population health. Since there is significant migration at retirement age among Parisians over sixty or seventy-five years, it is difficult to interpret our findings with regard to life expectancy.

Some studies suggest that over the course of a decade, more than a quarter of Parisians (with Paris defined as the agglomeration) leave Ile-de-France after retirement and settle in the provinces.[3] This proportion is more than double that of other large cities in France. Bad health can be one of the reasons for migrating around retirement age, just as it can be a reason for returning to the Ile-de-France region in later years (e.g., older persons seek the proximity of family, as well as recourse to prestigious hospitals).

Figure 13.1. Life Expectancy at Age 65+: Paris, Ile-de-France, and France, 1990

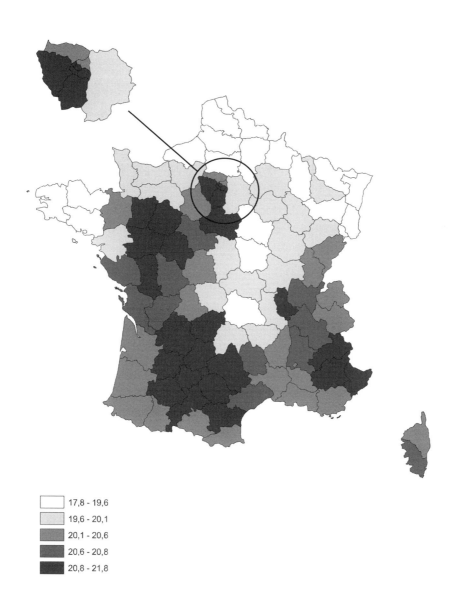

	17,8 - 19,6
	19,6 - 20,1
	20,1 - 20,6
	20,6 - 20,8
	20,8 - 21,8

Source: INSEE, 1990.

Part IV: Paris

Table 13.2. Correlations of Life Expectancy (LE) and Socioeconomic Characteristics by Gender: Paris and First Ring (136 communes), 1999

	Males			Females		
	LEB[a]	LE at 65	LE at 75	LEB[a]	LE at 65	LE at 75
Professionals	0.69	0.64	0.50	0.56	0.56	0.50
Workers	-0.77	-0.68	-0.51	-0.64	-0.59	-0.53
Households exempt from taxes	-0.78	-0.65	-0.45	-0.69	-0.57	-0.48
Mean taxable income	0.74	0.72	0.57	0.63	0.53	0.42
Population without a diploma	-0.76	-0.63	-0.45	-0.63	-0.57	-0.49
Population with higher degrees	0.72	0.69	0.55	0.58	0.57	0.51
Unemployment rate	-0.71	-0.57	-0.36	-0.64	-0.51	-0.42

Sources: ORSIF, 1999; INSEE, 1999.

Note: Each row provides the correlation coefficient between LE and the percent or rate of each socioeconomic characteristic, by commune. The correlations are adjusted for population size of the communes, which include Paris arrondissements. All communes with less than 30 deaths in 1999 were eliminated from the analysis, which is why the total number of communes is 136 out of a total of 143.

[a] Life expectancy at birth

Some studies suggest that retired Parisians who leave the Paris agglomeration are in worse health than those who stay. Evidence from one longitudinal study suggests that individuals leaving the agglomeration have higher-than-average mortality rates: "When one reclassifies the regional deaths according to previous residence, the low mortality rates of Ile-de-France disappear."[4] Data collected in a 1986 survey of a panel of 1972 retirees from the Paris agglomeration, some of whom emigrated and others of whom stayed, provide evidence in support of this conclusion: those who stayed were in better health.[5] Thus, despite the important distinction between the mortality measured in a given year and longitudinal observations, the results appear to be consistent.

With respect to the difference between Paris and its first ring, the presence of Parisians in nursing homes outside Paris can complicate interpretations of the health statistics for older Parisians. Thirty percent of Parisians in nursing-home beds reside in institutions that are under the city's jurisdiction but located outside Paris (see Chapter 15); this could have the effect of diminishing mortality rates among Parisians and augmenting them among residents of the first ring.

Whatever indicator is used—life expectancy at sixty, sixty-five, seventy-five, or eighty—it appears that older persons in Paris are in very good health, at least based on mortality criteria. To investigate this finding further, we present a typology of Paris arrondissements versus first-ring communes to refine the Paris versus first-ring comparisons. Finally, we present our recent analysis of perceived health status to test the reliability of our findings.

A Typology of Health Status for Paris and the First Ring

Based on the indicators in Table 13.2, data obtained from the 1999 census, and our analysis of the most significant correlations, we performed a factor analysis across our 143 units to explore the relationships between social characteristics and life expectancy and to classify groups of units with common features. We relied on a large number of variables that may be classified and defined as follows:

1. Social composition: share of workers, artisans, managers, employees, those involved in the agricultural sector, midlevel professionals, and retired persons
2. Employment: includes all fourteen classes of employment
3. Educational levels
4. Age structure: percentage of persons under twenty, from twenty to sixty, from sixty to seventy-five, and seventy-five and over
5. Economic status: average income of taxable households, average income of taxed households, percentage of households exempt from taxes, average income of these households
6. Diverse indicators of deprivation or social isolation, such as unemployment

rates, proportion of single-family households, proportion of foreigners, proportion of older persons living alone, rates of car ownership

In our factor analysis, we mapped the socioeconomic variables along the axes and used life expectancy and the density of general practitioners as supplementary variables. In this way, it is possible to show the social situations associated with high or low levels of life expectancy. We classified the principal components of the analysis in ascending hierarchy to synthesize all our data across sixty variables and 136 geographic units.

Based on this analysis, we arrived at a three-class typology that enables us to distinguish: (1) Paris; (2) the upscale suburbs; and (3) the average and working-class suburbs. This first result justifies our considering Paris apart from the rest of the first ring. The indicator of occupational mix provides an objective measure in our analysis.

In considering a typology within each class, we divided class 1 into three subgroups (1.1, 1.2, and 1.3); class 2 remains the same; and we divided class 3 into two subgroups (3.1 and 3.2).

Class 1. Paris. Each of the groups that constitute Paris is characterized by a large share of older persons who live alone. Distinguishing among these three groups, we find:

Class 1.1. The Heart of Paris. This group (Table 13.3) includes the arrondissements characterized by a large proportion of managers/executives and professionals, as well as persons who have completed a high level of schooling. In contrast, the proportion of workers is lower than the average. There are more single-person households and more older persons who live alone. Average net taxable income is higher than the Paris average. However, income from households exempt from taxes is lower than average. This is an indication of the enormous income inequalities among this group. The percentage of persons seventy-five and over is higher than average, as is life expectancy at sixty-five (for men and women). The density of general practitioners is slightly higher than average.

Class 1.2. Working-Class Paris. This group (Table 13.4) includes the arrondissements of eastern Paris, which constitute the former working-class neighborhoods of the capital. Socioeconomic indicators here reflect this situation, as this group is the most disadvantaged of those in Paris. Unemployment rates are high, as is the proportion of households exempt from taxes. Here the average income of households exempt from taxes is lower than the average, as is the average income of tax-paying households. Thus, the inequality of incomes among this group is less than in other Paris groups. The percentage of persons seventy-five and over is close to the aver-

Table 13.3. Socioeconomic Characteristics of the Heart of Paris, Class 1.1, 1999

	Group Average %	All Classes Average %
Managers/executives	20.7	12.4
Higher-education degree	30.3	18.0
Workers	4.2	8.3
Older persons living alone	60.0	51.0
Single-person households	53.0	40.0
Density of general practitioners	0.93	0.79
Persons 75+	8.4	6.6
Life expectancy at 65 (men/women)	18.7/22.6	18.10/22.1

Sources: ORSIF, 1999; INSEE, 1999.

Table 13.4. Socioeconomic Characteristics of Working-Class Paris, Class 1.2, 1999

	Group Average %	All Classes Average %
Unemployment rate	15.3	12.7
Households without cars	60.8	39.0
Foreigners	17.6	14.2
Households exempt from taxes	41.1	35.6
Older persons living alone	59.5	51.0
Single-person households	51.3	40.0
Density of general practitioners	0.77	0.79
Persons 75+	6.4	6.6
Life expectancy at 65 (men/women)	17.8/22.1	18.1/22.1

Sources: ORSIF, 1999; INSEE, 1999.

age, while life expectancy at sixty-five is slightly lower than the mean. This is true for the density of generalists as well.

Class 1.3. Upscale Paris Neighborhoods. These arrondissements, comprising most of western Paris, constitute the wealthiest neighborhoods (Table 13.5). All indicators demonstrate this fact—the percentage of managers/executives, average taxable household income, and the proportion of persons with higher educational degrees. In these neighborhoods, the share of households exempt from taxes is the lowest of all three Paris classes. They are therefore characterized by extreme income inequalities. The percentage of persons seventy-five and over is higher here than the average (11 vs. 6.6) and indicators for life expectancy at sixty-five are higher than in all the other classes. The density of generalists is much higher than the average.

Class 2. The Well-to-Do Suburbs. This class is comprised mostly of suburban neighborhoods in the western outskirts of Paris, which are characterized by high proportions of managers/executives, high net income for taxable households, and low unemployment rates (Table 13.6). In contrast to Paris groups (in class 1), the average income of households exempt from taxes is higher than the group average, which suggests greater homogeneity of income in these areas. The proportion of persons seventy-five and over is slightly higher than average, as is life expectancy at sixty-five (for men and women). The density of general practitioners, however, is close to the average.

Class 3.1. Middle-Class Suburbs. All the indicators for this group suggest that these neighborhoods are comprised of the middle class: the percentage of managers/executives is low, while the share of workers is high (Table 13.7). Net income for taxable households is lower than average and income for households exempt from taxes is higher than average. The income disparities are therefore lower than for Paris. The proportion of persons seventy-five and over is lower than average (5.4 vs. 6.6), while life expectancy at sixty-five is a little lower than average, as is the density of generalists.

Class 3.2. Working-Class Suburbs. All the indicators for this group reveal what we would expect to find in disadvantaged working-class areas—for example, high unemployment rates, and a high share (close to 50 percent) of households exempt from taxes (Table 13.8). The proportion of persons seventy-five and over is small (4.5 vs. 6.6) and life expectancy at sixty-five is the lowest among the six groups, for women and for men (a one-year difference in comparison to the average). Also, these indicators are lower than for all of Paris and its first ring, but higher than the average for France (Table 13.1). The density of generalists is lower than average, with a value identical to the preceding class.

Table 13.5. Socioeconomic Characteristics of Upscale Paris Neighborhoods, Class 1.3, 1999

	Group Average	All Classes Average
	%	%
Managers	21.2	12.4
Persons with higher degrees	37.5	18.0
Workers	2.6	8.3
Older persons living alone	54.1	51.0
Single-person households	50.5	40.0
Net taxed household income	396 KF	169 KF
Net income of households exempt from taxes	30 855 F	35 294 F
Households exempt from taxes	24.0	35.6
Density of general practitioners	1.2	0.79
Persons 75+	11.0	6.6
Life expectancy at 65 (men/women)	20.4/23.4	18.1/22.1

Sources: ORSIF, 1999; INSEE, 1999.

Table 13.6. Socioeconomic Characteristics of Well-to-Do Suburbs, Class 2, 1999

	Group Average	All Classes Average
	%	%
Managers/executives	15.8	12.4
Unemployment rate	8.7	12.7
Workers	5.5	8.3
Older persons living alone	49.2	51.0
Single-persons households	37.7	40.0
Net income of households exempt from taxes	37 554 F	35 294 F
Density of general practitioners	0.76	0.79
Persons 75+	7.2	6.6
Life expectancy at 65 (men/women)	18.5/22.5	18.1/22.1

Sources: ORSIF, 1999; INSEE, 1999.

Table 13.7. Socioeconomic Characteristics of Middle-Class Suburbs, Class 3.1, 1999

	Group Average %	All Classes Average %
Managers/executives	7.4	12.4
Employees	17.4	15.0
Workers	10.1	8.3
With CAP Diploma[a]	20.3	15.5
Older persons living alone	45.0	51.0
Single-person households	31.0	40.0
Density of general practitioners	0.70	0.79
Persons 75+	5.4	6.6
Life expectancy at 65 (men/women)	17.7/22.0	18.1/22.1

Sources: ORSIF, 1999; INSEE, 1999.

[a] A junior high school certificate

Perceived Health Status of Older Parisians

Every two years since 1988, the Centre de Recherche et de Documentation en Economie de la Santé (CREDES) has organized a survey of households on issues of health, social care, and social insurance. In essence, the survey consists of a panel of households, a quarter of which is surveyed every year. Every fourth year, the first quarter is once again surveyed; and so on. The sample is drawn from the Permanent Panel of Insurance Beneficiaries (PPIB) of the French National Health Insurance Fund for Salaried Workers. This sample is representative of 1/1200th of the beneficiaries. To assure that the sample is representative of the whole French population, additional samples based on the PPIB model were drawn from beneficiaries of the National Fund of Independent Professionals and from the national fund covering farmers and agricultural workers.[6]

As part of this survey, medical coverage and medical care use are studied. Questions are asked about the deferral of medical care because of financial barriers (cost sharing), about tobacco use, and about more general issues of perception and opinion. We completed the present analysis of perceived health status based on a sample of forty-three thousand throughout France from 1998 to 2000.

Unfortunately, the survey does not include individuals in institutions (hospitals or institutions for older persons). This represents an important limitation for our topic. However, these are the only individual-level data on perceived health status at our

Table 13.8. Socioeconomic Characteristics of Working-Class Suburbs, Class 3.2, 1999

	Group Average %	All Classes Average %
Managers/executives	3.7	12.4
Workers	14.3	8.3
Foreigners	20.6	14.2
Without CAP diploma	23.6	14.5
Unemployment rate	18.6	12.7
Households exempt from taxes	48.4	35.6
Older persons living alone	45.2	51.0
Single-person households	30.0	40.0
Density of generalists	0.68	0.79
Persons 75+	4.6	6.6
Life expectancy at 65 (men/women)	17.1/21.2	18.1/22.1

Sources: ORSIF, 1999; INSEE, 1999.

disposal. It is therefore tempting to analyze them to establish whether they support our general findings on health status of older Parisians based on mortality data.

Two years provide sufficient numbers to draw statistically valid conclusions for Paris, where the sample included 243 people aged sixty years and over, of whom 158 responded to the questionnaire. For the first ring surrounding Paris, the figure was 338, of whom 253 responded. The results are therefore sufficient to say something about the differences between the urban core and the first ring. All the tables that follow concern persons sixty years and older. The data were adjusted for age and sex differences.

Vital risk and severity. At the CREDES, we have developed two indicators of morbidity: vital risk and disability. These indicators provide information about the severity, evolution, and consequences of certain illnesses and are attributed to each individual by the doctors in charge of coding the surveys. The same scales of risk were used to define the minimal severity for each of the illnesses recorded in the survey. In this way, each observed illness is given two indicators of severity: minimum vital risk and minimum disability. These, in turn, provide an estimate of the probability of death or of disability risk for an individual who suffers from only one illness.[7]

From the survey records, an "indicator of vital risk" was constructed that measured the risk of death within the five years following the interview (Table 13.9). Clearly, the percentage of individuals at "very great risk or great risk" is smaller in Paris than in the whole of France (and higher in the first ring). However, the percentage of individuals with a "possible risk" is correspondingly higher in Paris. These observations therefore support the mortality findings for Paris.

However, since the table includes the population sixty years and over, it is necessary to perform an age adjustment, because those seventy years and older represent 29 percent of the sixty-and-over population of Paris and 26 percent of the sixty-and-over population of France as a whole. We therefore calculated an index standardizing for age and sex. These indices confirm the percentages obtained in Table 13.9.

Disability. Following the principle of "vital risk," an indicator of disability was constructed, with a scale from "not disabled" to "light restriction" to "very reduced activity." The score for this indicator is also given by doctors who analyze the survey records. The results here are also consistent with the findings on mortality (Table 13.10): the percentage of individuals for whom activity is very reduced is lower in Paris than the average for France. In fact, the percentage of individuals "without disability" is correspondingly two times lower in Paris than in the whole of France, and the median group in Paris (for light restriction or reduced activity) is more significant than for France as a whole. These figures do not contradict what we have seen about mortality: the extremes for mortality are less represented, with a parallel increase in median classes. The indices correcting for age and sex confirm these results.

Use of Medical Care among Older Parisians

Drawing on survey data on medical care use in France, we find that Parisians sixty years and over consult with physicians twice as often as do their counterparts in the

Table 13.9. Perceived Risk of Death by Respondents 60+: Paris, First Ring, and France, 1998–2000

	Paris	First Ring	France
	%	%	%
No risk	44.5	43.6	48.8
Possible risk	41.6	33.6	33.1
Very great or great risk	13.9	22.8	18.2
Total	100.0	100.0	100.0

Sources: PPIB, CREDES, 1998–2000.

Table 13.10. Perceived Risk of Disability by Respondents 60+: Paris, First Ring, and France, 1998–2000

| | Paris | First Ring | France |
	%	%	%
No disability	7.4	13.8	16.5
Light constraint	35.5	33.4	31.8
Restricted activity	42.5	33.5	34.6
Activity very reduced	14.6	19.3	17.1
Total	100.0	100.0	100.0

Sources: PPIB, CREDES, 1998-2000.

Table 13.11. Average Number of Annual Physician Consultations for Persons 60+: Paris, First Ring, and France, 1998–2000

	Paris	First Ring	Paris and First Ring	France
Specialist visits per capita	6.0	4.9	4.5	3.0
GP visits per capita	4.3	4.7	4.9	6.6

Sources: PPIB, CREDES, 1998-2000.

rest of France, and there is a clear gradient from Paris, the first ring, and the rest of the country.[8] Conversely, older Parisians consult with fewer general practitioners and the rate goes up in the first ring and beyond to the rest of France (Table 13.11).

In addition to higher expenditures on specialists, older persons in Paris spend more on pharmaceuticals, but 9.4 percent of these products are over-the-counter medications versus 4.3 percent in France. The small size of this age cohort makes it difficult to find any statistically significant differences in hospitalization.

Finally, as is always the case among those over sixty years old, 23 percent of the persons surveyed (versus 14 percent in France) declared that they had deferred medical care over the course of the previous year. This is consistent with the finding across all age cohorts in Paris before the implementation of universal coverage in January 2000.

In summary, the characteristics of medical care expenditures for older persons are not different from those for Parisians across all ages. These findings reveal stark contrasts and significant inequalities, regardless of age: expenditures on specialists are very high, but deferral of care and the percentage of individuals without complementary health-insurance coverage are also very high.

Concluding Interpretations

From a spatial point of view, Paris presents a striking contrast to London: there is a higher percentage of older persons in Paris in comparison to its outskirts, while in London the share of older persons in Outer London is higher than in Inner London. However, the heart of Paris is also the place where income inequalities are the highest, which is a feature it shares with the British capital. We have shown that the health of older persons in Paris and its first ring reflects a balance of contrasts. There are positive elements (high levels of life expectancy at sixty) and negative ones (a high proportion of persons living alone and large income disparities).

In Paris and its first ring, a large proportion of older persons reside in upscale, well-to-do areas. In contrast, only a small share of older persons reside in the deprived working-class suburbs and the neighborhoods of eastern Paris. Also, it is striking to note that income disparities are highest among the upscale neighborhoods, and 68 percent of persons seventy-five and over live alone in these areas.

The data we presented on perceived health status are consistent with the data on life expectancy in suggesting that older Parisians are in better health than their fellow citizens in the rest of France. Likewise, the study of Parisian retirees, which compared self-assessed health status of those who left the agglomeration with that of those who stayed, indicates that the latter are in better health.[9]

With respect to the use of medical care, our survey data indicate that Parisians, at all ages, use more specialist services, dental care, auxiliary personnel, and prescription drugs than the French average. We also know, based on residence-based hospital-admission data, that hospitalization rates for Parisians are lower than the average in France.

The good health reported by Parisians sixty years and over raises a number of questions. How can one disentangle the effects of relatively easy access to medical care in a world city with prestigious medical centers from frequent use of outpatient specialist care? Do patients who have more consultations with specialists merely reveal a selection bias based on higher social class and better living conditions? It is not easy to find data that can answer these questions. But the data we have examined do point to one clear trend. Population aging in the first ring around Paris, particularly among immigrants, will surely affect the so-called underprivileged and young municipalities. It is probably in these places that we must anticipate emerging needs for long-term care services.

Notes

1. De Kervasdoué, J., dir. 2000. *Le carnet de santé de la France.* Paris: Mutualité Française.

2. Observatoire Régional de la Santé d'Ile-de-France [Regional Health Observatory for Ile de France]. [ORSIF]. 2003. *La santé des Franciliens.* Paris: ORSIF.

3. Cribier, F., and A. Kych.1992. La migration de retraite des parisiens: Une analyse de la propension au départ. *Population* 3:677–718.

4. Desplanques, G. 1995. Le recul de la mortalité. In J. Dupaquier, dir. 1995. *Histoire de la population française.* Vol. 4, *De 1914 à nos jours.* Paris: Presses Universitaires de France, 240.

5. Cribier, F. 2003. La santé auto-estimée des hommes et des femmes à l'époch de la retraite. *Retraite et Société* 39:94–117; table 1, 102.

6. Auvray, L., S. Dumesnil, and P. LeFur. 2001. *Santé, soins et protection sociale en 2000: Enquête sur la santé et la protection sociale.* Paris: Centre de Recherche et de Documentation en Economie de la Santé (CREDES).

7. The minimum vital risk is made up of six categories of increasing risk: no indication of vital risk, very minor poor prognosis, minor poor prognosis, possible risk to vitality, probable poor prognosis (50 percent probability of death within the next ten years), and clear poor prognosis (death within the next five years). Minimal disability is comprised of eight categories of increasing severity: no difficulty, very little difficulty, little difficulty, difficulty but able to lead a normal life, has to somewhat restrict professional or domestic activities, slower or reduced activity, lack of domestic autonomy, bedridden or permanently confined to bed.

8. Permanent Panel of Insurance Beneficiaries (PPIB) of the French National Health Insurance Fund for Salaried Workers (CNAMTS). 1998–2000. Survey. Paris: CREDES.

9. Cribier, La santé auto-estimée.

14. Inequalities and Quality of Life among Older Persons in Paris

Marie-Eve Joël and Robert Haas

In France, the legal retirement age is sixty years. As a result, from a legal, administrative, or statistical perspective, sixty is considered an important threshold; it marks a significant change in status. Persons who have passed this threshold become "older persons," which introduces a number of changes in their rights and social benefits. The term "older persons" now includes an important and growing number of citizens over sixty for a period that can exceed forty years. This covers, in France, a wide variety of circumstances, the only common point being the departure from the world of work.

Although "older persons" typically refers to the statistical reference group of those sixty years and over, for the reasons we have just noted, two other age cohorts typically receive special attention, particularly in the areas of health and social services: persons seventy-five and over and persons eighty-five and over. These age groups coincide with periods in life when health problems emerge at disproportionately high rates and where the loss of autonomy begins to be most noticeable. Although they capture attention, the number of persons in these age groups is fortunately quite small.

What are the incomes and living conditions of Parisians in these age groups? How may we characterize their housing conditions? What can be said about their quality of life? This chapter aims to answer these three questions. However, it would be presumptuous not to emphasize, at the outset, the fragmentary nature of available information and the lack of routinely available and updated statistical profiles. For example, there is limited quantitative information on the cultural habits, transportation patterns, intergenerational ties, and neighborhood life of older persons. One explanation for these lacunae is that public consciousness of population aging has been late in coming. Another is that understanding population aging in cities requires information on spatial and intergenerational aspects of the process. After all, to be understood, older persons must be studied in the context of their relational networks—their family or their immediate proximity—and within their spatial confines, whether they are more or less livable. Ideally, it would be important to explore relationships between particular kinds of networks and neighborhoods or urban settings. Such data, however, are typically collected only in ethnographic case studies.

The Income of Older Persons

Pensions in Ile-de-France and France. A good approach to studying the income of older residents of the Ile-de-France region is to look at retirees who receive national old-age insurance. Although one can, due to one's professional career or that of one's partner, receive old-age benefits from a variety of sources, the general fund covers the largest number of formerly employed workers, primarily those in industry and commerce. As of 1996, the Ile-de-France region included more than 1.4 million retirees who received this benefit, 16.5 percent of the total population of retirees who receive benefits in France (excluding the territories).[1] In 2000, retirement benefits represented 17 percent of gross domestic product.

A study by the Institut National de Statistiques et des Etudes Economiques (INSEE; the National Institute for Statistics and Economic Studies) noted that in 1997 "the average monthly amount provided by national old-age insurance was raised to 3,840 F (585 euros) in Ile-de-France, as opposed to an average amount of 3,140 F (479 euros) for the entire country" (Table 14.1). Since more than a third of retirees are affiliated with many insurance schemes, the pension provided by national old-age insurance is complemented with those from other sources. As a result, in 1997 the overall amount of retirement increased in France to an average of 6,800 F (1,037 euros).[2] This average conceals striking disparities. One retiree in ten receives retirement benefits greater than 12,250 F (1,868 euros), while one in ten receives retirement benefits less than 1,800 F (274 euros).

There are also significant disparities among men and women: the average monthly amount for men in 1997 came to 8,800 F (1,342 euros); for women, 5,030 F (767 euros). Table 14.2 shows these gender disparities by age cohorts for Ile-de-France and France.

For Ile-de-France, the total pension payment exceeds the average amount for France by approximately 2,400 F (366 euros) per month (Table 14.1). This difference can be explained partly by the higher share of former managers/executives

Table 14.1. Components of Pension Payments: Ile-de-France and France, 1997

	Basic Allocation	Supplementary Allocation	Other Benefits[a]	Spousal Death Benefit	Total Pension
Ile-de-France	8,346	21	295	553	9,215
France	5,983	59	278	484	6,804

Source: SESI, sample across all public pension plans, 1997; includes pensioners 60+.

[a] For children or for a dependent spouse

Note: Figures are in French francs.

Table 14.2. Pension Payments for Persons 60+ by Gender and Age Group: Ile-de-France and France, 1997

	60–64	65–69	70–74	75–84	85+	All
Ile-de-France						
Men	10,641	12,418	13,496	12,313	11,219	12,228
Women	7,602	6,879	6,784	6,805	6,400	6,895
Ratio (men:women)	1:4	1:8	2:0	1:9	1:8	1:8
France						
Men	8,202	8,455	8,478	8,525	7,254	8,805
Women	4,903	4,149	3,779	3,567	3,087	5,034
Ratio (men:women)	1:7	2:0	2:2	2:4	2:3	1:7

Source: SESI, sample across all public pension plans, 1997; includes pensioners 60+.
Note: Figures are in French francs.

and professionals living in Ile-de-France, and partly by the higher wage levels there. As can be seen in Table 14.2, men received an average pension payment of 12,288 F (1,873 euros) and women received an average of 6,895 F (1,051 euros). The increase in the number of women in the work force over the past decades has led to significant increases in payments to those among the younger generations. That said, the higher average pension payment for retirees in Ile-de-France must be considered against the fact that living expenses there are also higher.

In comparison to inhabitants of the outskirts, Parisians with low incomes benefit from more subsidy programs to increase their pensions. Also, there are a wider range of services and amenities available in the city (e.g., subsidized or even free meals), thanks to the programs operated by the Paris authorities and the number of nonprofit organizations that attend to older persons in Paris.[3]

Income disparities in Paris. A survey of household incomes based on declarations to the Ministry of Finance provides valuable data on the incomes of older household heads across the arrondissements of Paris (Table 14.3). Comparison of their median incomes, by arrondissement, reveals strong income inequalities among the poorest household heads seventy-five years and over (in arrondissements 3, 10, 11, 18, 19, 20) and the most well to do (in arrondissements 6, 7, 8,16). The ratio of median income in the seventh to the second arrondissement is 2.3 (Table 14.3), higher than among the median incomes of households across all ages and higher as well than such income disparities among older households in the rest of France.

Income inequalities among arrondissements also vary greatly, as measured by the ratio of the ninth to the first income decile within each (Table 14.3). Profiles of different arrondissements vary according to the relative magnitude of low and high incomes within each. Thus, the income inequalities among household heads seventy-five and over are highest in the following arrondissements: 4, 6, 9, 16, 7, 1, and 8. In arrondissements 1, 4, and 9, the very center of Paris, the threshold for the lower incomes is the lowest. In these areas, older, relatively poor household heads continue to reside in old apartments, while another part of the housing stock was renovated by more well-to-do older household heads. In arrondissements 6, 7, 8, and 16, the threshold for low-income older household heads is much higher and the income disparities remain very high.

Arrondissements 8 and 20 represent both extremes of the income inequality distribution. Older households in the twentieth reveal low gaps among deciles because both low and high incomes are relatively low. The eighth arrondissement illustrates the opposite situation (the lower of the low incomes and the higher of the high incomes). Thus, the disparity among older household heads is the highest. The level of the high incomes is 13.5 times higher than that of the lower incomes. Thus, we see, older households across a wide range share the same neighborhood.

Such income disparities among older households are greater within Paris than among communes (jurisdictions) of the first ring. There, median incomes of older household heads are high in the western outskirts in the departments of Hauts de Seine and Yvelines (Neuilly-sur-Seine, Saint Cloud, for example). In contrast, they are far lower in the northeast outskirts, where more older household heads are likely to be working-class retirees with lower median incomes.

The growth of purchasing power. At the national level, estimates suggest that the purchasing power of persons fifty years and over is less than 30 percent of those under fifty, and that of retirees is, on average, equal to that of an active person. Over the past twenty years, the purchasing power of the average French household increased by 60 percent. The highest increase was for persons sixty years and over. At the beginning of the 1970s, one out of four pensioners lived under the poverty level; this proportion is no more than one of twenty-five today. Over the same period, in contrast, the poverty rate among active households (salaried and unemployed) has increased.

The Housing of Older Persons

INSEE's housing survey of 1996 provides a wealth of information on the French population's housing characteristics, by age cohort and place of residence. These data enable one to get a good sense of the housing of older persons for Ile-de-France, even if they are slightly out of date.

Table 14.3. Income Reported by Household Heads 75+: Paris Arrondissements, 2000

Arrondissement	Median in euros (€)	1st Decile Income Threshold (€)	9th Decile Income Threshold in 9th Decile (€)	Ratio (9th: 1st Decile)
1	21,272	7,169	76,745	10:7
2	15,398	6,025	41,790	6:9
3	16,616	6,117	51,785	8:4
4	21,041	7,214	65,964	9:1
5	23,982	9,185	69,042	7:5
6	31,544	10,150	93,974	9:2
7	35,393	10,418	105,059	10:10
8	34,011	8,161	110,539	13:5
9	19,012	5,886	56,903	9:6
10	16,946	6,585	44,892	6:8
11	16,526	6,534	42,947	6:5
12	20,884	9,107	50,746	5:6
13	19,555	7,879	47,257	5:9
14	22,315	9,529	55,070	5:7
15	23,839	9,441	59,847	6:3
16	35,757	10,190	99,523	9:7
17	23,051	8,412	67,012	7:9
18	16,836	6,884	40,807	5:9
19	17,305	7,089	41,614	5:8
20	17,067	7,212	40,439	5:6

Source: INSEE-DGI, Local Household Incomes Reported to Tax Authorities in 2000.

Home ownership versus rentals. When one examines the characteristics of housing units in Paris for household heads sixty years and over compared to those of all household heads, it is evident that homeowners are most often household heads sixty years and over (Table 14.4). Close to half of them succeeded in acquiring property, in contrast to one-third for all households. Renters, in contrast, represent young household heads with the exception of those in public housing (HLM—*habitation à loyer modéré*).

That older persons are most often homeowners is a great benefit when they reach the age where they must confront their increasing disabilities and eventually finance a range of home-care services. Homeownership also increases their sense of security and reinforces the desire to live at home. What is more, to be a homeowner means disposing of a certain capital and capacity for financial maneuvers in the event of the need for institutional long-term care. In contrast, payment of rent can be difficult to finance if it becomes necessary to cover the costs of increasing disabilities and sometimes leads older persons to retirement homes sooner than they would like. Renters in public housing (HLM) or rent-controlled apartments under the law of 1948 derive clear benefits from their status as renters, which then become difficult—almost impossible—to replicate should they need to move to a residential or nursing home, because the changes they would have to pay in such a case easily exceed their previous rents. Such situations can force older persons to apply for welfare support, which shifts responsibility to public authorities.

One might suppose a priori that living in an HLM is a sign of relative poverty; but this is not always true in Paris, because many beneficiaries of such housing have income levels well above the eligibility thresholds. In these cases, older renters do not typically wish to change their place of residence. As for older renters with rent-controlled apartments under the law of 1948, they can practically never

Table 14.4. Characteristics of Housing Units for Household Heads 60+ and All Households: Paris, 1996

	Household Heads 60+ %	All Households %
Homeowners	47.4	29.6
Unfurnished non-HLM rental units	28.0	41.8
HLM rental units	19.0	16.7
Furnished rentals	1.7	4.6
Units with no rent payments	4.0	7.3

Source: INSEE, Housing Survey, 1996.

be evicted. Since their rents do not correspond to market prices, they typically do everything in their power to maintain their apartments. These two factors exercise a strong effect on the housing situation of older persons in Ile-de-France, and more specifically, Paris.

Among older household heads that are homeowners, it is also possible to distinguish between those who are on the way to becoming property owners and those who are already owners. With the passage of time, as mortgage payments are paid off, those on the way to ownership become owners; thus, the rate of real homeownership is strongly correlated with age. As a share of all homeowners, 44 percent are on the route to ownership; for household heads sixty years and over, this share drops to 7 percent.

In Ile-de-France, the rental housing stock comprises close to half of all principal residences, and the distribution by age varies by the characteristics of the units. Over half of older renters live in public housing and over one-fourth live in private sector rentals. For rent-controlled units regulated by the law of 1948, in six out of ten households, the head is sixty years and over.

The problem of substandard units. Household heads sixty years and over in Ile-de-France, more often than the population of all household heads (6 vs. 4 percent), live in substandard units, defined in the INSEE study as those without toilets, showers or baths, and central heating within their apartment. Within Paris, slightly less than 75 percent of household heads sixty and over lived in housing that met all three INSEE standards, in contrast to 88 percent in the first ring.

To live in substandard housing as an older person, particularly one with emerging disabilities, can make it enormously difficult to maintain full autonomy at home. In some cases, the conflict between maintaining health and assuring hygienic conditions in one's apartment can make it impossible to stay at home. It is conceivable that the small size of an apartment and its deficiencies may lead an occupant to spend more time outside and thereby maintain stimulating activities and a rich network of friends.[4] Such circumstances, however, wherein problems that appear formidable are perceived as advantages, tend to be exceptions. They emphasize the need to take into consideration the full gamut of factors that affect the living conditions of older persons.

Quality of Life

Many neighborhoods have developed a range of services designed to improve the quality of life for their pensioners. These services typically cover housing improvements, meals on wheels, telephone assistance, free and subsidized transportation, travel accompaniment, and even cultural activities (both in the home and outside). These forms of solidarity organized by and around local governments should not be ignored. On the one hand, they depend on the density and dynamics of local civil society; on the other, they reflect a certain political tone and character—the personal charisma of local politicians and interests can orient and intensify the range of available services. In France, programs for older persons can differ depending on whether local government is aligned with the Left or the Right. The contrasts between those so aligned are very strong, and the range of services made available for older persons is emphatically heterogeneous.

Statistical surveys have not detected this diversity for several reasons. First, a centralized database does not exist. Second, programs do not last long. Finally, the structure of these programs is evolving and depends on the policies and organizations that support them. Every action initially undertaken by a mayor could be entrusted to a nonprofit organization and developed at the departmental level by the general council or one of its divisions. Conversely, it is also possible for local initiatives to engage the support of local governments.

Generally, population surveys show that older persons approve of their style of life, both in cities and in rural areas. However, the proportion of persons who say that they are not worried by any problem and feel that they are not lacking anything in their neighborhood is larger in the provinces than in the Paris region: 39 versus 25 percent.[5]

Cultural amenities for Parisians. Parisians and, to a lesser extent, the inhabitants of nearby suburbs enjoy an incomparable array of cultural activities. The concentration of theaters, cinemas, concert halls, and museums, not to mention cultural institutions, is particularly high in Paris. These institutions are easily accessible by Parisians and by most inhabitants of the first ring, who are well served by public transportation—the subway, suburban commuter rail or trains, and buses.

Retired persons benefit at reduced prices from numerous cultural institutions, where they can enjoy events reserved for them (for example, visits or special excursions). Free concerts are not rare and certain time slots are reserved for retired persons, which confer on them advantages not given to those engaged in full-time professional activities. Holders of the Paris Emerald card enjoy free access to certain institutions managed by the Paris administration, such as museums (permanent exhibitions), parks and gardens, pools and public baths, and outdoor sporting areas. Older persons may also dine in any of the forty-four Emerald restaurants operated by the Paris administration.[6] One can find at least one such restaurant in every arrondissement of Paris, and certain arrondissements (e.g., 5, 18, and 20) have as many as four.

At the level of communes outside of Paris, cultural initiatives are not missing from the lives of older inhabitants. As previously noted, an inventory of such activities remains to be made. An overview of the enormous array of cultural opportunities within Ile-de-France is hard to obtain, as is a panoramic view of the region's full resources devoted to older persons.

Transportation barriers between suburbs. Access to the wide range of cultural opportunities for older persons is facilitated by a dense network of public transportation and by the free access granted to persons sixty years and over who are holders of specific cards (Emerald, Amethyst, ONAC).[7] Nevertheless, it is important to note that if it is relatively easy to travel to and from Paris, traveling from one point in the suburbs to another can be very complicated and time consuming, even if the distances are shorter. The authorities and businesses involved are doing their utmost to correct these problems, but the transportation system remains oriented primarily toward the center of the region.

The disappearance of neighborhood shops. Paris today confronts a phenomenon that makes older persons the first victims: the disappearance of neighborhood shops. Despite their efforts, the Paris authorities have not managed to prevent this evolution, which is decidedly harmful to the quality of life and social interaction in many neighborhoods. One should not suffer the illusion that sixty-six thousand stores is a high number for some two million inhabitants. Over the last decade, nearly a quarter of small businesses in Paris have closed for good. Certain neighborhoods, such as the Eleventh Arrondissement, are more affected than others by a situation largely provoked by the increase in the price of a square meter of land and its development by what has come to be known as a "monoacitivity" (the regrouping in a particular geographic area of one kind of commerce, e.g., fashion design, clothing, furniture, jewelry shops, and so forth).

The high value of land is reflected in the rents of commercial enterprises in the center of Paris, which have become practically impossible to make profitable because businesses can add only a small amount of additional value. In the outskirts of the city, one can witness the progressive disappearance of grocery stores, which are now located some distance from the streets on which people live. Likewise, banks, medical practices, and real estate agencies have replaced butchers, fishmongers, newsagents, and even cafés.[8] Between 2000 and 2003, the number of butchers decreased by 12 percent; in three years, 15 percent of hardware stores and drugstores disappeared, as did 11 percent of newsstands. The lack of small shops is something that deeply disturbs older persons when asked about the inconveniences they suffered around their neighborhoods.[9]

The big city promotes solitude. The spatial separation of family life, notably due to changes in the workplace, and the disappearance of close relatives and friends, due to advancing age, contribute to the solitude and isolation of older persons in Paris and the Ile-de-France region. In Paris, 51.7 percent of persons aged sixty to seventy-nine years live as a couple, versus only 28 percent of those eighty years and over. Conversely, 39 percent of those aged from sixty to seventy-nine and 60 percent of those eighty years and over live alone. This phenomenon is not surprising, since the rate of living alone in France increases as a function of the size of one's commune of residence, reaching 20 percent in communes of over a hundred thousand inhabitants. In the course of thirty years, the population of persons living alone doubled, surpassing 6.1 percent of the total population in 1962 and reaching 12.6 percent of the population in 1999. In the Paris region, half of older households consist of people living alone, and women represent 80 percent of them.[10]

In the Paris region, 12.2 percent of persons sixty to seventy-nine years old and 5.1 percent of persons eighty years and over live with their children (Table 14.5). Thus, the degree of such cohabitation diminishes with the age of the parents. Cohabitation of older parents with their children has an impact on the volume of services given to dependent older persons. The time given by children living with their parents is notably higher than that of children who live in a separate home. Of course, it is not possible to know whether the cohabitation occurs in the home of the parent or the child.

The isolation of older persons has dramatic consequences in emergency situations, as was shown by the heat wave in August 2003. In such conditions, care for dependent older people relies principally on professional aides and is known to be difficult, in terms of both management and financing. The importance of informal networks of older persons should not be dismissed, yet they are not well known and their context remains largely conditioned by the stability and the intensity of social relations; it is thus, for example, with respect to the effectiveness of neighborhood help.

In the domain of home help, for instance, we counted 426 different services funded by the National Old Age Insurance for Salaried Workers or their local offices out of which specific services are delivered. Such services are organized in 376 communes of Ile-de-France, 20 of which make up the neighborhoods of Paris, 113 of which comprise the first ring, and 243 of which comprise the second ring.

Table 14.5. Characteristics of Households with Heads 60+, by Age Group: Paris, 1999

	60–79	80+
	%	%
Couple without child	42.8	26.4
Couple with child	8.9	1.6
Alone with child	3.3	3.5
Alone	39.2	60.6
Others	5.8	7.9

Source: Les personnes âgées à Paris: éléments de diagnostic socio-économique, Atelier Parisien d'Urbanisme, February 14, 2002.

What is more, most of the time local services do not go beyond the local commune in which they are organized. In such a manner, with only two exceptions, all the communes of the first ring are served. Likewise, in the second ring, only five communes are not served. As long as a neighborhood network of home helpers and other professionals, along with informal care, is not assembled and coordinated at the local level, care of dependent persons will remain fragile and subject to the hazards of unusual circumstances.

The idea of creating one-stop offices capable of bringing together in one place the information and professionals necessary for the organization and coordination of services for older persons found its expression in Local Centers for Gerontological Information and Coordination, commonly known as CLICs. Although the initial program was put in place late for budgetary reasons, the establishment of CLICs has progressed, notably in Paris and the Paris region.

Urban hostility and fear. Persons sixty years and over living in the city are far more concerned than are those who live in rural areas about the lack of security in their neighborhoods: 15 percent in provincial cities and 22 percent in the Paris region, compared with less than 5 percent in the rural areas. However, a general sense of insecurity is more often expressed by older persons living in cities in the provinces than in the Paris region. Although 2 percent of persons sixty years and over living in the city were victims of violent acts (that is, acts seen as such by the victim) in the last two years, the proportion of them who have witnessed such acts is larger: 5 percent of older persons in the provinces knew of at least one such situation, as compared to 14 percent of older persons in the Paris region.[11]

In cities like Paris, the organization of public places and their rhythm can themselves discourage older persons. Public spaces are primarily conceived for those who can travel quickly, can understand visual and more subtle signs, and have good eyesight. We all know that the majority of pedestrian streetlights change too quickly to allow older persons with difficulties to see the change from red to green, to decide whether to cross or not. That numerous sidewalks are not even smoothly paved is a source of apprehension for persons who do not travel well on foot and can discourage them from venturing out onto the street.

The example of large train stations in Paris is equally revealing. How, given that the departure-platform for trains is often posted less than fifteen minutes in advance, can older persons who move slowly and can get lost easily reach their train on time?[12] The accessibility of places and services is not created by people who have such difficulties. The pressure of numbers and of the crowd can itself discourage someone who feels vulnerable. For example, the work speed of cashiers in certain stores is often too fast for older persons, who need a little time to arrange purchases in their bags.

In this way, activities that for many seem innocuous and requiring of little effort can, in certain conditions, become treacherous for older persons and lead them not to undertake such activities. With a growing loss of autonomy, one can progressively slip into the inner recesses of oneself and become isolated.

The Future

One of the principal questions is how Paris and its surrounding region will respond to the challenges posed by the structural shift in the age pyramid. The growth in the number of persons sixty and over, and in particular those seventy-five and over, will have to become an occasion for reflecting on the adaptation of urban and periurban life for older persons, many of whom have their own needs, demands, and rhythms. This is particularly important given that the population of older persons will grow from 4.2 to 11.6 million by 2050.

It is necessary to rethink urban management and development as functions of demographic evolution. This is especially true given that Paris, with a concentration of 240 inhabitants per hectare, is the second-most-dense city of the four compared in this volume. The problem is complex because it concerns improving the quality of life for older persons while at the same time preserving the economic dynamism of Paris and the Ile-de-France region. To attract and retain businesses, whose financial contribution is essential for local governments; to maintain a housing stock that can assure decent conditions for the active middle class; and to conserve a quality of life for the large proportion of the population sixty and over constitute a formidable challenge for politicians and urban planners, who often must respond to competing demands.

When one speaks of people sixty and over, it is important to count the entire population of such persons, and not just those who are fragile or less autonomous because of special needs. There is often a tendency to consider problems of aging as primarily concerned with issues related to the older old and to persons with disabilities. However, such issues concern only a small proportion of persons seventy-five and over. To focus only on them would tempt us to mistake the trees for the forest.

Also, questions related to the prevention of aging-related pathologies are rarely tackled, or only in a narrow sense, such as the prevention of falls. In this regard, the matter of guidelines for good hygiene should be noted. At times these are uselessly restricting, for example, when they are used for the preparation and pricing of meals. *Program for Prevention and Organization of Services for Frail Older Persons, 2002–2005*, published by the Minister of Health in the spring of 2002, illustrates this tendency well. On the one hand, under a general plan, prevention programs are restricted to older persons who are already frail; on the other, the causes of frailty are not examined as part of the dysfunctions of the organism, prevention not being conceived of as a function of these dysfunctions. Thus, such programs focus on problems with stairs and falls, malnutrition, urinary incontinence, or difficulties related to multiple drugs and their possible adverse effects. But is the universe of older persons summed up in their weakened bodies?

This preoccupation with the body, of which the limitation of the environment of older persons in their domestic space is one of the expressions, finds a certain component of explication in the successive meanings given to the words "cure" and "care." The evolution of meaning generates confusion between two functions—one therapeutic, the other related to caring—the first clearly taking precedence over the second.[13] To care is also to be concerned about someone and to take their needs into account, to care for them, to be focused on them with attention, to advise, and to warn them. The needs of a person do not add up only to the needs of the body; to be engaged with someone implies therefore to be interested at least in everything that affects his or her conditions of life. As a consequence, all true prevention of needs, in the sense of providing for them in advance, constrains the consideration of a range of interventions as broadly understood as possible.

It is true that questions about the principle of prevention, taken in its broadest sense—regarding the objectives and the hierarchy of needs and priorities of persons concerned and of society as a whole—are practically absent from reports and action programs. Health and sociomedical dimensions of intervention alone seem only to circumscribe possible public action in support of older persons. The problems of the environment and of lifestyle, as well as the repercussions of older persons living in an environment and an urban milieu poorly adapted to the advance of age, are not taken into consideration; yet the living conditions of older persons depend heavily on doing so.

This kind of essential reflection does not appear to be supported at this time. Will the persons most concerned succeed in provoking such thinking? Will they make their voices heard? The awareness on the part of retirees of their social and political importance is hardly apparent in France, compared to their counterparts in the United States, which seems somewhat of a paradox when one considers the rate of aging of the French population and the age of a good number of French politicians and opinion leaders. There is little doubt that the evolution of living conditions of older persons and their future quality of life will depend, in no small part, on this awareness and their capacity to make their expectations known to and understood by decision makers.

Notes

1. Institut National de Statistiques et des Etudes Economiques [INSEE]. Ile-de-France. 1998. *Les personnes âgées en Ile-de-France*. No. 34, p. 51.
2. This average-income figure was calculated by the *Service des Statistiques, des Etudes, et des Systèmes d'Information, Ministère du Travail et des Affaires Sociales* on the basis of a sample of sixty thousand retirees.
3. The Division of Public Affairs (Direction générale de l'information et de la communication) of the mayor's office in Paris and the Center for Social Action for the City of Paris (Centre de l'Action Sociale de la Ville de Paris [CASVP]) publish *Solidarity Guidebook*, which is periodically updated with contact information for institutions that provide a variety of services and social assistance.
4. See, e.g., Guillet, P. 1989. *L'aventure de l'âge*. Paris: Syros; and Guillet, P. 1985. *Le sens à la vie*. Paris: Syros.
5. Michaudon, Hélène. 2001. *Le cadre de vie des plus de soixante ans. INSEE Première*, no. 760. February.
6. The Emerald card is available to all Parisians sixty years and over, and to persons above a certain disability threshold. Eligibility requires that they have spent at least three of the previous five years in Paris and that their income taxes do not exceed a certain ceiling set by the Council of Paris (2,028 Euros in 2003, with an exemption for veterans and their widows, sixty-five years and over). This card is given to eligible beneficiaries for a period of one year and is renewable. It can also be given to Parisians living in retirement homes managed by the CASVP, which are located in the first and second rings of Paris.
7. The Emerald card provides free public transportation in Paris. In addition, one can purchase, on a means-tested basis, the Amethyst card, which provides free public transportation across the entire Paris region. Also, the Office National des Anciens Combattants (National Office for Veterans) card is available to all veterans for public transportation in Paris.
8. De Chenay, Christophe. 2003. Paris voit peu à peu disparaître ses commerces de proximité. *Le Monde*. September 16.
9. Michaudon, *Le cadre de vie*.
10. Boutin, Christine. 2003. *Pour sortir de l'isolement, un nouveau prôjet de société*. Rapport parlementaire au Premier ministre. September.
11. Ibid.
12. Ibid.
13. Béraud, Claude. 2000. Apprendre à soigner. In Pascal-Henri Keller Janine Pierret, dirs. *Qu'est-ce que soigner ? Le soin du professionnel à la personne*. Paris: Syros. One may find such approaches in the British and American literature, e.g., in the distinction between "care" and "cure." See, e.g., Winnicott, Donald. 1988. Cure. In *Conversations ordinaires*. Paris: Gallimard.

15. Living Arrangements and Long-Term Care for Older Persons in Paris

Florence de Maria, Victor G. Rodwin, and Marc Esponda

In France, since 1997, there have been significant efforts to improve and rationalize long-term care services for older persons. Some reforms promoted under the banner of "aging and solidarity" have increased resources to finance more home help for the most dependent older persons—and assist their caregivers. In this regard, the replacement of the disability allowance (PSD) by the more generous personal autonomy allowance (APA) in 2002 is the most important. Others have aimed to rationalize payment for institutional services, taking into account their client "case mix" based on measures of dependency. In addition, there have been central initiatives to encourage healthy aging (*bien vieillir*) through exercise and nutrition programs. One consequence of the 2003 heat wave (*canicule*) has been to strengthen political resolve to implement these reforms.

The Paris administration—both the city and the *département* (see Chapter 12)—was a forerunner in implementing these reforms following its general master plan of 1999–2004. For example, its experimentation with the Emerald Coordination Centers for each arrondissement led the central government to require localities throughout the nation to establish "local centers for gerontological information and coordination." The Paris city government, in particular, because of its relative prosperity, the magnitude of its older and vulnerable population, and its relatively low density of nursing-home beds, has pursued an active policy of supporting vulnerable older people in their homes.

In Paris, as in the rest of France, most older people live at home—97.3 percent of those aged sixty years and over, according to the 1999 census. At the age of eighty, this becomes a little more difficult for frail older persons. But even at this age, the lion's share of older persons lives at home, and there is a much higher proportion living at home in Paris (94 percent) than in the first ring (88 percent) and in the rest of France (84 percent).

We therefore begin this chapter with an overview of the state of Paris housing and the characteristics of the units occupied by older persons. We go on to describe the Parisian home-care service system for frail older persons, with special attention to the operation of home-nursing services. Finally, we present the distinctive features of long-term institutional care for older Parisians—residential/retirement homes and nursing homes for those with higher levels of disability.

Overview of Housing for Older Persons

Most of the built environment that people come to admire in Paris goes back to the nineteenth century.[1] Nearly two-thirds of its housing stock was erected before 1949. Half was built before 1915, in contrast to 28 percent of the first ring. These proportions are similar for the share of housing units occupied by household heads sixty years and over. In the city's historic center, the proportion of older housing stock rises to 90 percent. In the outer arrondissements, the older housing stock does not exceed 66 percent, except In the seventeenth and eighteenth, where it is around 80 percent. The housing units built since 1949 are concentrated in five outer arrondissements: the thirteenth, fifteenth, sixteenth, twentieth, and nineteenth.

Another characteristic of Paris's housing stock is the small size of the units. Units with one or two rooms are the norm and represent 58 percent of all units, in contrast to 34 percent in the first ring. This proportion never falls lower than 45 percent in areas of western Paris and often exceeds 65 percent in the north. As for public or social housing (HLMs, this represents only 17 percent of all housing units in Paris. Two-thirds of it was built since 1945 and is relatively comfortable in comparison to the older housing stock in Paris.[2] The other third, mostly low-cost housing (HBM) represents the housing built between 1918 and 1939. In the peripheral arrondissements of eastern Paris (the thirteenth, nineteenth, and twentieth), social housing represents around 3 percent of all housing units; in the twelfth and fourteenth arrondissements, 20 percent; and in the most central arrondissements and the sixteenth, never more than 9 percent.

In summary, Paris has an old housing stock dominated by small units, which is undergoing gradual transformation as older units are progressively renovated. For older Parisians, a number of characteristics stand out (Table 15.1). First, their homeownership rates are higher, although they drop slightly after the age of seventy-five. Second, although they have significantly more space (share of units with more than 40m^2), still, of all units with less than 40m^2, one-fourth of households with heads aged sixty or over have less than 40m^2 of space. Third, although the share of private unfurnished rental units is lower for older household heads, slightly over a quarter live in such units, which are, on average, in far worse shape than the newer social housing.

Paris, like New York, London, and Tokyo, has a strong tradition of protecting its population from the exorbitant rises in land and housing costs. As a consequence, these cities' share of rental and social housing stock is dramatically higher than in their respective nations as a whole. In Paris, where only 30 percent of housing units are owned, older household heads stand out because they own close to half

(47 percent) of all units (Table 15.1). In the first ring, the equivalent figure for older household heads is 56 percent. For the most part, these units were acquired to raise their families, and after the departure of children, or separation from or death of a spouse, the household heads have "aged in place." In Paris, given the small size of the units, it is harder to raise a family.

Older household heads in Paris who rent their homes (53 percent in contrast to 70 percent for all ages in Paris; and 43 percent for older household heads in the first ring) have, on average, higher rates of access to social housing. Of all units rented by older Parisians, close to 40 percent are in social housing.[3] These units are typically larger than the private ones and therefore better adapted to families. After their children have gone, many of these household heads decide to stay in the public sector because of the low rent. That is why as many as 40 percent of older Parisians still live in social housing. In contrast, for older household heads living in the first ring, over half (56 percent) are in social housing. That is because social housing is more available there and represents close to half of all HLMs in Ile-de-France.

Given the share of older Parisians who live in small and often unfurnished private apartments and those who rent and live in social housing, it is important to raise a question, to which we do not have good answers. How many older Parisians live in substandard conditions that might endanger their health and place them at disproportionate risk in the event of another heat wave?

Since indicators of substandard housing conditions are often tied to the age of the housing, we presume that these conditions are worse in Paris than in the first ring. Also, since conditions tend to be better in social housing than in private unfurnished rentals, there is reason to believe that substandard conditions are significantly higher in Paris. Based on common indicators of poor housing conditions, which we will refer to here as "substandard," there is good reason to be concerned about many older household heads in Paris (Table 15.2).

In 1999, twenty-seven thousand housing units occupied by household heads sixty years and over had no bathroom (i.e., neither shower nor bath) and twenty-two thousand had no toilet. With respect to bathrooms, older household heads (8.7 percent) are worse off than the average for all household heads (5.6 percent); for toilets, they are slightly better off (7.1 vs. 8.0 percent). The age of the Paris housing stock, as well as its low share of social housing, can explain these high levels of substandard housing. The share of housing units without a bathroom is much lower in the first ring for all household heads, as well as for those sixty years and over (respectively, 4 and 2.3 percent). Likewise, the share of units without a toilet is lower (respectively, 3.4 and 3.5 percent).

The share of housing units without bath or shower occupied by older persons is particularly high in roughly half of Paris arrondissements, where it varies between 8.9 and 19.5 percent—over four times as high as in the well-to-do parts of the city. For units without a toilet, the variation is even higher—from 8.1 to 20.9 percent—in roughly half of Paris arrondissements and five times as high as in the more well-to-

Table 15.1. Characteristics of Households Headed by Persons 60+, by Age Group: Paris Arrondissements, 1999

	All Households	% of Total	60–74	% of Total	75+	% of Total	60+	% of Total
Total housing units	1,110,912		174,388		133,496		263,349	
Number of homeowners	329,113	29.6	84,007	48.2	61,821	46.3	145,828	46.8
Number of units with less than 40m2	421,593	38.0	45,322	26.0	33,786	25.3	79,108	26.1
Number of private unfurnished rental units	463,966	41.8	45,416	26.0	40,668	30.5	86,084	27.8

Source: Census 1999, INSEE; obtained from APUR.

Table 15.2. Substandard Housing Conditions for Households Headed by Persons 60+: Paris and Arrondissements, 1999

Arrondissement	Household Heads 60+ %	Housing Units without Bath/Shower %	Housing Units without Toilet %
1	7.7	11.6	11.3
2	5.7	19.5	20.9
3	5.9	14.3	13.2
4	8.3	12.7	10.9
5	8.5	9.5	7.7
6	9.8	7.1	7.7
7	10.8	5.6	6.3
8	8.7	6.2	8.5
9	7.5	11.3	10.5
10	5.9	15.9	14.1
11	6.6	13.9	11.4
12	8.8	8.2	5.7
13	7.2	7.3	3.9
14	8.4	7.3	4.8
15	8.9	5.9	4.3
16	11.5	4.3	5.8
17	8.8	8.9	8.1
18	6.9	13.3	9.6
19	5.7	6.3	5.0
20	6.7	9.2	5.9
Paris	7.9	8.7	7.1

Source: Census 1999, INSEE; obtained from APUR.

do parts of the city. These substandard housing conditions are concentrated in the center north of Paris (first, second, third, fourth, ninth, tenth, eleventh, seventeenth, and eighteenth arrondissements). Among these areas, 80 percent of units are small, 60 percent have fewer than two rooms, 80 percent were built before World War II, and half include a share of older persons close to or higher than the Paris average. In the second arrondissement, one-fifth of older persons live in units without a toilet. This area, more than most others, is characterized by a high concentration of small and old units.

The persistence of substandard housing conditions reflects technical as well as socioeconomic factors. First, units are for the most part very small. There is often no space in which to install plumbing. Second, bringing these units up to standard can raise complex problems for landlords, some of whom do not have the resources to improve their units or have no incentive to renovate because of the low returns from renting in the neighborhood, lack of interest in their property, or ease in renting the property as is. The recent evolution of substandard housing conditions between the last two census years (1990–1999) confirms a decrease in substandard housing due largely to demolition of pre-1949 housing units or renovations by landlords (often with government subsidies).[4] Such renovations have transformed the structure of housing units by progressively eliminating single-room occupancies, for example, hotel rooms, maids' rooms, and small furnished rooms. Thus, housing conditions are improving for the younger old. For example, with regard to the absence of a shower or bath, rates of substandard units (7.5 percent) occupied by persons sixty to seventy-four years are, on average, lower than for those seventy-five years and over (10.3 percent).

Such progress, however, should not make one lose sight of the fact that 6 percent of all housing units occupied by older persons, and considered adequate by Parisian standards, do not have central heating (in contrast to 5.8 percent for all units), and 19 percent of all units in buildings with five stories or more have no elevator (in contrast to 24.3 percent for all units) (Table 15.3). The latter indicator underestimates the problem of walk-ups for older persons, for it does not capture their number in buildings with fewer stories.

In light of the effects of the canicule on the population of older persons living at home, it is now critical to reflect on the design of appropriate indicators and the collection of data that will enable local decision makers to get a handle on the distribution of vulnerable older persons who reside not just in officially sanctioned "substandard" units but also in walk-ups and units without central heating. Given that air conditioning is rare in Paris housing units, and even in residential and nursing homes, one cannot expect that there will soon be information on its prevalence across the city. But it is no surprise that the government has already allocated funds and issued a regulation calling for all institutional long-term care providers to provide a cooling room in the event of another canicule.

Older Persons Living at Home

Most older persons live at home. As they grow older, their proportion in various forms of residential care, and eventually in nursing homes, increases significantly. A recent study suggests that two-thirds of Franciliens sixty years and over run into minor difficulties for certain activities of daily living, and that just over one-quarter seek some kind of assistance due to a health problem.[5] In France, the two principal centrally financed programs to support people who have difficulties with the activities of daily living in their home environment were designed to support home help and home nursing. There are, of course, people who rely on both kinds

Table 15.3. Housing Units in 5-Story Buildings or Higher without Elevators, by Age of Household Head: Paris and Arrondissements, 1999

Arrondissement	All Ages %	60–74 %	75+ %	60+ %
1	46.7	44.0	37.8	41.8
2	55.2	54.2	48.5	52.0
3	45.3	42.0	39.0	40.8
4	42.4	38.8	35.6	37.5
5	31.3	25.3	23.8	24.6
6	34.1	28.2	26.1	27.3
7	20.0	13.7	13.5	13.6
8	18.4	13.7	11.4	12.6
9	43.2	40.3	38.7	39.6
10	43.9	40.5	38.6	39.7
11	35.0	29.6	28.9	29.3
12	21.3	17.3	17.2	17.3
13	13.2	9.3	11.5	10.2
14	20.6	15.7	17.4	16.4
15	14.8	10.3	11.5	10.8
16	7.7	5.7	5.3	5.5
17	25.9	19.6	19.1	19.4
18	37.8	32.3	34.1	33.0
19	13.7	10.1	11.9	10.8
20	17.2	13.9	14.5	14.1
Paris	24.3	19.1	18.9	19.0

Source: Census 1999, INSEE; obtained from APUR.

of services. Given the complexity of multiple programs and funding streams supporting each form of home care, and the absence of information on the numbers of people receiving different kinds of services, it would be a perilous task to calculate the proportion of older persons receiving various forms of home help versus those receiving long-term home-nursing services.

A 1995 survey from a sample of Parisians seventy years and over living at home sheds some light on this black box.[6] It suggests that some thirty-two thousand older Parisians (15 percent) were either homebound or needed assistance leaving their homes. Ninety-one percent of them depended on services—either from professional home-care aides and nurses or from the informal sector of family, friends, and neighbors. Since some twenty-three thousand older Parisians (66 percent) received formal care services for either nursing, home cleaning, or both, this survey provides a rough estimate of the share of homebound older persons seventy and over that relied only on informal services—44 percent.[7] Here we are concerned with the organization and magnitude of formal services for older persons living at home.

Another survey of persons aged sixty and over receiving home-nursing services in Ile-de-France indicates that 46 percent of Parisians enrolled in the home-nursing program also receive some supplemental home-help services.[8] For the most part (90 percent), a range of these services are provided by roughly twenty nonprofit organizations (*associations*) represented since 1967 by a federation of home-care organizations that has recently contracted with Paris authorities to maintain a range of standards in personnel and procedures for covering all twenty arrondissements of the city. In essence, the heart of home care, which relies so heavily on the "kindness of strangers," has become institutionalized in a kind of public-private partnership with the city.

Home help. This universal program consists in paying a home helper to assist older persons who are unable to perform household tasks (shopping, housecleaning, etc.) on their own. Payment is means tested, so that higher-income persons receive a smaller benefit; but everyone over a certain level of dependency is eligible for a minimal contribution. Since 2002, for people over sixty years who meet the dependency criteria, the APA contributes toward the costs of daily home-help services.[9] Payments are made directly to the organizations that employ these workers. Before the implementation of the APA, persons under a low income ceiling and with severe levels of disability could qualify for financial support to pay for a home helper: caretaker allowance (*allocation compensatrice pour tierce personne* [ACTP]). In contrast to the APA, the ACTP was a cash payment to the beneficiary and could be used to pay a spouse, who would thus be considered a home helper. That is why some older persons have preferred to maintain this benefit rather than switch to the APA (combining the two is prohibited).

The effect of the new APA has been to increase demand massively for home care. This, in turn, has placed a burden on local authorities and nonprofit organizations to respond to eligibility requests and deliver the services. In this context, and faced with a market in which it is difficult to find qualified personnel (in 1999 only 9 percent of home aides had completed training certificates in home help in France),[10] the state has embarked on a vast reform to make careers in home help more attractive. It has created a new certification in the field, initiated a process to validate previous work experience, and established a fund to modernize the profession.

For people over sixty-five years and above the levels of disability required for eligibility to receive the APA, home help is also financed by local pension funds or local welfare programs, the French equivalent of Medicaid home care in New York.

As in the case of the APA, these programs pay the same nonprofit organizations for their beneficiaries.

Taking all these programs together, close to twenty thousand Parisians over the age of sixty-five (6.2 percent of the population in that age cohort) received publicly financed home care on a regular basis in 2003. Not only is Paris a generous provider of such services in comparison to Ile-de-France and the rest of the nation, but also the city administration operates a public service, the Center for Social Services (CASVP), with a local headquarters in each Paris arrondissement. In addition, at least half of the twenty nonprofit organizations that deliver home care in Paris have more than a hundred full-time employees.

Home nursing Services. We present home nursing after home help because these services are needed mostly by a population that is seventy-five years old and over (80 percent of requests for these services come from Franciliens of this age).[11] As a general rule in France, home-nursing care can be prescribed by physicians, provided on a fee-for service basis, and reimbursed under the national health insurance program.[12] In addition, for persons over the age of sixty, nursing care may be delivered daily by nonprofit organizations that specialize in home-nursing care. Such a care plan also must be prescribed by a physician and requires a more arduous authorization process by the local health insurance fund (Caisse Primaire d'Assurance Maladie de Paris). In this case, services are usually provided daily for an average period of two years. They include assistance with personal hygiene and other activities of daily living.

In contrast to home-help services, it is possible to present a geographic analysis of home-nursing services, since their catchment areas are defined contractually (Figure 15.1).

A look at the spatial distribution of people seventy-five years and over who receive daily nursing care indicates that most of the peripheral arrondissements are less well served (less than fourteen persons per thousand) than those in the center (seventeen per thousand).

It is striking to note that arrondissements that are least well served correspond, on average, to those with a higher proportion of persons seventy-five and over (Table 15.4). For example, the sixteenth arrondissement, which has the highest share of older persons in Paris (11.5 percent of persons seventy-five years and over), has the lowest rate of persons receiving home-nursing care (10.8 persons per thousand). In addition, there is a gap between arrondissements that resemble one another in socioeconomic characteristics. For example, the nineteenth and twentieth arrondissements have similar shares of older old, of average household income, and of substandard housing; yet the nineteenth arrondissement provides more than twice as many older old with home-nursing care (Table 15.4). After phoning the local home-nursing services organization for the twentieth arrondissement in the spring of 2004, we learned that the previous director was not terribly energetic and

Figure 15.1. Persons 75+ Receiving Home-Nursing Care: Paris, 2002

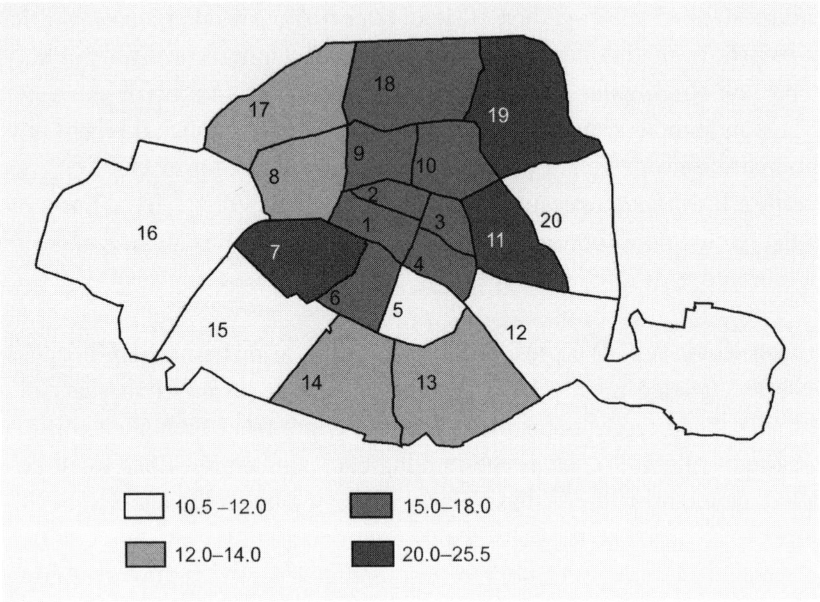

Source: Les services de soins infirmiers à domicile pour personnes âgées en Ile-de-France–Bilan au 31 décembre 2002," CRAMIF; and ORSIF.

that the new director had just obtained authorization from the local health-insurance fund to increase the level of home-care nursing.

Why are there such service disparities, and what is the right amount of home-nursing care for an older population? A cynical hypothesis might be that there is a negative correlation between the arrondissements with many older household heads living in walk-ups and the number of older persons receiving home nursing (simply because nurses want to climb stairways no more than anyone else). Fortunately, this does not appear to be the case. But one could hardly conclude based on the limited indicators we have examined that home-nursing services are in fact approved on the basis of apparent need. Consider, for example, the second arrondissement, in which the older heads of households have some of the highest rates of substandard housing (Table 15.2), the highest rate of walk-ups (Table 15.3), and the lowest median income (Chapter 13). The rate of persons seventy-five and over receiving home-nursing services there is still below the Paris average.

Since 2001, the Ministry of Social Affairs has decided to reduce disparities in home-nursing service rates across all French regions by increasing the rates in "underserved" regions and extending the benefit to twenty thousand more older persons before the end of 2005. The "optimal" service rate is supposed to be 18.48

Table 15.4. Persons 75+ Receiving Home-Nursing Care: Paris and Arrondissements, First Ring, and France, 1999

Arrondissement[a]	Population 75+	Share of Total Population	Persons 75+ Receiving Home-Nursing Services	Per 1000 persons 75+
1	1,293	7.7	23	17.8
2	1,113	5.7	19	17.1
3	2,025	5.9	35	17.3
4	2,534	8.3	43	17.0
5	4,974	8.5	58	11.7
6	4,389	9.8	70	15.9
7	6,183	10.8	125	20.2
8	3,404	8.7	45	13.2
9	4,191	7.5	66	15.7
10	5,305	5.9	84	15.8
11	9,871	6.6	202	20.5
12	12,039	8.8	126	10.5
13	12,302	7.2	148	12.0
14	11,184	8.4	150	13.4
15	19,979	8.9	220	11.0
16	18,549	11.5	200	10.8
17	14,162	8.8	180	12.7
18	12,824	6.9	219	17.1
19	9,886	5.7	251	25.4
20	12,337	6.7	134	10.9
Paris	168,544	7.9	2,398	17.7
First Ring	237,919	5.9	3,359	14.1
France	4501,804	7.7	67,404	15.0

Sources: Census 1999, INSEE; for Paris and the First Ring : "Les services de soins infirmiers à domicile pour personnes âgées en Ile-de-France–Bilan au 31 décembre 2002," Caisse régionale d'assurance maladie d'Ile-de-France; for France "STATISS 2003 : Les régions françaises (places installées au 1er janvier 2002)," DREES, DRASS (Direction régionale des affaires sanitaires et sociales). Data obtained from the Observatoire régional de santé d'Ile-de-France (ORSIF).

[a] One home-nursing agency serves arrondissements 1, 2, 3, and 4 (the center of Paris); another serves 9 and 10; a third serves 9, 10, 11, 18, 19, and 20 (northeast Paris). For these three agencies, the number of older persons served in each arrondissement was determined, in principle, in relation to the share of population 75+ in each arrondissement.

for 1,000 persons seventy-five years and over. Using this measure as a standard, it would seem that Paris is "underserved," albeit less so than the first and second rings. Within Paris, however, Table 15.4 indicates that many arrondissements (for example, the fifth, twelfth, fifteenth, sixteenth, and twentieth) appear vastly "underserved" in comparison to others (the seventh, eleventh, and nineteenth). In fact, it is not possible, based on existing data, either to set a meaningful standard or to evaluate the disparities among Paris arrondissements. Without a better understanding among arrondissements of levels of disability, home help, institutional alternatives to living at home, and levels of informal support, setting a standard is much like making policy in the dark. Nonetheless, it is noteworthy, in comparative perspective, that the Paris authorities are so actively engaged in supporting a large number of older persons living at home. Whether this reflects a shortage of institutional long-term beds in Paris, or better health of older Parisians, or simply a greater capacity to care for older dependent persons in an urban core is hard to know.

Arrangements for Institutional Long-Term Care

Along with aging and increases in rates of disability, when it becomes difficult to care for a frail older person at home, Parisians face the following choices. They may select a residential, congregate housing kind of arrangement where they would have their own individual units with kitchens and a variety of common services such as meals, security, and sometimes even twenty-four-hour nursing care—*foyers-logements.* Such living arrangements could be considered different levels of assisted living. Alternatively, they may find a bed in a total institution that provides room and board, but no nursing care—a residential/retirement home. Or more typically, if their level of disability is higher, they may try to be admitted to what would be called a nursing home in the United States. This includes "medicalized beds" in congregate housing/assisted-living arrangements—a term meaning that twenty-four-hour nursing care is available. Alternatively, it includes long-term care beds in hospitals.

According to the 1999 French census, 4.5 percent of persons seventy-five and over are institutionalized in Paris, much less than in the first ring (7.7 percent).[13] This gap may reflect a healthier population of older persons in Paris (see Chapter 14). Or it may reflect the many Parisians who are admitted to residential, especially nursing, homes outside the city, since there is a shortage within Paris. In Ile-de-France, there are 20.6 retirement-home nonmedicalized beds per thousand persons sixty-five years and older; in France, the equivalent figure is 28.9. For Paris and the first ring, the equivalent figures are lower for retirement beds— 9.1 and 15.3. Likewise, for nursing-home beds, the number per thousand persons sixty-five years and older is much lower in Paris (12.8) than in the first ring (22.7). In Ile-de-France, the equivalent figure is 22.9, in contrast to 24.8 for France as a whole.

In comparing living arrangements across countries or cities, it is useful to broaden the census definition of institutionalization to include the full range of institutions and services available to frail older persons, for example, residential/retirement homes, of which the foyers-logements are the most common in Paris.

Foyers-Logements. This form of congregate housing/assisted living consists largely of individual housing units with a set of collective services ranging from meals to security and alarm systems. It is the most distinctive aspect of institutional long-term care in Paris, simply because it is more developed there than in any other department of Ile-de-France. Over the past two decades, the city's Center for Social Services (CASVP) has increased their number of beds by 75 percent. This has brought the Paris ratio of foyers-logements for one thousand persons aged sixty-five and over (19.4) close to that of the first ring (19.7) and much higher than in France (15.8). Thus there are six thousand units in this kind of living arrangement for older Parisians; most of them (87 percent) are managed by the CASVP, the remainder by nonprofit organizations (Table 15.5).

Nursing homes. In 2001, there were 13.9 nursing-home beds per thousand persons aged sixty-five and over, 57 percent in the retirement homes that provide nursing services, 35 percent in long-term care beds of hospitals, and less than 10 percent in foyers-logements that provide nursing services. In the first ring, there were more nursing-home beds: 23 per thousand persons aged sixty-five and over, with two-thirds in retirement homes with nursing services, almost one-third in long-term care beds of hospitals, and none in foyers-logements. Since 1997, the central government has decided that it should not matter where these nursing-home beds are located, so long as the institutions that house them are reimbursed on the basis of their clients' levels of disability. Thus, all nursing-home beds are now considered to be located in institutions for older people with disabilities, EHPADs (*établissement d'hébergement pour personnes âgées dépendantes*).[14]

So far, the effect of this reform has been to extend nursing-home bed capacity by giving providers an option to use "nonmedicalized" beds for older persons who require nursing care. Not surprisingly, there has been a "statistical" increase in the rate of nursing-care beds and a decrease in "nonmedicalized" beds. In 2002, the first year that the reform was implemented by various providers, the rate of nursing-care beds increased from 13.9 to 15.1 in Paris and from 23 to 26 in the first ring.[15] Over the course of 2001–2002, however, there were no increases in the number of units/rooms in foyers-logements or other residential/retirement homes for older persons. Thus, these increases should be interpreted with caution. Whether they were accompanied by additional resources for frail older persons, let alone by any improvement in the quality of care, remains an open question.[16]

To obtain a deeper understanding of the current supply of nursing-home care and a better assessment of future needs, the Regional Observatory for Health in Ile-de-France relied on the results of a national survey to estimate the number of frail older persons in the region.[17] For 2000, estimates based on national self-perceived assessments of disability suggest that the number of persons seventy-five years and over with significant disabilities comes to eighty-nine thousand.[18] For the first ring, the equivalent figure is thirty-three thousand, and in Paris, twenty-four thousand.[19] Based on such estimates, Paris and the first ring will provide, respectively, 169 and 343 nursing-home beds per thousand persons seventy-five and over.

The Role of the City in the Provision of Institutional Long-Term Care for Older Parisians

As noted in the introduction to this chapter, Paris has played a distinctive role in providing institutional long-term care to its older population. Not only does its Center for Social Services (CASVP) manage a network of foyers-logements within the city; but also it provides a range of such institutional options for Parisians in the first ring. Its Paris facilities are filled only with Parisians, and its facilities in the first ring are filled almost entirely by Parisians (90 percent).[20] With respect to nursing-home care, Paris is exceptional because most of its nursing-home beds (93 percent) are provided by its municipal public hospital system—Assistance Publique–Hôpitaux de Paris (AP-HP)—in long-stay hospital wards. AP-HP, like the CASVP, manages hospitals not only in Paris but also in the rest of Ile-de-France. All these long-term care beds are available to Parisians, who fill 90 percent of them in Paris and 30 percent outside, mostly in the first ring.

Over the years 1991 to 2001, the proportion of Parisians residing in hospital nursing-home beds diminished slightly, and this trend may be reinforced by the projected increase of frail older persons in the first and second rings. Nonetheless, a recent study of the region indicates that Paris still stands out in comparison to all other departments of Ile-de-France, because (as can be seen from Table 15.5) even its residential/retirement homes not managed by the CASVP accommodate a large share of older Parisians (76 percent). Likewise, even its long-term care beds not run by AP-HP accommodate 79 percent of older Parisians.[21]

The Paris authorities typically argue that such data underestimate the number of beds occupied by Parisians. But even if one dismisses this position, as do the regional authorities of Ile-de-France, it is clear that there is presently a relative shortage of institutional long-term care beds in Paris.

Taking into account the number of older Parisians who spent their older years in institutional long-term care outside Paris (Table 15.5), one ought to adjust the rates of residential/retirement-home beds as well as nursing-home beds per one thousand for Parisians sixty-five years and over. This brings the rate for residential/retirement beds from 26.4 to 27.7 and the rate of nursing-home beds from 12.4 to 16.5.[22] In light of these adjusted figures, it is clear that a large number of Parisians (30 percent of those in nursing-home beds) are forced to leave Paris to find a nursing-home placement. Another regional study indicates that of Parisians who sought some form of institutional long-term care, between 55 percent and 62 percent (depending on the kind of institution) could find beds only in the first and second rings.[23]

Table 15.5. Number of Units/Beds Occupied by Parisians in Residential Units, Retirement Homes, and Nursing Homes: Paris and the Rest of Ile-de-France, 2000

	Units/Beds in Paris			Units/Beds outside Paris in Ile-de-France			
	Reserved for Parisians	Occupied by Parisians (n)	%	Reserved for Parisians	Occupied by Parisians (n)	%	Total
Residential/retirement-home beds							
CASVP-managed *foyers-logements*	5,256	5,256	100	404	351	87	5,607
Other residential units	822	822	100				822
CASVP-managed retirement-home beds	93	93	100	62	55	89	148
Other retirement-home beds	2,748	2,088	76				2,088
Total		8,259			406		8,665
Nursing-home beds							
CASVP-managed residential units	342	342	100	104	90	87	432
Other residential units	0						0
CASVP-managed retirement-home beds	1,135	1,135	100	984	876	89	2,011
Other retirement-home beds	1,345	1,022	76				1,022
Beds in AP-HP long-stay hospital wards	1,422	1,280	90	1,129	339	30	1,619
Other long-term care hospital beds	110	87	79				87
Total		3,866			1,305		5,171

Sources: ORSIF, December 31, 2000 ; CASVP, 2000; AP-HP, 2000.

Concluding Observations

Over the next thirty years, given the population projections for older persons in the first and second rings (see Chapter 12), one may wonder whether older Parisians will continue to be accommodated in residential/retirement homes outside the city and, more importantly, in nursing homes there. Even if older Parisians do continue to be accommodated outside Paris, as a result of further growth of institutional long-term care beds in areas with lower land values, there will be no way to escape the policy issues raised by the patterns of living arrangements and long-term care for older persons in Paris. What determines which Parisians get to stay in their city and which leave? Does the system of home help and home nursing provide older frail Parisians with substitutes for institutional long-term care; or do persons with the highest rates of disability emigrate, leaving the healthiest in Paris?

If one reads the mayor's report on the canicule, or the report of his committee charged with evaluating its consequences, one comes away with the impression that the city's response has been timely, effective, and above all, political.[24] A closer reading of the evidence suggests that the heat wave revealed the impotence of French public authorities' responses, including those of the Paris authorities. More importantly, it pushed into public view some critical concerns about the vulnerability of the oldest old, who have typically been swept beneath the surface—their social isolation and neglect, compounded by inadequacies of staffing in institutional long-term care facilities. This is all the more true in Paris, where despite the high levels of services available to older persons living at home alone and the relatively high number of foyers-logements, the number of excess deaths was greatest.[25]

In the current context, the task of assessing the needs of vulnerable older Parisians in relation to the programs dedicated to supporting them has taken on a new urgency. The pervasive ignorance about the characteristics of vulnerable older persons—their exact location, the extent of their social isolation, their housing conditions and levels of disability—has become conspicuous. Yet, all these characteristics could be helpful in devising an indicator of vulnerability as a guide to appropriate interventions. The challenge for the future may be posed precisely in these terms: Will Paris emerge as an innovator in designing the range of necessary support systems for its frail older persons, or will it take another canicule to spur needed reforms?

Notes

1. Esponda, M. 2002. L'habitat parisien reste marqué par la prépondérance de petits logements. *Le logement.* Vol. 2 of *Atlas des Franciliens.* Paris: IAURF-INSEE.

2. "Comfortable" here is used in the sense that the French population census defines minimal conditions of housing comfort: units with a toilet and at least a shower or bath. We use the term "substandard," in this chapter, to denote housing units that do not satisfy these minimal conditions.

3. The population census does not allow one to relate social housing units to the older population that is poor except for those HLM units that are vacant. Also, information on the number of HBM rent-controlled units inhabited by older persons and regulated under the law of 1948 is, unfortunately, not available.

4. The programs to renovate housing (OPAH) are urban-planning procedures that began in 1977 and seek to renovate older housing units in a specified geographic zone, within which an effort is made to coordinate public and private policies.

5. Qualite, L. 2002. 700 000 Franciliens ont un besoin d'aide lié à leur état de santé. INSEE, *Ile-de-France à la page*, no. 208.

6. Fontaine, D., et al. 1995. Conditions de vie des Parisiens âgés vivant à domicile en 1995. INSERM, ORS Ile-de-France.

7. Fior, Sylvaine. 1997. Quotidienneté de l'aide professionnelle è domicile auprès des personnes âgées à Paris. *Revue Française des Affaires Sociales.* Special issue. October, 81–95.

8. Recours aux services de soins infirmiers à domicile Franciliens, UFASSAD (Union des fédérations des associations de soins et services d'aides à domicile), URHIF (Union régionale de l'hospitalisation d'Ile-de-France), URIOPSS, and FEHAP (Fédération des établissements hospitaliers et d'assistance privé à but non lucratif d'Ile-de-France), 2001.

9. Since 1997, the Autonomie Gérontologique Groupe Iso-Ressources scale has become the national instrument for evaluating levels of disability among older persons. It defines six categories of people with disabilities. At one extreme (#1), the totally dependant individual; at the other extreme (#6), the fully autonomous one. This scale is used to determine eligibility of older persons for the APA. Persons classified from #1 to #4 are eligible for the APA, which covers a range of services for persons with high levels of dependency (#1–#3), as well as for persons with lower levels of dependency (#4).

10. Dutheil, N. 2000. Les services d'aide à domicile en 1998 et 1999. DREES [Direction de la Recherche, des Etudes de l'Evaluation, et des Statistiques] Etudes et résultats, no. 91.

11. Recours aux services des soins infirmiers à domicile Franciliens, op cit. note 8.

12. Unfortunately, it is not possible to obtain data on the number of older persons receiving services from nurses in private fee-for-service practice. Thus, we analyze only services for older persons who have gone through the more arduous process of preauthorization for an extended period of regular nursing care.

13. The census defines institutionalization as living in group quarters, from those for migrant workers, students, retirees, religious communities, and nursing homes to all

other forms of institutional housing. Of persons seventy-five and over institutionalized in Paris, 69 percent live in retirement homes, 15 percent in long-term hospitals beds, and 16 percent in religious communities.

14. Levels of disability are evaluated for each long-term care institution on the basis of a global indicator for the average level of dependency of each institution's residents. Each resident is evaluated on the basis of the AGGIR scale.

15. From dataset on long-term care institutions for older persons on December 31, 2002, ORSIF, Paris. Local population estimates are for January 1, 2001, INSEE.

16. In the future, each EHPAD will be required to sign an agreement that specifies the conditions under which it operates—financial, service coverage, quality, and frequency of case-mix classifications.

17. The Handicap, Disability, and Dependency Survey—Handicaps-Incapacités-Dépendance (HID)—completed by INSEE between 1998 and 2001 aimed to establish, for the first time in France, an estimate of the number of persons with different kinds of disabilities, including disabilities associated with aging. The AGGIR scale was used as a measure of disabilities.

18. The HID survey referenced in the preceding note, like its predecessors, demonstrated that the frequency of disabilities becomes important between the ages of seventy-five and eighty years. It is for this reason that a floor of seventy-five years was chosen.

19. The HID survey is based on self-declared disabilities and therefore measures only individual perceptions of dependency.

20. According to the CASVP, in 2001, the proportion of older Parisians in institutions owned and operated by the City of Paris and located in the first ring was respectively 87 percent in foyers-logements and 89 percent in retirement homes (*maisons de retraite*).

21. *Etude comparative entre les résidants en maisons de retraite et les patients en unités de soins de longue durée en 2000—Enquête spécifique Ile-de-France.* 2003. Paris: DRASS [Regional Office for Health and Social Affairs].

22. In contrast to the rates presented for Paris and the first ring, those noted in this paragraph take into account the occupancy rates indicated in Table 15.5.

23. See the preceding note.

24. See *Mission d'Information et d'évaluation sur les conséquences de la canicule à Paris.* See the city's Web site, www.paris.fr/fr/solidarite.

25. *Conséquences sanitaires de la canicule d'août 2003 en Ile-de-France-Premier bilan.* 2003. Paris: ORSIF (ORS). October. (www.ors-idf.org).

16. Tokyo: A Pathbreaker in Long-Term Care?

Naoki Ikegami

Over the course of the past century, among the four cities studied in this book, Tokyo has undergone the greatest physical changes. Very few buildings survived the great earthquake of 1923 and the carpet bombing of 1945. More recently, the economic boom years of the 1980s, and efforts to heat up the economy in the 1990s, have led to massive urban construction projects.

Of the four, Tokyo is also the city that has experienced the least social change. The population is still primarily composed of ethnic Japanese, and except for small enclaves around exclusive apartments where wealthy expatriates live, Tokyo lacks the cosmopolitan atmosphere of the other cities. The ethnic homogeneity has contributed to the more equal distribution of income and also to higher costs in providing long-term care (LTC), due partly to the high hourly wages of home helpers and to the high costs of institutional care, which reflect high wages as well as high land costs, particularly in the urban core of Tokyo (see Chapter 19). Moreover, strict immigration policies have prevented the large-scale introduction of foreign live-in workers in the homes of older persons in Tokyo.

Tokyo prides itself on being a strategic location for the LTC insurance program, because it was one of the centers in which the seeds of the program were first sowed. After all, the governor of the Tokyo Prefecture, Ryokichi Minobe, established a program of "free" medical care for older persons in 1969, which forced the central government to make it available for the whole nation by 1973.[1] This, in turn, led to an influx of older patients to hospitals, thus exacerbating what was known as "social hospitalization" (see Chapters 20 and 21) and turning many hospital wards into de facto nursing homes. Public resentment in response to providing free inpatient care for "social" (nonmedical) reasons and corporate leaders' worries about the rising costs of health insurance were crucial factors that allowed the passage of Japan's new LTC insurance program (LTCIP) in 1997 and its implementation in April 2000.

Both Governor Minobe and his successor, Shunichi Suzuki, greatly expanded Tokyo's social welfare programs, including services for older persons. Since the economy was in such good shape in the 1980s, Governors Minobe and Suzuki could both afford to finance these expansions without having to wait until 1989, when the implementation of the Gold Plan provided generous national subsidies for increasing and upgrading the supply of long-term care institutions. However, although the supply of long-term care infrastructure expanded more in Tokyo than in other prefectures, demand was also greater because of the more rapid increase in older persons living alone.

The difficulty faced by municipal-level social welfare offices in handling complex LTC situations was one important factor that explains why Japan enacted a universal LTC entitlement program based on the social insurance model. Thus, I would argue that Tokyo played a leading role in social policy development and could be said to have been the harbinger of the future. Now, Governor Shintaro Ishihara's allegiance to the right wing does not bode well for the expansion of social welfare programs in Japan, though he has not yet cut back benefits on his own initiative (cuts have been made in accordance with national decisions).

Tokyo continues to take the lead with regard to LTC. It is doing so by reacting to the structural weaknesses of LTCIP, the foremost being the acute shortage of institutional LTC beds, which has been exacerbated by the implementation of LTCIP. Although 75 percent of nursing homes' capital expenditures are funded by the government, there are no allowances for purchasing land, the most expensive factor, by far, in Central Tokyo. Before implementation, ward governments had purchased beds in nursing homes built in outlying areas (at $100,000 per bed) for the exclusive right to admit residents from their wards. After implementation, however, admission to nursing homes became an entitlement based on the amount of functional support needed, regardless of the amount of family care or income available.

If an older person meets the eligibility criteria, except for the lowest level of need, she or he can go directly to a nursing home and demand to be admitted. That, at least, is the theory. In practice, waiting lists are so long that the prospects of dying seem higher than the prospects of being admitted, especially in Inner Tokyo. (Whether nursing homes have continued to honor the agreement to admit residents from a ward that made capital contributions, on a per-bed basis, is not always clear; officially, they are not supposed to do so.)

Because the shortage is so acute, Tokyo has been in the forefront of establishing both officially certified private nursing homes and de facto nursing homes that are legally no different from residential housing. The advantage of the latter is that they do not have to adhere to the statutory requirements of staffing and physical standards. Some have been converted from dormitories for unmarried employees whom companies are now eager to get rid of in order to reduce labor costs. The first floor may now be the home-helper station that sends its helpers to the upper floors, though not necessarily on an exclusive basis. Ward governments within Tokyo have a hard time regulating such facilities because they are technically "housing." The approval to open a home-helper station is left to the prefectural government, not to the ward. On one hand, these official and nonofficial nursing homes may decrease the pressure for real nursing homes and save ward governments from having to pay any of their capital expenditures. On the other hand, there is no assurance that their residents would be admitted from their own local area. Therefore, such projects are not a panacea for wards overloaded with demand for institutional LTC. Indeed, some wards are actively trying to restrict their establishment, because more official nursing homes would lead to premium increases under LTCIP for older persons living within their jurisdiction. So far, however, these wards have been unable to stop the building of these new types of nursing homes.

As Tokyoites grow older, nursing-home beds increase, and the demand for all forms of LTC expands under LTCIP, a new policy issue is emerging—how much is society willing to pay for aging in place, or in the same neighborhood, especially in the inner part of large cities where land and other expenses are so high? Home and community care may not be so much a problem, because the higher labor costs may be compensated by a larger workforce attracted to large cities. Institutional care, however, will surely be much more expensive. If older persons own their homes, they may be able to finance the admission fee for assisted living. But reverse mortgages, however attractive in theory, appear to be far less attractive in practice. Even if they do work, such a financing scheme is useful only for homeowners, who represent a minority of households in the urban cores of large cities.

So, what is to be done? Since publicly funded resources are limited and will be increasingly stretched in the future, the only solution may be the Paris model (see Chapter 15) of dispersing frail older persons out of the urban core. However unpalatable a solution this may appear, the issue must be confronted in all four world cities. The one bright spot is that the practice of moving an older single parent from her hometown to join her child living in Tokyo, usually after the death of her spouse, may decrease as LTC services expand in rural areas. Expansion of LTC services in rural areas, however, will take some years. In the meantime, it is likely that Tokyo will continue to be a pathbreaker in the organization and financing of LTC, which makes the chapters that follow of special interest to all those concerned with the future of LTC in large cities.

Note

1.   After World War II, the position of the mayor of Tokyo, who had jurisdiction over the twenty-three wards of Central Tokyo, was abolished and the governor took on that role. The wards (*ku*s) became quasi-cities in administration, but they tended to depend more on the prefecture than did the municipalities within the Tokyo Prefecture. However, they have since become more autonomous, as symbolized by the change made in the English translation of *ku* from "ward" to "city."

17. Aging, Socioeconomic Status, and Neighborhood Differences in Tokyo

Yukiko Kudo

Introduction

What is it like to grow old in Tokyo? How different is it from growing old in New York, Paris, or London? Is it different from growing old in other parts of Japan? To answer these questions, it is important to start by comparing the demographic, socioeconomic, and health status of the older persons in Japan, Tokyo Prefecture, and Central Tokyo's twenty-three wards. Next, I compare the differences in people's characteristics among the neighborhoods in the twenty-three wards, and finally, the socioeconomic status and living arrangements of older persons living in Inner and Outer Tokyo.

Tokyo is still young compared to the nation as a whole (Table 17.1). In 1985, only 8.9 percent of the population was sixty-five and over in Tokyo and only 9.5 percent in the twenty-three wards, as compared to 10.3 percent in Japan. Although population aging is increasing in every district, the ratio of population aged sixty-five and over was 15.4 percent in Tokyo and 16.7 percent in Japan in 2000. Inner Tokyo, on the other hand, is aging faster than the rest of Japan (Table 17.2).

When population aging in Tokyo and in the twenty-three wards is compared, every year it is higher in the twenty-three wards than in the rest of the Tokyo Prefecture. Although Tokyo is still young compared to Japan, the city's population is aging rapidly. The dependency ratio in the twenty-three wards is lower than in Japan and in the Tokyo Prefecture, as the population of the group fourteen and under is low in the twenty-three wards.

Japan's low fertility rate accounts for the increase in the proportion of older people in the country. Table 17.2 shows the change in the total fertility rate (TFR) by year. Each year, TFR is highest in Japan, followed by Tokyo and the twenty-three wards. Especially in the nine inner wards (Chuo, Minato, Shibuya, Nakano, Toshima, Bunkyo, Shinjuku, Chiyoda, and Meguro), TFR is extremely low: 0.82 percent in 2000, which is less than two-thirds of the average in Japan and approximately 80 percent of that in Tokyo. Since this tendency is predicted to continue, population aging is likely to accelerate.

The income indices of the nine inner wards, the twenty-three wards, and Tokyo Prefecture all exceed that of Japan (Table 17.3). The index is highest in the inner nine wards, second highest in the twenty-three wards, and third highest in Tokyo. In 1990, the index of the twenty-three wards was 160 and that of the nine inner wards was 231, compared with 100 for Japan. While the gap among the income indices

Table 17.1. Changes in Total Population, by Age Group and Dependency Ratio: Japan, Tokyo, and Wards, 1985–2000

	Population	0–14 %	15–64 %	65+ %	Dependency Ratio[a]
Japan					
1985	121,048,923	21.5	68.2	10.3	46.7
1990	123,611,167	18.2	69.7	12.1	43.5
1995	125,570,246	16.0	69.5	14.6	43.9
2000	126,686,000	14.8	68.5	16.7	46.0
Tokyo Prefecture					
1985	11,829,363	18.0	73.1	8.9	36.8
1990	11,855,563	14.7	74.7	10.6	33.8
1995	11,773,605	12.7	73.9	13.0	34.8
2000	11,944,048	12.2	72.4	15.4	38.1
Central Tokyo (23 Wards)					
1985	8,354,615	16.8	73.7	9.5	35.7
1990	8,163,573	13.7	74.4	11.2	33.4
1995	7,967,614	12.0	73.9	13.7	34.8
2000	8,134,688	11.1	72.0	16.4	38.1
Inner Tokyo (9 Wards)					
1985	1,975,868	14.5	74.7	10.8	33.9
1990	1,782,475	12.1	74.9	13.0	33.5
1995	1,679,515	10.2	74.3	15.5	34.6
2000	1,736,067	9.1	72.8	17.3	36.3

Sources: Japan Census 1985, 1990, 1995, 2000; *Tokyo Statistic Yearbook on Public Health*, General Affairs Bureau, 2000.

[a] Ratio of persons <15 and >65 years to the population 15-64 years.

Table 17.2. Fertility Rate: Japan, Tokyo, and Wards, 1995–2000

	1985	1990	1995	2000
Japan	1.75	1.54	1.42	1.36
Tokyo	1.46	1.23	1.09	1.04
Central Tokyo (23 Wards)	NA	NA	1.02	1.00
Inner Tokyo (9 Wards)	NA	NA	0.84	0.82

Sources: Vital Statistics 2000; *TMG Yearbook on Public Health* data 2000, from Statistical HP of TMG on Public Health.

**Table 17.3. Income Index and Per Capita Income:
Japan, Tokyo, and Wards, 1985, 1990, 1995**

	Income Index			Per Capita Income		
	1985	1990	1995	1985	1990	1995
Japan	100.0	100.0	100.0	933		
Tokyo	140.0	154.0	138.5	1,306	1,968	2,101
Central Tokyo (23 Wards)	143.0	160.7	142.5	1,334	2,054	2,162
Inner Tokyo (9 Wards)	181.7	231.7	184.9	1,695	2,961	2,804

Source: Individual Income Index, Japan Marketing Education Center, 1986, 1991, 1997.

**Table 17.4. Labor Force Participation among Persons 65+:
Japan, Tokyo, and 23 Wards, 1985, 1995, 2000**

	1985	1995	2000
Japan			
%	26.0	26.5	23.1
(n)	(3,242,860)	(4,836,490)	(5,081,747)
Tokyo			
%	30.4	29.7	25.6
(n)	(321,075)	(454,205)	(488,127)
23 Wards			
%	32.8	31.8	27.5
(n)	(259,676)	(347,575)	(367,887)

Source: Japan Census 1985, 1995, 2000.

narrowed in 1995, per capita income in the twenty-three wards is more than 1.4 times larger, and in the inner wards 1.8 times larger, than that in Japan. In terms of income gaps in the twenty-three wards, there is a significant difference between the highest per capita income, ¥3,904,000, and the lowest, ¥1,684,000.

As for the average disposable income per household member, for households headed by those sixty-five and over, it is about ¥1.76 million yen, which is similar to that of other age groups.[1]

It is well known that labor-force participation among Japan's older persons is high. As shown in Table 17.4, the rate is higher in the twenty-three wards and Tokyo than in the nation as a whole.

The lowest number of older persons aged eighty and over living alone occurs in Japan as a whole, followed by Tokyo, the twenty-three wards, and the nine inner wards (Table 17.5). In every group, the ratio has been gradually increasing since 1985. Further study will be needed to clarify how the higher ratio of those aged eighty and over living alone is related to the level of service in each region. It is notable that the figure in the nine inner wards in 1995 shows quite a high level, 22.1 percent.

Health and Welfare Status

Average life expectancy at birth is highest in Tokyo (Tables 17.6, 17.7, 17.8). In 1995, the average for males was 76.4 years in Japan, 76.7 in Tokyo, and 76.4 in the twenty-three wards. The average for females was 82.9 years, 83.1, and 83.0, respectively. Compared with the figures in 1975, all average life expectancy has increased. In Tokyo, from 72.9 to 76.7 for males, from 77.4 to 83.1 for females, and in the twenty-three wards, from 72.7 to 76.4 for males, from 77.4 to 83.0 for females.

Table 17.8 shows the percentage of older persons in long-term care institutions or hospitals. In 1995, the ratio of those aged sixty-five and over in hospitals was 2.3 percent in Japan, 1.6 percent in Tokyo, and 1.0 percent in the twenty-three wards. In contrast, the figures for those aged eighty-five and over were 7.9 percent, 5.7 percent, 3.8 percent, respectively. The hospitalized ratio is decreasing in every group, while the ratio of institutionalized older persons in the same period is increasing in every group. The ratio of those aged eighty-five and over rose from 6.4 percent to 7.3 percent in Japan, 6.1 percent to 6.8 percent in Tokyo, and 3.2 percent to 3.3 percent in the twenty-three wards. When comparing the differences among the three groups, it is noteworthy that the ratios of both hospitalization and institutionalization are low in the twenty-three wards. Tokyo's rate of institutionalization among older persons is still low compared to the other prefectures in Japan, but it is rising rapidly.

Table 17.5. Persons 80+ Living Alone: Japan, Tokyo, and Wards, 1985–2000

	1985 %	1990 %	1995 %	2000 %
Japan	7.4	9.4	11.6	14.5
Tokyo	11.0	14.0	16.9	22.6
Central Tokyo (23 Wards)	12.3	15.5	18.7	25.1
Inner Tokyo (9 Wards)	14.2	18.0	22.1	28.9

Source: Japan Census, 1985, 1990, 1995, 2000; *TMG Basic Survey on Social Welfare,* TMG Social Welfare Bureau, 1980, 1985, 1990, 1995, 2000.

Table 17.6. Average Life Expectancy at Birth, by Gender: Japan, Tokyo, and 23 Wards, 1975–2000

	Japan		Tokyo		23 Wards	
	Male	Female	Male	Female	Male	Female
1975	71.73	76.89	72.87	77.40	72.76	77.42
1980	73.35	78.76	74.17	78.90	74.04	78.83
1985	74.78	80.48	75.60	80.85	75.37	80.69
1990	75.92	81.90	76.05	81.94	75.72	81.79
1995	76.38	82.85	76.73	83.12	76.35	82.96
2000	77.72	84.60	77.96	84.46	77.68	84.30

Sources: The TMG Life Tables (1995, 1985), The 18th Life Table, The 16th Life Table, TMG Bureau of General Affairs.

Table 17.7. Life Expectancy at 65 by Gender: Japan, Tokyo, and 23 Wards, 1980, 1995, 2000

	Japan		Tokyo		23 Wards	
	Male	Female	Male	Female	Male	Female
1980	15.52	18.94	15.89	19.28	15.84	19.22
1995	16.48	20.94	16.67	21.15	16.50	21.06
2000	17.43	22.44	18.47	22.38	17.68	22.30

Sources: The TMG Life Tables (1985, 1995), The 18th Life Table, The 16th Life Table, TMG Bureau of General Affairs.

Table 17.8. Institutionalized Persons 65+ and 85+: Japan, Tokyo, and 23 Wards, 1990, 1995

	Patients in Hospitals		Patients in Social Institutions		Others	
	65+ %	85+ %	65+ %	85+ %	65+ %	85+ %
Japan						
1990	2.6	7.6	1.7	6.4	0.0	0.0
1995	2.3	7.9	1.8	7.3	0.0	0.0
Tokyo						
1990	2.0	6.8	1.5	6.1	0.1	0.0
1995	1.6	5.7	1.6	6.8	0.1	0.0
23 Wards						
1990	1.4	5.1	0.7	3.2	0.1	0.0
1995	1.0	3.8	0.9	3.8	0.2	0.0

Sources: 1990 & 1995 Population Census of Japan, Vol.2, Nos. 1, 2.

Neighborhood Differences among the Twenty-Three Wards

Health and socioeconomic status. The differences among the wards of Tokyo with regard to health and socioeconomic status are striking. For example, there is quite a difference between the higher-income wards (such as Chiyoda, Chuo, Minato, Shinjuku, Bunkyo, Meguro, and Shibuya) and the lower-income wards. According to the ratio of population aging in the year 2000, there is a 7.5 percent difference between Taito Ward, the highest, and Edogawa Ward, the lowest. Moreover, the increase in population aging is highest in Kita Ward, over 4.1 percent, whereas population aging decreased by 0.2 percent in Chuo Ward between 1995 and 2000. Persons aged eighty and over who live alone represent 23.8 percent in Minato Ward, the highest, and 13.4 percent in Edogawa Ward, the lowest.

It is generally assumed that Tokyo is a city with great uniformity compared to other big cities in the world. However, a detailed analysis reveals considerable differences across wards. This is an important point and will greatly influence the development of long-term care insurance by municipalities. Municipalities are required to respond to local characteristics, so they must have the capacity to be flexible and innovative.

As of December 2000, about 10 percent of those sixty-five and over in Tokyo were determined eligible for long-term care insurance (197,964 out of 1,904,789 people). An additional 6.7 percent are provided with institutional care services (36,992) and home-care services (95,799).[2] Looking at individual wards, the ratios of those assessed as eligible for long-term care vary from the lowest at 8.13 percent in Katsushika Ward to the highest at 13.5 percent in Chuo Ward.

Several questions require further analysis. Does each ward within Tokyo have adequate beds in special nursing homes to meet the needs of the growing older population? To what extent has the government realized its goal of transitioning older persons from institutional care to in-home care? Does the policy adequately meet the needs of populations whose health, economic, and social status can vary widely? To address these questions, we must first examine the socioeconomic status, housing conditions, and living arrangements of older persons. I address each of these issues in the sections that follow.

Socioeconomic Status of Older Persons: Comparison of Inner and Outer Tokyo

Inner Tokyo is characterized by greater inequality, higher land prices, less home ownership, and a larger percentage of older people living alone than Outer Tokyo. As a result, older residents of Inner Tokyo are more likely to need long-term care services.

Affluence and poverty. Tokyo is more homogenous than New York City, London, or Paris, but income variance in older households, as reflected by local household tax burdens, suggests significant differences among the twenty-three wards. For example, I calculated the annual local tax per household insured by the municipal NHI Program in 1998, which bases its premiums on taxable income. Three inner wards— Chiyoda, Minato and Shibuya—are by far the most affluent areas, and the concentration of income there largely accounts for the variance across Central Tokyo.

Generally, the municipal NHI beneficiaries have lower income levels and wider variation than have the employed population. In addition, local taxes are progressive and comprised of three brackets: 5 percent for taxable incomes up to 2 million yen, 10 percent for incomes up to 7 million yen, and 15 percent above that. This means that a resident with an annual taxable income of 7 million yen will pay exactly double the amount in taxes that a resident with 4 million yen would pay (600,000 yen versus 300,000 yen). As a result, comparisons based on local taxation may exaggerate the degree of variance.

One should also be cautioned that the figures for Tokyo are most likely the annual taxable incomes of "individuals," as opposed to "households," because tax is levied on the former rather than on the latter. On the other hand, NHI premiums levied on household and individual incomes are combined for households with more than one member. With these cautions in mind, it seems safe to conclude that the geographic variance of incomes for older households is much wider than for younger households.

In addition to having wards with some concentrated wealth, Tokyo includes wards with high concentrations of poverty. The indigent population is entitled to the means-tested poverty allowance, which also pays for medical care. When one looks at the number of means-tested poverty-allowance recipients per population, one easily realizes that one ward, Taito, has a conspicuously high concentration of poverty. This reflects the fact that the ward contains a particularly poverty-stricken district. The indigent population under the poverty allowance is not covered by NHI and does not affect income level calculated from NHI data.

Housing. As with any large city, housing is a serious problem for Tokyo. For older persons, particularly disabled older persons in need of care, housing can be a key determinant in the ability to age in place. Tokyo, as the largest and most crowded city in Japan, is always ranked worst in housing conditions, in terms of both cost and space.

According to the national census conducted in 1995, the rate of ownership among households in Japan is approximately 60 percent. However, Tokyo was ranked the lowest of the forty-seven prefectures, with an ownership rate of only 42 percent. The size of housing in Tokyo is also the smallest of the prefectures—57.6m^2 as opposed to the national average of 85.9m^2 per household. The average size of housing is even smaller for the twenty-three wards (55m^2). Moreover, the variance in the size of housing is not related to whether the ward is inner or outer. Although Chiyoda Ward has a conspicuously large housing size per household among the inner wards, this may be partly explained by the fact that Chiyoda Ward is where the imperial family resides.

Older households in Japan have higher rates of ownership—86.1 percent in 1995.[3] and according to the latest survey of older households performed every five years by the Tokyo Metropolitan Government, more than 70 percent of older persons in Tokyo own their own homes.[4]

However, there is some variance in home ownership among the twenty-three wards. For example, the centrally located wards, Chiyoda, Chuo and Minato, have the smallest rate of ownership (approximately 65 percent), despite their large housing size. The predominantly residential western part of Tokyo, consisting of Meguro, Setagaya, Nakano, Suginami and Nerima Wards, has a high rate of ownership, near the national average of 80 percent.

Another limiting factor of housing with respect to home care is the availability of elevators. In Japan, buildings of up to five stories do not require elevators. Older persons who live in such high buildings and who are at risk of becoming disabled face great challenges. The 1995 Tokyo survey gathered information about the housing conditions of the older persons and found that about a third of the population sixty-five years and over live on the second floor or higher, without elevators.

Land prices. The central part of Tokyo serves as a hub of both political and financial activities for the whole of Japan. Its activity is most vividly reflected in the price of real estate. Residential real estate prices are a good indication of how desirable it is to live in Tokyo.

The inner wards generally occupy the most expensive part of Tokyo. The land prices of Chiyoda Ward are staggeringly high (the average is 1.3 million yen, or over $10,000 per square meter), even after a decade of constant land-price decline. However, some of the inner wards, namely Koto and Sumida Wards, have lower land prices than most other wards have, while Meguro and Shinagawa, both located in the western suburbs, have real estate prices as high as those in the inner wards. This reflects the history of development in Tokyo, in which the western part of the city was developed before the residential area.

Given the high percentage of home ownership by the elderly in Tokyo, high real estate prices translate into "wealth" for older homeowners. However, this wealth does not translate directly into cash income. Moreover, correspondingly high property taxes may make it difficult for older homeowners to continue to live in their homes. There have been some attempts to institutionalize "reverse mortgages" in order to turn dormant real estates values into cash flows. Unfortunately, many of these attempts have ended in failure because of the real estate "crash" since 1990.

Living alone. Family conditions are an important determinant of home-care use. There is a clear distinction between the inner and outer wards with respect to older persons who live alone. Except for Koto Ward, the inner wards have a uniformly higher rate of older persons living alone (by 7–9 percent) than the outer wards.

Heavy reliance on external social services, like home help for older persons who live alone, is shown clearly by a national survey conducted by the Ministry of Health, Labor, and Welfare in 2000.[5] Recipients living alone are more than six times as likely to use home-help services as recipients living with families. Demand for visiting nursing services, however, does not appear to be affected by family conditions. Visiting nursing services are medical services whose demand is dependent upon medical conditions, while home-help services are alternatives to family caregiving.

Growing Old in Tokyo

The most recent national census shows that Japanese society is more complex than ever. Although it used to be common to get married, the country's unmarried ratio has risen over 10 percent. The age of first marriage is also rising. Tokyo is at the forefront of these changes; more than half the group between thirty and thirty-four are not married. In Tokyo, too, a decline in the fertility rate due to late marriages is striking. Such attitudes among the young will certainly increase the ratio of old to young in the future. Before long, it will no longer be the common experience to grow old in the shelter of one's family.

The changes in employment circumstances are making young people more economically unstable than their parents were. As a result, the young are more likely to live with their parents for longer periods, delaying their independence. Today's older generation is economically and socially stable compared with previous generations—partly the result of the improved social welfare system, including pension and medical insurance, that arose after World War II. Eventually, conflict between generations could erupt over limited social resources.

Diversity of lifestyle is remarkable even among older people. By the end of the decade, the country is certain to see profound transformations in relations between young and old, and in choices both groups make on how to live and how to grow old. If Tokyo's municipal government can respond to the needs of its citizens in this time of unprecedented change, the city may well be a vital, safe, and hospitable place for young and old to live.

Our comparison of inner and outer wards suggests lessons that will be valuable for policy makers. While housing conditions in the inner wards are not any worse than those in the outer wards, the high prevalence of older persons living alone in the inner wards will cause an increase in the demand for home help. In addition, older patients from the inner wards are likely to be sicker and hence to spend more on medical costs than those in the outer wards. The inner wards of Tokyo are by no means plagued with what sociologists call "inner-city" problems, but the growing need for long-term care services presents significant challenges to these inner wards. Still, the inner wards of Tokyo remain the wealthiest in Japan, amply evidenced by their higher incomes and real estate prices.

Notes

1. Comprehensive Survey of the Living Conditions People. 2002. Tokyo: Ministry of Health, Labor, and Welfare.
2. Business Statistics Monthly Report. 2000. TMG Welfare Bureau. December.
3. National Household Survey, Ministry of Health and Welfare. Tokyo, 1995.
4. Household Survey. Tokyo: TMG, 2000.
5. National Household Survey.

18. The Challenge of Aging in a Global City: Tokyo

Yasuo Takagi

Characteristics of Aging in Tokyo

I conducted a comparative analysis on the availability and use of social and medical services in Tokyo and its various districts: Minamitama, where middle-class businesspeople live; the southeastern area, which includes Meguro Ward, Setagaya Ward, and Shibuya Ward, where wealthier people live; and the more solidly lower- and working-class district (made up of what the Japanese call *shitamachi*—good old working-class neighborhoods)—in the northeastern area, which includes Arakawa Ward, Adachi Ward, and Katsushika Ward.

Families and the Older Persons in Tokyo

With respect to income levels in these three areas (Table 18.1), the income level in the upper-class area is 1.4 times the average of the entire country; in the lower-class area, almost the same as the average; and in the middle-class area, almost the same as in the Tokyo metropolitan area. The income level in the lower-class area of Tokyo is nearly the same as the national average. As is common in big cities, there are more households on welfare with incomes below the national average. This is particularly true in the lower-class areas, where the percentage of households receiving welfare is twice the national average.

Tokyo and other large cities in Japan have dramatic new family and lifestyle characteristics. These trends are most noticeable in the wealthier neighborhoods of Tokyo but cut across class boundaries. The image of the traditional Japanese family, where children care for their elderly parents, has virtually disappeared in upper-class areas and is showing signs of vanishing in the middle-class areas as well.

Changes in Tokyo include a sharp increase in young men and women living alone. While there has been an increase in the number of nuclear families all over the country, the percentage of households consisting of only husbands and wives in Tokyo is below the national level. On the other hand, the percentage of Tokyo households comprised of couples sixty-five and over is as high as 35.1 percent and accounts for about 40 percent in the upper-class areas. Similarly, the percentage of households consisting of people sixty-five or older living alone is as high as 18.4 percent in the upper-class area and as high as 14.9 percent in the lower-class area, which indicates that about half the older persons in Tokyo live alone or as part of a couple. The percentage of older people living alone in the upper-class area is 56.8 percent. Eighty percent of the older persons who live alone are women.

Table 18.1. Socioeconomic Characteristics of Persons 65+: Japan, Tokyo, and Selected Areas, 1997–1999

	Per Capita Income[a]		Families on Welfare (per 1,000)[b]	Persons 65+	Aging Ratio (%)
	In thousand yen	Standard Value			
Japan	3,673.4	100.0	14.90	20,138,786	15.9
Tokyo Prefecture	4,364.0	118.8	17.67	1,685,171	14.5
Southwestern / upper-class area	5,313.0	144.6	9.49	183,378	15.4
Meguro	5,212.6	141.9	12.34	38,073	16.0
Setagaya	5,161.5	140.5	8.31	113,879	14.7
Shibuya	5,988.2	163.0	10.53	30,426	16.5
MinamiTama / middle-class area	4,390.6	119.5	11.44	145,721	11.8
Hachioji	4,257.6	115.9	13.68	61,647	12.3
Machida	4,596.9	125.1	10.50	44,654	12.3
Hino	4,323.6	117.7	10.25	20,130	12.4
Tama	4,521.2	123.1	8.51	13,116	9.2
Inagi	4,148.2	112.9	8.72	6,174	9.6
Northeastern / lower-class area	3,635.5	99.0	26.06	176,887	14.6
Arakawa	3,673.4	100.0	30.74	31,135	18.4
Adachi	3,613.1	98.4	33.57	83,407	13.5
Katsushika	3,653.3	99.5	17.36	62,345	14.8

Sources: Census of Japan, 1997–2000; Ministry of Health, Labor, and Welfare, 2000; Tokyo Metropolitan Government (Fukushimap), 1997. Available at http://nenrin.or.jp/chpju/fukushimap.

[a] As of 1997 per taxpayer

[b] As of 1999 per taxpayer

Provision and Use of Social Services by Older Persons

The use of home-care services by older persons in Tokyo is higher than the national average (Table 18.2). The level of institutional long-term care, however, is far below the national average, because land prices are high and it is difficult to acquire property. In addition, since the cost of facility improvements is enormous in both upper- and lower-class areas of Central Tokyo, upgrading has been slow to happen. However, in the middle-class area, where there are many nuclear families and communities are not connected strongly with each other, people tend to rely more heavily on institutional long-term care. As a result, the total number of institutional long-term care beds for frail older persons remains at just half the national level (Table 18.2).

The number of fee-charging retirement homes for older persons, in which public funds are not invested, is three times as high (per population 65 and over) in Tokyo as at the national level. A quarter of fee-charging retirement homes are located in Tokyo. In addition, private companies provide facilities for wealthier older persons in Tokyo. However, these facilities are constructed mainly in the suburbs and in the lower-class area, not where upper-class people live. Clearly, the number of facilities for older persons is now and will continue to be insufficient as Tokyo's aging population increases. The public and private sectors have their work cut out for them. Private companies must expand their service facilities of every kind; and the welfare system must be reformed.

Provision and Use of Medical Services for Older Persons

In Tokyo, hospitals and clinics make up for the shortage of institutional long-term care beds for frail older persons. Many people, however, frequently use hospitals outside their district. Of those in the central area, where both upper- and lower-class

Table 18.2. Use of Home Care Services for Persons 65+: Japan and Selected Tokyo Areas, 1997

	Home-Help Services	Day-Care Service
Japan	144.2	175.1
Tokyo Metropolitan Area	204.3	190.2
Upper class	208.3	198.7
Middle class	192.7	134.9
Lower class	205.4	170.9

Source: TMG, Fukushimap, 1997.

people live, more than half go to hospitals outside their district. In the middle-class suburbs, many people gravitate to local hospitals.

Furthermore, because of the small number of institutional long-term care beds for frail older persons, many older persons in Tokyo go routinely into general hospitals for long periods, even when their needs are not acute and are not suited to hospital services. This has become a serious problem. In the suburban middle-class areas, where there is an abundance of long-term care institutional beds for frail older persons, the rate of patients in long-term care institutions is well above the national average. These areas are characterized by more use of institutional care than of home-care services. As policy evolves, it will be necessary to consider the service patterns and needs of the middle class.

Changes in Living Arrangements of Older Persons and Social Supports

Tokyo has undergone radical changes in recent decades and will see further shifts as the population rapidly grows older. Special consideration must be extended to older persons who live alone, most of them women, and to the increasing homeless population. It is reported that about 30 percent of the homeless in Japan—5,700 people—live in Central Tokyo's twenty-three wards, a 70 percent increase from five years ago; 10 percent of them are sixty-five and over. Without intervention and improvements in social supports, the older homeless population will continue to grow.

As we look ahead at the shortage of facilities and the changes in family configurations, it is imperative that we increase facilities and services. Because the costs will be enormous, the public and private sectors must work together methodically and innovatively to meet upcoming needs. How should responsibilities be allocated between individuals, families, local and municipal governments, and the national government? The answers to this question are critical to Tokyo's survival, with its distinction as the fastest-growing population of older persons in a country that is aging faster than any other in the world.

19. Growing Old with Tokyo

John Creighton Campbell and Ruth Campbell

We first came to Tokyo from New York in the summer of 1965. John had just graduated from college and was about to embark on a year of Japanese-language training before graduate school; Ruth was the mother of a two-month-old boy and for a year or so had been working with older people in East Harlem. As we drove in the dark from Haneda Airport to our new home in Western Tokyo, we were struck by the endless busy sidewalks and the rows of small shops still doing business in midevening. Ruth had grown up in a small grocery store, and she immediately felt at home—a feeling that we both still have in Tokyo, almost forty years later.

Small Stores and Social Networks

Small stores in fact play a big role in the lives of older Japanese. They are the core of a neighborhood, giving residents daily contact with a small number of people known for years. Such a social network gives many urban neighborhoods the quality of a small village. Japanese women have typically visited the same vegetable, fish, and meat shops almost every day, and gone every week or so to the local hardware, flower, liquor, notions, confections, drug, stationery, electrical, and other small stores that make up the set of shops found nearby almost everywhere.

And that is just shopping. While around the neighborhood, people often stop at the local three-table coffee shop, which always seem to be run by two or three ladies of a certain age. The housewife who didn't have a chance to get out that day might well call out to the local noodle or sushi shop for a quick delivery. When we did that in our first Tokyo neighborhood, the scooter-riding delivery boy always stuck his foot into one of John's shoes and marveled at this gigantic new addition to the neighborhood social network.

Small stores provide much of the texture of daily life for many customers, mostly women but also older men, who might add a tobacco stand and the local "snack" (actually a bar) to their list of stops. They also keep a lot of older people employed. Forty years ago, and even more so today, the proprietor and anyone helping in a small neighborhood shop is over sixty-five (or at least looks it). If the owner is lucky, one of his children might be willing to carry on the business, in which case the wife would probably be helping in the store while her husband holds down an outside job for additional income (either could be the proprietor's child). One does not so often see a man between high-school age (except a part-timer or maybe a grandson) and retirement age in these small shops.

This pattern is reflected in the macropicture of employment. On the one hand, a very high percentage of the Japanese labor force works in small and medium enterprises, especially very small enterprises, of which the majority are tiny retail shops. On the other, many more older people work in Japan than in any other industrialized country, and more older people work in Tokyo than in the other world cities examined in this book (Chapter 2).

These two observations are not unrelated. That is, what foreigners and Japanese alike usually see as "typical" Japanese workers, the "salarymen" and industrial workers who are "permanent employees" of big corporations, are actually a minority of the labor force. They are predominantly male, and they are young—for much of the postwar period, the normal "retirement" age (*teinen*) in big organizations was fifty-five. Many men and most women are not guaranteed a permanent job, but yet they need not "retire." They work on and on, as small proprietors or employees in small enterprises (in manufacturing as well as retail and other services). They are joined in the gray labor force by those who "retired" from their primary job and then found a second job.

In looking at income statistics, according to a recent OECD comparative study, the standard of living of elderly Japanese is among the highest in the world, partly because of substantial employment income.[1] Pensions are not very high for people who had been self-employed, and so the continuing modest revenue from a small shop keeps the household going. On the other hand, retirees who are eligible for the Employees' Pension do quite well, and their second-job incomes are often an extra.

Living arrangements also differ substantially between these two groups. The salaryman household is more likely to be a nuclear family, and after retirement the older couple will probably live alone, at least until one dies or becomes quite ill. Shop owners and other self-employed are more likely to be in a three-generation household.

Change and Variation

The foregoing description was even more accurate forty years ago, around the time David Plath delineated the great differences of lifestyle between salaryman and shopkeeper families in his book on leisure.[2] In the ensuing decades, many more Japanese have come to live in suburbs and shop by car in big supermarkets, malls, and superbox stores. The aspiration for that kind of life was well expressed in a catch phrase of the 1960s—a man would want to live *kaa tsuki baba nuki* (with car, without grandma). This ideology of modernity has long contended with the "traditional" ideal of family solidarity, and it has certainly gained over the years. Still, to a visitor from the West, the enduring strength of the older way of life, in which older people are imbedded both in the household and in a neighborhood social network, is striking.

While naturally the most-urban areas have seen the fastest rate of change, these generalizations hold even in the metropolis of Tokyo. In fact, the contrast is quite stark between the downtown *shitamachi* wards (good old working-class neighborhoods) of the city, which despite the encroachment of apartment buildings still look quite villagelike, and the affluent urban-suburban lifestyle of the affluent western wards of Setagaya or Nerima. But the *shotengai* (shopping streets) of small shops are still to be found in most areas. They are under increasing economic pressure, not least from the ubiquitous *konbine* (convenience stores), far more than are their erstwhile models in the United States, along with other more modern and efficient retail outlets. But so far, at least, they survive.

How has this pattern endured for so long in Japan's postindustrial society? Partly it is simply the tenacity of cultural reproduction. Partly it is a result of government policy. An array of tax breaks and protectionist regulations both international and domestic—for example, requiring the assent of local shop owners before a big store can move in, or can keep late hours—have helped keep the small-business sector alive. Why this retrograde set of policies, in a country once famous for its dedication to super-high growth via constant expansion of the export-oriented big-firm sector?

One answer is politics. The urban "old middle class," along with farmers, has long been the core of the Liberal Democratic Party's constituency. It is a source of votes, and of political campaign support via the neighborhood small-store associations and resident groups. These interests (along with the empire of public works projects) have built walls that so far have largely withstood the pressures for widespread American-style "reform," even through the long decade of economic malaise in the 1990s.

Another answer is social policy. From the early postwar period, Japanese policy makers chose to emphasize full employment as the route to national welfare. Part of that policy was to expand big business, and to encourage "permanent employment" for stability of the modern-sector labor force. Another big part was the maintenance of the traditional small-business sector to take care of the others. In terms of government spending and other direct supports, in fact, far more resources went into the latter, because the benefits of high economic growth flowed into the modern sector via the market. What Kent Calder called "compensatory policy" was needed more and more, so the shopkeepers and farmers would not fall behind.[3]

This all worked fine for quite some time. However, even before the bubble burst and the pressures of globalization put the entire system under strain, policy makers and indeed the general public came to realize that this formula would not work for the most rapidly growing segment of the Japanese population, older people.

Care for Frail Older People under the Old System

To return to the personal: for many years John has been studying the evolution of old-age policy at the national level in Japan, while Ruth carried out various projects involving interviews with hundreds of older people and their families, social workers, managers of institutions, and others at the grassroots level of old-age care in Tokyo and elsewhere. Here is one story.

Together with a visiting nurse, Ruth visited a sushi shop in the Okubo residential area of Shinjuku in the mid-1990s. This was owned by a three-generation household living above the store. The patient was the grandfather, who had severe Parkinson's disease and was going to adult day care three times a week, as well as having the visiting nurse at home. When he went to day care, his son carried him up and down the steep, narrow stairs on his back. Much of the weight of this difficult situation was born by the *yome,* the daughter-in-law, who had to take a hand in her father-in-law's care, manage her baby and two-year-old, and play a big role in the business. She had grown up in the neighborhood and knew what she was getting into. She felt quite stressed, but she thought her mother-in-law had worked hard all her life and deserved some help.

The grandmother realized her daughter-in-law's difficult situation (she had probably lived through a similar time herself), and she tried to help by doing most of the cooking and watching the children a bit. She was grateful that she and her husband could live together above the store. Her husband had been prominent in the local *shotengai* association—the shop had several plaques on the wall attesting his many services—and she remembered the big parties they threw when everyone got drunk. She had come from the country to marry into this *sushiya* (sushi shop) and had clearly enjoyed the active social life. She also remembered how hard the work was, and was glad she now had some time to relax, even though her share of caring for her husband was certainly a burden.

The grandmother's main relaxation was playing with the children, and her husband's biggest satisfaction was lying on the tatami floor—he was almost immobile—and having the children crawl all over him. The children were clearly very fond of both of them. The household did not have much income, since a neighborhood sushiya does not generate much profit and their pensions as former self-employed people were quite small. They did have a lot of assets, in that the property the shop stood on had become quite valuable, but that didn't help their current situation.

In reflecting on this case, it is evident that without substantial services this family would not have been able to continue in this pattern, which, for most of them at least, was the best choice in a difficult situation. They certainly could not easily have paid for such services on the private market. In fact, although we lack detail on this point, they probably got all the services free.

That is, before Kaigo Hoken (the public, mandatory Long Term Care Insurance system) began in 2000, both institutional and community-based services were managed under the old *sochisei,* sometimes translated as "administrative placement system." This system had originally centered on public assistance and, in effect, poor houses, but it had gradually been extended to cover an expanding variety of social welfare provisions. In particular, from the initiation of the Gold Plan or Ten-Year Strategy for Health and Welfare of the Elderly, promulgated by the central government in 1990, community-based services for frail older people had been expanding at a rapid pace.

Under the sochisei, someone desiring services would go to the Welfare Office run by the local government and apply. A caseworker would evaluate the situation and order up whatever services thought necessary. These were subsidized by the national and prefectural governments, but not on an open-ended basis, so budgetary constraints could be important. Even when funds were available, the services could still be quite expensive for the municipality because the subsidies were based on prices, including wages, that were adequate in rural areas but not in the high-cost cities.

Tokyo, of course, had the highest wages and other costs, including real estate (crucial for nursing homes and for community facilities like day-care centers). But Tokyo also had far more tax resources than had any other prefecture, and it had a history of generous welfare provision. Even in the 1920s and 1930s, voluntary groups (including activists from the super-elite Tokyo University) had opened clinics and other facilities for the poor and feeble.[4] More recently, Tokyo led the way with "free" medical care for the elderly in 1969. Accordingly, the Tokyo metropolis, as well as many of its constituent wards and cities, had the will and the means to top off the national subsidies generously. Despite the economic downturn from 1991, this general pattern continued well into the 1990s, and even intensified with the Gold Plan expansion of old-age welfare services.

How were the services delivered? Tokyo was different from other prefectures, for several reasons beyond having more resources, including an old and tangled relationship with municipal labor unions. In most of Japan, most service delivery, including home helpers (the earliest and main component of community-based care), had come to be contracted out to local nonprofit agencies (particularly the public-private Social Welfare Councils) who could hire nonunion workers. In Tokyo, the strength of the unions slowed this process, so that relatively more services were provided by public agencies, which had to give annual and seniority-based raises in line with those of other local civil servants. It was at least rumored that some very senior home helpers or nurse aides in nursing homes earned salaries of some $100,000 a year.

Another aspect of the sochisei heritage in public assistance was that most services were provided free. In principle, clients and their families were supposed to be charged on a sliding scale based on income for anything up to the full cost of both institutional and community-based care. In practice, the fees were very low and in most cases nonexistent. Any fees paid simply flowed into the municipality's general revenues, and service provision was budgeted as part of overall municipal expenditure (including the subsidies from above). Officials or agencies who had any contact with the client thus had no incentive to worry at all about fees; they just allocated services within their budgets.

The Okubo shushiya family was perhaps lucky both in living in Shinjuku, among the most generous municipalities within the generous metropolis, and in the timing of the grandfather's illness. Ten or fifteen years earlier, the municipal caseworker might well have turned them down for services on grounds that family care was available; what's more, adult day care, which probably was the biggest help to the family, barely existed then. The Gold Plan (and Tokyo's extra efforts) had expanded services both in the sense of higher volume and by accepting ordinary, middle-class frail older people rather than concentrating only on the poor and the childless as before.

Why the New LTCI System?

Six or seven years later under LTCI, the family would have been eligible for many more services—and by this time "night" or respite care, weeklong stays in nursing homes, had become widely available—but also would have had to pay a 10 percent co-pay rather than (probably) getting all the services free. That could be burdensome for families in a delicate financial position.

Why the switch to LTCI? John has been following this decision-making process since its origins in the early 1990s.[5] Some of the key reasons have already been mentioned. The swift rise in demand for services that followed announcement of the Gold Plan indicated that needs were great—relying on family care would not handle the rapidly growing numbers of frail elderly people. More old people were living apart from their children. More and more women were working. Moreover, attitudes had changed—younger women were increasingly unwilling to bear the traditional burdens of caregiving even if they had the time. The sushiya wife did not really have the time, and although she was willing to put up with her multiple burdens for a while, she perceived the overall situation as unfair, and perhaps as old-fashioned.

Such feminist concerns were well represented in the early deliberations about LTCI in the first half of the 1990s, and they help account for why Japan did not opt to include a cash benefit to cover family care (in Germany, which initiated an LTCI system in 1995, some 70 percent of noninstitutionalized clients opt for the cash rather than for direct services, even though the value is considerably lower).

Although the idea of a cash benefit was popular among the general public (and conservative politicians), the view prevailed that simply getting more money would not really transform patterns of care and liberate women caregivers. Note, for example, this remark at a meeting in late 1995 of the Long-Term-Care Benefits Subcommittee of the Advisory Council on Health and Welfare of the Elderly, the official Ministry of Health and Welfare (MHW) committee for drawing up plans for LTCI : "In some cases, by receiving cash, the pattern of family caregiving would become fixed [*koteika*], and in particular there is the danger that women will be tied down [*shibaritsukareru*] to family caregiving. A cash benefit is allowed in German LTCI, but the family situation is different in Japan and Germany."[6]

LTCI in Germany was aimed at propping up the traditional family caregiving pattern. In Japan, for many participants in the process, the goal was to dismantle it.

Another reason for the switch, also implicit in the story of the sushi-shop family, was that the administrative apparatus of the sochisei was not up to managing a complex set of programs that went beyond a safety net for the poor and childless. In particular, there were no clear criteria for eligibility, no effective mechanism for charging fees (many older people much better off than the sushiya family were now getting services), and not much in the way of accountability for quality in service provision. Beyond such practical problems, distaste was growing (particularly among U.S.-influenced officials in the MHW) for the bureaucratic and arbitrary sochisei itself.

Yet another important reason was cost: everyone believed that Japanese would not tolerate a tax hike, and spending on Gold Plan programs was going up and up. Half the costs of the LTCI system would be covered by a new social insurance premium paid by everyone aged forty and older (including the elderly) but perceived as acceptable because it was directly tied to a solution of the pressing problem of how to care for all the frail elderly. Moreover, responsibility for the new program, including its financing, now rested unambiguously with the municipal government as the insurer—its total spending for LTCI was linked, by a complex but strict formula, to the premium level it was willing to charge its population sixty-five and over.

Financing of service provision was transformed. Instead of the municipality directly paying contracted providers (or doing the work itself), clients would contract with providers—which now included for-profit companies for noninstitutional services—and could change them when they wished. This is a consumer-based approach to accountability and quality control. The client could receive as much service as desired, from a single or multiple providers, up to a monthly limit determined only by his or her physical or mental condition as measured by an objective test based on Assistance in Daily Living indicators, devised and scored by the MHW. No longer could a local Welfare Office official decide who was worthy and for how much. Six categories of need provided services worth from about $400 to over $4,000 per month (though all with a 10 percent co-pay).

That the Japanese LTCI law was passed in 1997, two years after Germany had started its program, has led many observers to assume that Japan had simply picked up this idea from the West (as had been true over the years for many policy changes in Japan). John's research reveals that this was not the case. Although Japanese officials did study the German case, as well as other aspects of long-term care in Scandinavia, the United Kingdom, and elsewhere, the logic of the new system was mainly homegrown. In fact, the fairly detailed proposals for LTCI that emerged from official committees as early as 1993, before the German system had been enacted, turned out to be quite close to the final product. The main role of the German model was legitimization, easing the eventual passage of the law, rather than determining the content of the new program.[7]

The Reaction to LTCI

We spent a year in Japan (albeit in Kyoto rather than Tokyo) shortly after the start of LTCI, and since then have visited several times for a week or two. We are most struck by the change in tone in the media coverage of the new program and in how professionals talk about it. Newspapers and television paid enormous attention to LTCI in the months before and after it started. Nearly every story used the catch phrase "mountain-of-problems Kaigo Hoken."

The Tokyo-based *Asahi Shinbun* was most vociferous. Its tone had been set years before by a well-known reporter, Okuma Yukiko, who was a leading spokesperson for oppressed women caregivers and an unabashed enthusiast for Scandinavian-style welfare—a view widely shared by most social workers in the field. The *Asahi* and other outlets ran many stories about impoverished old people who could afford neither the new premiums nor the co-pays, or who despite great need somehow did not pass the computerized test and had their services stopped. Much was made of the point that many eligible people either did not apply for certification or, once certified, did not actually start using services or used only a small portion of their entitlement.[8] One result was that several large companies that had opened many local home-care agencies in anticipation of a rush of business had to scale back their plans and lay people off, gaining more headlines.

By a year or so later, coverage had calmed down in both volume and critical tone. What in a way was the most striking point—that this massive new system had in fact started up quite smoothly—had come to be generally accepted. People were paying their premiums without much complaint, and there was a steady upward trend in applications for certification and in actual use of services. The problem of unaffordable co-pays came to appear overblown: in Tokyo, for example, in a small survey (N=843) of certified older people who were not using services in Shinjuku, carried out fifteen months after the start of LTCI, only 3.4 percent mentioned cost as the reason for not participating.[9]

Perhaps the biggest surprise to officials after Kaigo Hoken started was that many more people than expected decided they wanted to go to an institution rather than receive services at home—or, as was widely assumed, the families rather than the older person made that choice. LTCI was supposed to offer free choice, and rather than having to apply to the local Welfare Office for placement, people now could just approach an institution directly. The result was long waiting lists—longest in Tokyo.[10]

Why the underestimate? As had happened before, the authorities had been too sanguine about how well the traditional family worked.[11] It turned out that given the chance, many families would be happiest to say goodbye to their aged parent. But causes aside, the demand for institutional beds was a tough policy problem for the government. Institutions are expensive to build, and in practice the benefits paid by LTCI for people in institutions cost far more than services they received at home.

The short-run response has been to backtrack on the principle of free choice by establishing priorities for admission to institutions to favor people with heavy needs, or for whom family caregiving was not feasible because no one was available or the situation in the household was too tense. Excluding such criteria was a key policy change under LTCI: the eligibility questionnaire is based strictly on physical or cognitive disability, and the review committees that make the final decision are not supposed to take into account either income or the availability of family care.

The new criteria are similar to those of the sochisei era, but the decisions are in the hands of the individual institution rather than of the local Welfare Office, Many have set up committees with community participation to make these decisions, and it is possible that via this route or some informal channel, local officials have a voice. It is also the case that without an explicit rule that the waiting list should be followed in order, institutions are able to "cherry pick" to select applicants who would be less trouble or more "profitable," though so far this practice does not seem to be widespread.[12]

In the longer run, the biggest part of the answer probably lies in housing policy. That topic takes us back to Ruth's experiences in Tokyo over the years.

Housing and Care for the Frail Elderly

As noted earlier, many Japanese old people live with their children (happily or not), and many who do not, particularly retirees from the large-firm sector, have enough money to live comfortably on their own. That often means staying in their house or selling it to buy an apartment. Strolling around affluent and fashionable neighborhoods like Aoyama, Roppongi, or Meijiro, one often sees slightly frail but quite well-dressed couples, or a lady, perhaps with a small dog and looking quite self-sufficient. It is not unlike New York's Upper East Side. Tokyo is one of the world's great centers of wealth, and such advantages do not disappear with age.

A small number of these people might eventually move into a "fee-paying old people's home" (*yuuryou roujin homu*), a remarkably inept term to describe something like an up-scale assisted-living facility in the United States. These residences vary widely, but most are extremely expensive, if only because they guarantee lifetime care, which is both expensive and highly risky with the small insurance pool of a single facility.

However, many older people had neither the family nor enough money to make such reasonably satisfactory arrangements. Prospects for an old-age couple, or especially an elderly widow with low income, whose children are nonexistent, distant, or estranged have long been grim, particularly in Tokyo's high-cost housing environment. Years ago, Ruth met a divorced woman in her late sixties in Shinjuku who was on public assistance. She had been living in a terrible room in an old wooden apartment building, and her caseworker from the Welfare Office had taken months to find her a decent apartment. Landlords were unwilling to take an old single person for fear they would somehow be responsible if she became frail.

More recently, Ruth made several assessment visits with a caseworker in Shinagawa Ward. One frail elderly woman was living with her son in a terribly run-down small apartment. Her son was gone all day and in any case seemed to have no concern for her. She relied heavily on her neighbors, who took turns bringing her meals. The caseworker offered her meal-delivery service, which is available in Shinagawa, but she turned it down because she didn't want to lose the human contact with her neighbors. However, at the strong urging of one neighbor (apparently the person who had called City Hall about her), she did finally agree to accept home-help service to maintain herself and her apartment.

Even when the actual living quarters are not so bad, rental housing in Tokyo is not very well suited for frail older people. The lower-priced apartments are mostly in three- or four-story buildings without elevators. Private houses, built on tiny plots because of high land costs, are often two or three stories with exceedingly narrow staircases; the deep bathtubs of Japan are also difficult for people with even moderate frailty. If a hospital bed is needed, the only place it can go is the living room or dining room–kitchen. Wheelchairs are often impossible indoors; older people who cannot walk well often simply creep around on hands and knees (and indeed will spend nearly all their time in a single small room).

Another of Ruth's assessment visits in Shinagawa was to a man badly incapacitated by stroke. He lived with his wife in a small apartment; she had called to try to get some services. She was mostly interested in day care, and she and the caseworker discussed whether someone would be able to carry him up and down the steep stairs.

Why is there little appropriate housing for frail older people? Even the United States has built a lot of public or government-assisted senior housing, often of high quality. A "cultural" explanation might be that Japanese still assume that living with children is normal. A political explanation would observe that the government has often announced plans for dealing with the aging society that included more senior housing, including "care houses" with services attached, so the need has long been recognized. However, little has been built, partly because the Ministry of Construction, which has little institutionalized interest in aging and is strongly attached to large-scale public works, is in charge of housing.[13]

Some time ago, policy was changed to give older people priority entry into regular public housing. One motive seems to have been to fill up old and small apartments that were no longer attractive to younger people. Many old couples or singles did move into these buildings, which were inexpensive and often in rather central locations. However, not only had they not been adapted for frail seniors, but also most are rather unpleasant physically, as well as isolating. Tokyo social workers tell stories about old people who moved from quite poor housing in a neighborhood into these large buildings and soon succumbed to sadness.

Although it was not much recognized when Kaigo Hoken was initiated, the new LTCI system holds some promise for invigorating old-age housing policy in Japan, both directly and indirectly. Some information from Katsushika Ward in the Shitamachi area of Tokyo, where John spoke with some administrators in March, provides illustrations.[14]

First, the direct effects. LTCI can cover care in two kinds of facilities that are intermediate between institutions and housing. One is the Alzheimer Group Home (AGH), a "house" (sometimes an apartment or part of a bigger institution) with up to nine residents and three staff. Patterned on Scandinavia's, these group homes are now seen as the best solution for caring for moderately demented older people, who need constant supervision but often not much direct care. The LTCI benefit is the same as for people living in the community; it covers the costs of care but the "rent" is paid by the resident (or family).

Katsushika had not thought it would have anyone in such facilities when it drew up its plan for the first year of LTCI, but in fact, one place got started during the first year and another in the second year. It is now planning to have 103 residents in AGHs by 2007—a figure that may be exceeded well before then. Nationally, the number of AGHs grew from 266 in 2000 to 2,832 in March 2002.[15]

According to a MHLW official John interviewed in May, the explosive growth of AGHs has two causes. On the demand side, the difficulties of caring for demented people at home, plus the long waiting list for regular institutional care, has sent many families looking for some new solution. On the supply side, AGHs are small and often use an ordinary house so do not require much financing; moreover, since the idea came along at a time when the spirit of deregulation was in the air, they are easy to start—a license from the prefectural government is needed but the requirements are not severe. There are minimum qualifications for the director and other staff, but in effect, nearly anyone can open one.

There is concern about AGHs; because they are isolated and the residents are not in a position to complain (or even be fully aware they are not being cared for well), oversight is a problem. The central government is currently training prefectural officials to make site visits, but by March 2003 only 398 had been investigated.

The other type of intermediate facility is the aforementioned fee-paying old-people home, where residents can have their care covered by LTCI instead of either paying a large lump sum at the beginning or paying out of pocket when needed.[16] That makes true assisted living with guaranteed continuity of care quite realistic, even for middle-income families, since the finances required are only to buy or rent the apartment (often with the proceeds from selling one's house). Katsushika anticipated that about 50 people would be covered in this way in the second year of Kaigo Hoken, but in fact 94 had signed up; it is now forecasting 268 by 2007, but again this number might be exceeded. It is not a difficult business to get into for a real estate developer.

Another direct effect of LTCI on housing policy is that beneficiaries are eligible for up to about $1,800 worth of home reconstruction (with a 10 percent co-pay), once in a lifetime. This program was hard to administer at first because welfare specialists know little about home building, but it has been very popular, and in the slack economy some construction firms are making a specialty of installing ramps, railings, and special bathtubs.

Finally, among direct effects, the MHW is now planning to move nursing homes toward a more residential model. Newly built nursing homes are to provide private rooms and what is called the "unit" system, which means a cluster of rooms around a shared living and dining area with homelike furnishings. Residents are to have more freedom to organize their lives, including when they eat and go to bed. The extra cost of this higher standard of living, including the additional staff required, would be borne by the resident (or family). Existing nursing homes, with their four-bed rooms and highly institutionalized routines, would still be available for low-income people.

The indirect effect of LTCI on housing comes from a new incentive for municipal governments. For a person at a given level of need, LTCI must pay at least $700–$800 more per person per month for institutional care compared with the bill for community-based care. If the mayor of a Tokyo ward could arrange for a hundred people to live in some sort of housing with community-based services, rather than in an institution, it would save about $1 million (note that Katsushika had about nineteen hundred people in institutions in 2002).

It is therefore not surprising that Katsushika officials told John they were talking with private developers and looking into various ways to encourage senior citizen housing, as by donating land. These need not be fee-paying old-people homes or any particular type of facility, the service provider (home helpers, day care) might or might not be in the actual building, and no onerous regulations need be met. .

Whether this sort of approach will take off or not remains to be seen, though it seems quite promising as a source of appropriate housing (often with services) at affordable prices where older couples and singles can live comfortably on their own. Whether that would appreciably ease the demand for institutional care is a tougher question.

The difficulty is that Japanese tend to equate living in the community with family care. Admission to an institution seems to many family members the only way to get their aging parent off their backs, literally or figuratively. It seems unlikely that very many older people would move from a three-generation household into an assisted-living facility; a move to a hospital or nursing home would seem much more natural. However, as the Japanese family continues to evolve, housing-based strategies may look more attractive.

Concluding Remarks

For the most part, the impact of Kaigo Hoken has been similar in Tokyo to the rest of Japan. Despite a barrage of negative media reports about problems and injustices in the first year—actually, from about six months before implementation to about six months afterward—in fact the program has worked pretty well as designed. In particular, community-based services have been expanding rapidly, and although no comprehensive assessment has yet appeared, there is considerable fragmentary evidence that the lives of many frail elderly people have been improved and the burdens on their family caregivers relieved.

It is the institutional rather than the community side of LTCI that is still quite problematical, and here Tokyo is somewhat distinctive. The main reason is the high price of land. Up to a decade ago, when land prices were in the stratosphere, it was extremely difficult to build nursing homes and other facilities, so the available stock was much lower than in most other areas.

The problem is now not as acute, in that housing prices have declined sharply in absolute terms and moderately relative to other areas. In fact, as the current building boom in central Tokyo attests, canny developers have been betting on future prosperity and investing in major innovative projects. The most entrepreneurial is the Mori organization, which recently opened the amazing Roppongi Hills project of offices, luxury stores, restaurants, and a big hotel.

As argued earlier, the initiation of LTCI, which in effect takes the risk out of housing frail elderly people, provides an incentive for developers to think creatively about a newly attractive market. At the same time, the fiscal pressures of the new system (and the economic situation more generally) give municipalities a strong incentive to find ways to make noninstitutional living more attractive to the consumers who now can choose for themselves.

Will this trend develop, and it what direction? It is too early to say. It is, however, possible to hope that both municipal officials and private developers will think hard about what makes for a satisfactory life for frail older people. We think that means some kind of connection with their families in a way that is helpful without being oppressive in either direction, and also something like the sorts of social networks of the traditional Japanese neighborhood we described at the start of this chapter. That many relatively healthy older people are eager to work suggests they could play a role here, whether in small retail shops or various service organizations.

This rosy picture cannot be called more than a hope right now, but there are some good possibilities and perhaps a few positive signs.

Notes

1.   See www.oecd.org.
2.   Plath, David W. 1964. *The After Hours: Modern Japan and the Search for Enjoyment.* Berkeley: University of California Press.
3.   Calder, Ken E. 1991. *Crisis and Compensation: Public Policy and Political Stability in Japan.* Princeton: Princeton University Press.
4.   Hastings, Sally. 1998. *Neighborhood and Nation in Tokyo, 1905–1937.* Pittsburgh: University of Pittsburgh Press.
5.   Campbell, J. C., and N. Ikegami. 2000. Long-term Care Insurance Comes to Japan. *Health Affairs* 19(3): 26–39.
6.   Kôseishô Kôreisha Kaigo Taisaku Honbu Jimukyoku [Office of the Old-People-Care Countermeasures Headquarters, Ministry of Health and Welfare]. 1996. *Kôreisha kaigo hoken seido no sôsetsu ni tsuite* [Regarding the establishment of the long-term-care insurance for the elderly system]. Tôkyô: Gyôsei, 129.
7.   Other Japanese social programs were more directly borrowed, in the past and quite recently—Alzheimer Group Homes, the fastest-growing program under LTCI, was clearly an import from Scandinavia.
8.   For community care, virtually everyone already institutionalized applied for and used all their benefits right away.
9.   The main reasons were that they were in a hospital or another institution (38 percent) or that they were being cared for adequately by their family (30 percent). Many of these people applied for certification because it is required for application to a nursing home.
10.   According to Ministry of Health, Labor, and Welfare (MHLW) officials, a study in Tokyo showed that people were applying for an average of 2.7 institutions at once, so the actual number of people waiting is much smaller than the official figures.
11.   In the early 1970s, the advent of free medical care for the elderly led to an unanticipated rush to enter hospitals, often without much medical justification (called "social admissions").
12.   For the first three years of LTCI, selection of people at lower levels of need was attractive for institutions because the fee schedule was relatively flat for institutional care: the additional revenue for taking heavy-care people was quite modest. However, in 2003 the MHLW adjusted the schedule to reflect actual costs more accurately.
13.   In fact, the Ministry of Construction appeared most interested in senior housing in the 1980s, when other public works spending was being tightly constrained. Even then, there was not much progress, partly because of the difficulties of integrating

care services, since those were under the MHW—bureaucratic sectionalism (*tatewari gyousei*) has long been the plague of Japanese governance.

14. The data that follow are from the *Katsushika-ku Dainiki Kaigo Hoken Jigyou Keikaku* (Work plan for the second period of Kaigo Hoken). 2002. Intermediate Report. October.

15. Kousei Roudousho Rouken Kyokuchou. 2003. *Kaigo Hoken Tantousha e no Kitai* (Expectations for those in charge of LTCI). Presentation materials. May 14.

16. The government then required the companies to refund much of the lump-sum payments to the residents who qualified for LTCI, apparently causing some financial hardships.

20. Creativity under Uniformity: Implementation of Japan's New Long-Term Care Insurance in Central Tokyo

Etsuji Okamoto

Before Long-Term Care Insurance

Before Japan's new long-term care insurance (LCTI) system went into effect, medical and nonmedical aspects of long-term care (LTC) had been financed by distinct schemes: medical services by health insurance and nonmedical services by general revenue. While medical services were well financed, the budget for nonmedical welfare services was restricted.

This imbalance in funding is the major reason Japan developed an oversupply of medical services and a paucity of nonmedical welfare services. This imbalance has led to lengthy hospital stays among older persons. Japan has many nursing homes, but they have always been in great demand, as evidenced by long waiting lists. The construction of nursing homes has also been subject to budget restrictions. Moreover, for patients to be admitted to nursing homes requires means testing and red tape. Because of this, and because many older disabled persons did not have access to adequate home care, they often turned to geriatric hospitals, admission to which requires only the order of attending doctors.

To remedy this situation, the government in 1988 created "skilled nursing facilities" (SNF). SNFs are essentially an amalgam of geriatric hospital and nursing home: they are similar to geriatric hospitals in that they are funded by health insurance (so there is no means testing) but are similar to nursing homes in terms of their facilities and amenities. The number of new SNFs increased rapidly, but the anomalous situation remained in which older persons of the same level of disability were institutionalized in different types of facilities.

There were also restrictions on access to home-care services under National Health Insurance, which covers physicians' house calls and visiting nursing services but does not regard home-aide help as a medical service. Home-aide services are similar to respite care, in that municipal governments support them to help relieve the burden placed upon family caregivers. Some municipal governments volunteered to provide home-aide services and to subsidize "short stays" (temporary relocation from home to nursing home, usually for one to two weeks, to give respite to family caregivers) for disabled older persons living in the community, but this was also subject to means testing based on household income. As a result, people often relied on hospitals for these services, because hospitalization does not require means testing.

Drawbacks of Japan's Health Insurance System

Although Japan has a long-standing "national" health insurance system, it is by no means a consolidated system. The entire population is covered, but the insurers are fragmented into the Employees' Health Insurance (EHI) system and the National Health Insurance (NHI) system, which is run by municipal governments and which provides for the nonemployed population, including pensioners. Since retired older persons will eventually migrate to the municipal NHI, there has been a growing imbalance between the two as the percentage of enrollment by the older population increases. A small number of older persons are insured by EHI, most of whom are dependent family members of younger workers.

Consequently, the municipal NHI system has been plagued with chronic financial difficulties because of the growing cost of health care for older persons, which is sustained by massive governmental subsidies. A call for total unification of the two systems has so far been unsuccessful, mainly because of strong opposition from employees' health insurance firms and from industries. As a patchwork remedy, the Elderly Health System was created in 1983 to develop a financial redistribution mechanism. This was to help equalize the enrollment by older persons between the two systems, but it too failed to provide a complete resolution.

The LTCI system was created not only to help family caregivers but also to consolidate the hitherto fragmented health-insurance system, at least for older persons. Consolidation was to be achieved by separating medical care for chronic conditions of older persons (e.g., in geriatric hospitals) from the benefits of health insurance and integrating it with welfare services under a single umbrella of municipal governments.

Innovations of the New LTCI System

Japan's LTCI insurance was influenced by the German LTC insurance, Pflegeversi-chrung, with respect to the use of needs assessments and by the British Community Care Act of 1990 with respect to care management, both of which are practices intended to allocate resources rationally and equitably. The goal of the needs assessment is to measure objectively a beneficiary's level of need. Care management is designed to allow for the most rational and equitable allocation of resources through professional coordination of the services offered by different providers.

This approach reflects lessons learned from the government's experience with health insurance. Under the former health-insurance scheme, the government respected doctors' freedom of practice and took a laissez-faire approach with respect to hospital construction, at least until the late 1980s. Although all medical claims were subject to audit and review, hospital claims for medically unjustifiable hospitalization were seldom denied payment. Because there was a lack of uniform control, more hospital beds than were warranted by evidence were constructed, leading to a severe geographical variance across the country.

Only in the 1990s did the government depart from this laissez-faire approach and adopt a certificate-of-need standard when permitting hospital construction in oversupplied areas. LTCI also departs from the laissez-faire approach by requiring that actuarial plans be established by every municipal government.

Responses of Tokyo's Twenty-three Wards

The creation of the new LTCI system effectively consolidated the fragmented sources of funding for health insurance. This enabled municipal governments to develop regional plans to cover their entire jurisdiction.

The role of municipal governments as insurers. Before the LTCI came into effect, LTC in community settings was provided by municipal governments, supplemented by a national governmental subsidy. Although this system respected the initiative of municipal governments, it inevitably led to a large variance in the amount of services enjoyed by the residents of each municipality. In addition, since the system was basically a means-tested "welfare" system, eligibility and co-payment rates were largely determined by income and family conditions.

As a result, older persons who were middle class and disabled found it more convenient and less expensive to be hospitalized for a long time, as hospitals were financed from health insurance with no restrictions related to income or family conditions. Such medically unjustifiable hospital stays largely account for an extraordinarily high number of hospital beds per capita. The LTCI system launched in April 2000 has effectively restructured the system to equalize the service level throughout the country. Under the new system, eligibility for benefits, as well as reimbursement levels, became subject to a national standard set by the central government. A uniform assessment tool was developed to evaluate the level of care needed by beneficiaries, to ensure that beneficiaries of the same disability level were entitled to the same level of care.

New restrictions on municipal governments. In some respects, the new LTCI system placed restrictions on municipal governments by standardizing the scope and level of benefits. In particular, the new LTCI law stipulates that additional benefits (LTCI Act, sec. 62) and preventive activities (sec. 175) described as "optional" must be provided under municipal governments' initiatives. However, the law also stipulates that these additional benefits be financed exclusively from a premium levied on older persons and prohibits municipal governments from allocating budgets based on their general revenue, as was their practice before the LTCI law. These restrictions, which discourage additional benefits, were put in place to avoid increasing the premium that the older population must assume.

The restrictions were also intended to distribute the government subsidy equitably among municipal governments. Like all forms of social insurance, Japan's LTCI system is far from being an "insurance" system. As illustrated by the revenue structure of Minato Ward, premium contributions from the elderly population constitute only 4 percent of the revenue of the LTCI budget, as compared to 23 percent from government subsidies, 30 percent from working-population premiums, 11 percent from the Tokyo Metropolitan Government subsidies, and 32 percent from general revenues. The remaining revenue comes from subsidies from the central and prefectural governments, plus premium contributions from working-class individuals between the ages of forty and sixty-four.

Local discretion under LTCI. Although LTCI places some new restrictions on municipalities, it also affords them a great deal of local discretion. This is illustrated by examining Nakano Ward, the only ward that included the additional benefits pursuant to section 62 of the act. Four wards—Nakano, Shinagawa, Ota, and Shibuya—provide preventive activities pursuant to section 175, but these activities are essentially emergency loans used to help pay for the high co-payments for care rather than for preventive activities.[1]

The additional benefit from Nakano Ward subsidizes half the transportation costs of commuting for day services. The ward is known for its encouragement of the active and direct participation of residents in policy making. It sometimes clashes with the central government over such matters as direct election of education board members, which in most municipal governments are political appointees.

Nakano's independent political culture is also reflected in the LTCI system: Nakano's LTCI ordinance established a blue-ribbon committee to supervise the insurance operation. This is ironic, because such blue-ribbon committees were required in all municipal governments under the National Health Insurance Act but were eliminated in the new LTCI Act. However, the LTCI Act does encourage the direct participation of beneficiaries as a matter of policy.

The elimination of blue-ribbon committees from the LTCI Act may reflect the aversion of the central government to such an apparatus, which tends to be dominated by radical parties. It may also reflect the historical fact that such committees were absent in the original NHI Act, which was enacted in the prewar period, and were added only at the behest of the U.S. occupation army as part of democratization and demilitarization in the postwar era.

The actuarial plan of Nakano Ward reads: "After elaborate discussion on the financial effect on premiums and insurance operation, we decided to include a subsidy for transportation costs for the following reason: providers of day service are expected to fund their own transportation to and from the home but such conveniences may not be feasible when beneficiaries opt for providers who reside far away, in which case beneficiaries will be responsible for the transportation cost. In view of the extra cost for specially equipped automobiles required for transportation of the disabled, it makes sense that this burden be shared among all beneficiaries."

Evidence-Based Policy Development: Actuarial Plans

Before the LTCI, there was a large variance in the use of short-stay, day-care, and home-care services within the various municipalities, and Tokyo was no exception. Between 1993, when local planning for the care of older persons was decentralized, and 1998, the variance in the use of these services among the twenty-three wards of Tokyo remained high, .[2]

The geographic variance in the provision and use of services was attributed to a lack of regional planning, so in the early phase of LTCI development, it was agreed that regional planning was necessary to ensure the balanced development of LTC services. To provide a baseline for evidence-based planning, and to evaluate the needs and interests of the elderly population in using LTC services, the government decided to require all municipal governments to conduct surveys of the older population. In addition, all municipal governments must develop actuarial plans to ensure sound financial operation over a five-year period. The mandate to survey not only the level of care need of potential recipients but also their interest in using the services reflects the unique nature of LTC.

In comparison to medical care, LTCI is influenced to a greater degree by personal preference and by social factors such as housing and family conditions. For example, Nakano Ward developed its actuarial plan on the assumption that 52.2 percent of eligible recipients would be interested in using home-help services in 2000. The ward projects that the interest in using the services will increase gradually and reach 60.6 percent in 2004.

Actuarial plans will be based on two factors: the estimated number of disabled older persons and their interest in using services. Municipal governments are required to encourage the entrance of service providers who provide the kinds of services for which a mismatch is expected between supply and demand. Actuarial plans also set the premium level levied on the older population.

Under the mandate, all municipal governments nationwide conducted preliminary surveys to assess potential need for long-term care in 1998. The central government set strict guidelines concerning the survey design: simple sampling surveys were to be conducted of the entire elderly population (primary survey) and then more detailed surveys designed for the population of disabled and institutionalized older persons were to be implemented (secondary surveys). An outline of the sample size of the surveys of Tokyo's twenty-three wards appears in Table 20.1.

Although all municipal governments publish their actuarial plans, their formats vary considerably. At a minimum, municipal governments are expected not only to estimate potential demand for services but also to project how the growing demand will be met. Some wards project the demand-supply relationship for a five-year period. Generally, the demand for home-help and bathing services is well met and the "market" appears already to be saturated. On the other hand, visiting rehabilitation services seem to be in great demand. Nakano Ward has a bold plan to meet the

Table 20.1. Summary of Persons 65+ and Preliminary Survey Samples for Japan's Long-Term Care Insurance Program: Central Tokyo, by Ward, 1998

Wards	Persons 65+	Primary Sample (all persons 65+)	Secondary Sample (disabled persons)	Institutionalized Population
Chiyoda	8,175	4492	825	155
Chuo	13,129	4012	1109	330
Minato	27,174	3000	1787	655
Shinjuku	46,282		3922	567
Bunkyo	30,634	4000	1474	484
Taito	30,689	5000	626	338
Sumida	37,635	3600	3009	
Koto	53,092	3500	350	100
Shinagawa	72,677	5000		
Meguro	39,375	5960	1292	771
Ota	101,089	4369	3365	1490
Setagaya	118,632	14499	3668	460
Shibuya	31,335		500	
Nakano	49,124	14670	1504	695
Suginami	81,093	7000	3014	493
Toshima	41,513	11000	3928	553
Kita	59,880	3000		
Arakawa	32,756	4000	3276	442
Itabashi	74,686	10000	1535	758
Nerima	91,773	9379	6178	965
Adachi	88,955	5146	5203	
Katsushika	65,316		305	
Edogawa	70,582	5000	3003	649

Source: TMG: www.nenrin.or.jp/center/fukushi/fukushimap/h10/index.html (accessed November 2001).

Note: Inner wards appear in bold.

demand for all services by 2004, the end of the planning period, while Kita Ward is pessimistic about the prospects of meeting the demand for three kinds of services—visiting rehabilitation, day-care, and short-stay services. Kita Ward projects that only 25 percent of the demand for these three services will be met, and the gap will not be closed by the end of the planned period.

New Initiatives: Satisfaction Survey

The new LTCI system advocates extending the role of insurers or municipal governments. They are encouraged to do more than simply fulfill their financing roles. For example, they are asked to provide quality assurance, establish an ombudsperson system, and conduct periodic satisfaction surveys. One year after the launch of the new system, some wards conducted satisfaction surveys on service recipients of the LTCI system. The most comprehensive of such surveys is that conducted under the auspices of the Tokyo Metropolitan Government. The survey includes both an institutional component and a home-care component; I analyze here findings from latter.

The Tokyo survey was conducted on a self-selected sample of 4,827 noninstitutionalized older persons from seven wards, six cities, and one village during September and December 2000. The names of the participating municipalities are withheld in the report, but one ward, Taito, voluntarily published its findings on its official Web site. Five other wards not included in the Tokyo survey, Shinjuku, Minato, Toshima, Setagaya and Bunkyo, all of which are inner wards, conducted satisfaction surveys on their own. Their target populations, sample sizes, and response rates appear in Table 20.2.

Respondents. Since the target population is older disabled persons who require care, it is in some cases impossible to obtain responses from the recipients themselves, particularly from those who are severely disabled. In these cases, responses had to be obtained from a family member or neighbor. Understandably, the more disabled the recipients are, the more likely it is that respondents are not themselves recipients. Caution should therefore be taken in interpreting the responses, because responses for the severely disabled reflect the satisfaction of the caregivers and not necessarily that of the recipients of care. The Tokyo and Bunkyo surveys provide details about this tendency.

Toshima Ward took a unique approach toward this problem, with the guidance of health sociologists from the Tokyo Metropolitan Institute of Gerontology. From the beginning, they separated the recipients into two groups: level 2 or "severe disability," and level 1 or "borderline disability." They asked all recipients with borderline or level 1 disabilities to respond themselves and asked others to respond for those with level 2 or more severe disabilities. The results were then analyzed separately.

Although it is not methodologically sound (since the level of care need is not adjusted), this approach yielded some interesting results. To the question "Do you

Table 20.2. Results of Satisfaction Surveys Conducted by the Tokyo Metropolitan Government and by Wards, 1998

	Target	Survey Method	Sample	Respondents	Response Rate (%)
Tokyo	Home	Interview/questionnaire	4,827	4,281	89.00
Taito	Home	Interview	958	505	52.70
Shinjuku	Home	Mail questionnaire	4,345	2,647	60.90
Setagaya	Home	Mail questionnaire	2,367	1,634	61.96
Minato	Home	Interview	390	344	88.20
Bunkyo	Home/institution	Mail questionnaire	2,395	1,575	65.80
Toshima	Home	Interview	1,500	1,018	67.90

Source: TMG: www.nenrin.or.jp/center/fukushi/fukushimap/h10/index.html (accessed November 2001).

want to enter a nursing home?" only 11.1 percent of the recipients replied yes, while 23.5 percent of caregivers admitted that they would like to send those they cared for to nursing homes. However, to the additional question asked of caregivers, "Do you think the recipient would like to enter a nursing home?" only 7.4 percent of caregivers admitted that the recipient would agree.

For the next question, "Do you mind being taken care of by nonfamily members? (Do you think he or she minds?)," the responses were split similarly for recipients and caregivers: 44.9 percent of caregivers and 46.3 percent of recipients replied yes (recipients without family members are excluded from the denominator). Similarly, slightly less than half of both the caregivers and the recipients felt that LTC should be provided by family members without resorting to social services.

The Toshima survey reveals a certain amount of ambivalence on the part of caregivers: while caregivers believe that recipients feel happy living together and being taken care of by them, many still wish they could be freed from the duty of caregiving by sending recipients to nursing homes.

Household structure. LTCI recipients in Tokyo are characterized by a high rate of older persons who live alone. In Tokyo, 24.4 percent of the LTCI recipients live alone. The rate is the highest in Shinjuku, where 30 percent of the elderly in need of care are living alone. This figure is conspicuous when compared with national data from the 1995 census, which show only 5.5 percent of the elderly in need of care living alone.

As previously demonstrated, disabled older persons who live alone use six times more home-help services than older persons who live with younger family members. Consequently, the observed high rate of older persons in Tokyo who live alone implies a high demand for home-help services.

Use of home-care services. Japan's LTCI requires that beneficiaries who want to receive services undergo a needs assessment. Beneficiaries who become eligible will be entitled to services that fit their monthly "budget," which is determined by the level of care need. Eligible beneficiaries may opt to exhaust the "budget" or not to use the services at all. However, unspent funds may not be used the following month.

All surveys included a component that measures the use of home-care services. Caution should be taken in comparing the results, however, because some surveys asked about home-care services overall while others inquired about specific kinds of services. In Shinjuku, more than 30 percent of the beneficiaries who were assessed as eligible for the services were not using them. When the ward then asked why these services had not been used, 30 percent of the respondents attributed their lack of use to reliance on family members.

Even those who use services do not spend their entire allocated budget. Surveying this, Bunkyo Ward found that 60 percent of recipients did not use up their entire budget. When asked why budgets had not been exhausted, recipients' most common reason was that there was "enough" in the budget for all their services. However, 18 percent of respondents to this question also cited heavy co-payments as a reason.

Claims and worries. Tokyo, Taito, Minato, and Shinjuku Wards all surveyed how many of the recipients had claims or worries for which they wanted to ask for help or consultation. For these four wards, respectively, 25, 20, 32, and 39 percent of the respondents had claims or worries. Further surveying revealed that recipients were most likely to bring up such claims or worries with care managers: 30–45 percent of the respondents in these four wards said that these claims were brought up with care managers, suggesting an important role for care managers as key elements in ensuring the satisfaction of recipients.

Satisfaction with needs assessments. The initial step in using the LTCI is the needs assessment. All beneficiaries who claim to be disabled and who wish to receive services must undergo a needs assessment to determine that they are disabled enough to warrant services. The needs assessment is also important because it sets the budget within which services are provided in proportion to the level of care need (e.g., borderline and levels 1–5, with level 5 the most disabled). Understandably, needs assessments can sometimes become sources of contention.

Municipal governments, upon receipt of an insurance application, contract care managers in the private sector to visit the beneficiary and conduct an on-site inspection using a uniform assessment tool much like MDS (Minimum Data Set). These care managers are subject to strict rules that ensure against conflicts of interest and guarantee privacy protection. In addition, municipal governments are concerned about how beneficiaries view the inspecting care managers.

Fortunately, the majority of beneficiaries feel that inspecting care managers understand their situations well: on average, 80 percent of the respondents felt that the surveyors "fully understood" or "understood" their situation. However, these surveys are targeted toward beneficiaries who are determined to be eligible for services. On average, nearly 10 percent of the beneficiaries who applied for services are dismissed and are not included in the satisfaction survey. It is natural for beneficiaries who have been dismissed to feel that inspecting care managers did not understand their situations. As one might expect, many disputes involving the validity of the needs assessment arose after the implementation of the LTCI.

Satisfaction with the care plan. The care plan is the itinerary of home-care services and includes the selection of services that can be chosen. Timing is a crucial factor in determining the success of home care. The care plan is also important from the insurers' standpoint: it is a yardstick against which insurance claims submitted by providers will be adjudicated. For claims to be fully reimbursed, not only must the total amount claimed be within the budget set by the level of care need, but also the cost of category-specific services must remain within the monetary limit speci-fied by the particular care plan.

Because of its importance, the care plan is far more complicated than a simple itinerary and requires professional skill to complete. Care managers are profession-als who are qualified to assess, develop, manage, and submit care plans to insurers after determining if providers have done as directed by the plans. Care-management fees are fully reimbursed by the LTCI. However, the LTCI legislation also permits recipients or family members to act the part of care managers, completing the pa-perwork for the care plans.

Given the complexity and cumbersomeness of the paperwork, the majority of recipients contract with care managers to do everything for them. The surveys confirm that nearly 90 percent of care managers—almost 98 percent in the case of Minato—"completed the care plan." Shinjuku appears to have a relatively large number of recipients who fill out their own care plans, but even this number may involve some misunderstanding: according to the official Web site of the Shinjuku government, only one self-made care plan has ever been submitted. There is a pos-sible explanation for this discrepancy. Care managers discuss in depth with recipients and family members the nature of the "itinerary" of care plans. Consequently, recipi-ents and family members may well feel that they completed the plan by themselves, even though the paperwork is being taken care of by care managers.

Just as satisfaction with a vacation is determined by the quality of the itinerary, satisfaction with LTC heavily depends on the quality of the care plan. Although different categorizations of responses make it difficult to display results in the same graph, surveys from all the wards indicate that care plans are received favorably. However, an alarming fact related to the satisfaction with care plans was revealed by the Tokyo survey. According to the practicing rules of care managers, recipients should have the freedom to choose among available service providers; care managers are required to give a full list of providers from which recipients can choose. This rule is intended to encourage competition among providers to ensure better quality of care and better recipient satisfaction. Unfortunately, the rule is not strictly enforced, because the majority of care managers are also employed by service providers whose interests they are inclined to serve, rather than act as neutral agents. Although Japan's care-management program was deeply influenced by the British Community Care Act of 1990, in which care managers employed by local governments act as neutral agents to "purchase" services from competing providers, Japan's care managers are not employed by insurers, even though their fees are paid by them.

Care managers acting as sales agents are not likely to inform recipients of rival providers, even when they are more suitable. In fact, surveys show that only half the respondents replied that they had been given the freedom to choose from among the available providers.

Whether such lack of choice affects the satisfaction of recipients has so far remained open to question. However, the Tokyo survey explicitly dealt with this issue and revealed that restrictions on freedom do affect satisfaction. Recipients who were given freedom of choice among providers showed higher rates of satisfaction (nearly 65 percent) than those who were not given such freedom (50 percent). Unfortunately, other surveys, while asking whether recipients were given freedom of choice, failed to cross-tabulate with the rate of satisfaction.

Burden of family caregivers. For the question "Was the burden on family caregivers reduced?" yes answers outnumbered no's in all the surveys. Shinjuku Ward had the highest approval rate, nearly 60 percent. Moreover, close to half the respondents admit that the new LTCI system helped reduce the burden of family caregivers.

Overall rating of the LTCI system. The final component of the surveys asked respondents to rate the LTCI overall. The reply "neutral" was the most common answer—an average of 40 percent of respondents, with the exception of Toshima Ward. However, Japanese respondents are generally reluctant to express a definite yes or a definite no and are more inclined to respond with "neutral." As a result, researchers familiar with social surveys prefer to omit "neutral" from the available choices.

Possibly due to suggestions from Tokyo Metropolitan Government sociologists, the Toshima survey did not provide "neutral" as a choice. The result of the Toshima survey shows an equal split between "satisfied" and all the other response choices. It is noteworthy that the Toshima survey shows such a large share of negative responses. If one interprets "no response" as "somewhat dissatisfied," the overall response to the new LTCI may be evenly split between satisfaction and dissatisfaction.

Conclusions

LTCI involved the implementation of several new policy tools, including needs assessments, budgeting calibrated to the level of care need, care management, and a complaints-resolution system. As a result of these changes, adapting to the new system has been a struggle for both recipients and municipal governments.

With the new system firmly in place, municipal governments are beginning to look beyond their minimally required role as insurers. The next challenges they must face are how to secure enough services to meet the growing demand for long-term care, and how to satisfy recipients and improve the quality of care from providers. To achieve this second goal, municipal governments need to monitor recipients and providers. Some of Tokyo's twenty-three wards have already begun to do that. Effective and skillful care management is a crucial means of achieving recipient satisfaction, as well as a cost-effective use of financial resources. To establish care managers as independent professionals, municipal governments, as insurers, must see that they are independent from providers or from any conflicts of interest.

The results of the various wards' surveys showed that while most recipients and family caregivers appreciated the new system for reducing the burden on family caregivers, they are not overwhelmingly enthusiastic about the new system. In addition, there was a sharp difference in satisfaction between recipients who had the freedom to choose their providers and those who did not.

The creation of the new LTCI consolidated what had been a fragmented health-insurance system into various municipal government organs, empowering them to play a larger role as insurers and to take initiatives in guiding both providers and recipients. As an insurer, each municipal government is given the power to tax. It can, as a representative of local residents, choose between a "high tax and high welfare" and "low tax and low welfare" approach to long-term care policy.

Local politicians may feel hesitant to ask for more taxes or higher premiums for fear that this request will backfire on them. This may be a principal reason why none of the wards except Nakano dared to include additional benefits at the expense of elderly beneficiaries. Still, the demographic characteristics of the older population of Tokyo, particularly that of the inner wards, suggest that there is a large demand that is not being met under present conditions.

Notes

1. Confirmed by contacting the Tokyo Metropolitan Government, November 2001.
2. Elderly Health and Welfare Map, Longevity Society Welfare Center 3-8-21, Toranomon, Minato-ku, Tokyo. Available (in Japanese) at www.nenrin.or.jp/center/fukushi/fukushimap/h10/index.html (accessed November 2001).

21. Long-Term Care in Tokyo: Home or Institutional Care?

Keiko Honda

Introduction

Urbanization, modernization, and the increasing participation of women in the labor force are transforming the traditional role of the Japanese family, once rooted deeply in Confucian family values. I explore here the policy implications of the changing role of the family for older persons in Central Tokyo's twenty-three wards. Specifically, I document the efforts to address the decreasing capacity of families to care for older persons through a combination of more formal home- and community-based services, as well as institutional long-term care facilities.[1] Unlike the other cities discussed in this volume, the challenge for Tokyo is not how to shift older persons from nursing homes to home- and community-based settings, but how to build its capacity for the full continuum of formal long-term care services.

Policy Highlights

Increased amount of home-care services. Tokyo may experience the most intense aging trend in Japan during the next decade. In keeping with the goals of the Gold Plan to shift investments from nursing-home to home care, the Tokyo Metropolitan Government (TMG) proposed to increase home-care services considerably more than institutional long-term care services—a strategy based on the goal of "better quality of life" and "cost effectiveness." As the Japanese population ages, the government is pursuing changes that will alter greatly the current practice of keeping too many older persons in long-term care beds of general hospitals—so-called social hospitalization—and begin to improve the current strategy of providing "life-style support."[2]

Local disparities in institutional long-term care within Tokyo. TMG has set a goal to reduce the proportion of Tokyo's older persons' institutional service use by residents outside Tokyo and thereby increase the capacity for Tokyo metropolitan residents. It also seeks to reduce disparities among areas within the Tokyo Prefecture, which is a vast self-governing unit consisting of Central Tokyo's twenty-three wards and its surrounding twenty-seven cities, five towns, and eight villages. TMG's policy initiative to narrow these disparities is well supported in a study indicating that local variation among Tokyo's local jurisdictions was greater than among all prefectures in Japan.[3] While evidence examined in the study supported TMG's concerns about disparities in the provision of institutional long-term care, such variation itself does not imply any problems of "access" to long-term care, partly because of the higher rates of sharing resources with Tokyo's seven surrounding prefectures: Saitama, Kanagawa, Chiba, Gunma, Tochigi, Ibaraki, and Yamanashi. Furthermore, the potential preexisting differences in the need for care and the extent of available informal care among Tokyo's jurisdictions may well account for the observed local disparities in use.

In 1996, 15.5 percent of Tokyo residents chose hospitals outside the Tokyo Prefecture for inpatient care, and 15.1 percent of all inpatient beds in Tokyo were used by non-Tokyo residents, a much higher proportion than the national averages, both at 6.6 percent.[4] Under the current system, Tokyo's older population, as well as older persons in neighboring prefectures, can use any institutional care services in any of these prefectures—not just long-term institutional facilities but also services such as short-stay institutional care and day care at nursing institutions.

In 2000, approximately 12 percent of Tokyo's older persons who used Special Nursing Homes, 33 percent who used Health Facilities for the Elderly, and 33 percent who used Long-Term Medical Facilities chose institutions outside the Tokyo Prefecture. These proportions, however, are decreasing as TMG implements its plan..

Demographics

Demographic factors have been important determinants in the sweeping changes experienced by the family in Tokyo. Fertility, already declining, continued to fall to 1.29 children per family as of 2003, a drop that, coupled with increased rates of longevity, has increased the burden placed on family members in supporting older persons. These trends have led to a weakening in the physical capacity of families to provide such care. Shifts from extended to nuclear families lead to diminished roles for family members as caregivers for older persons and, at the same time, reduced roles for older persons as caregivers for young children. Such changes can marginalize older persons, weaken their traditional sources of social support, and eliminate purposeful social roles.

Aging and living alone. Tokyo Prefecture's current population is 11.75 million, of whom 15.5 percent (1.82 million) are sixty-five years or over.[5] According to the latest projections, the percent of older persons will increase 1.6-fold, to 25.2 percent (2.9 million), by 2015.[6] Although in 1997, Tokyo's ratio of older persons was below the national average proportion of 15.9 percent, a closer look at the wards in Central Tokyo reveals a higher rate of aging (17 percent) in Inner Tokyo. Moreover, the proportion of the oldest old (aged eighty-five and over), as a share of those sixty-five years and over, is slightly higher in Inner Tokyo (6.5 percent) than in Outer Tokyo (6.1 percent). In 2000, rates of aging increased throughout Tokyo and remain higher for Inner Tokyo (Table 21.1)

Table 21.1. Persons 65+ and 85+: Tokyo and Japan, 1997–2000

	Persons 65+ as Percent of all Persons		Persons 85+ as Percent of Persons 65+	
	1997	**2000**	**1997**	**2000**
Tokyo	14.5	15.8	6.2	9.7
Inner	17.0	17.7	6.5	10.0
Outer	14.6	16.0	6.1	9.5
23 Wards	15.2	16.4	6.2	9.
Japan	15.9	17.3	9.3	10.2

Sources: Tokyo Metropolitan Government, Fukushimap 1997, available at *http://nenrin.or.jp/choju/fukushimap;* Statistics Bureau (Ministry of International Affairs and Communications).

At the same time, the proportion of "(self-rated) healthy" older persons in Tokyo has steadily increased, exceeding 80 percent in persons between sixty-five and sixty-nine and 70 percent in those age seventy and over. Almost half of adults aged between fifty and seventy-nine who live in Tokyo consider "senior" to apply to persons aged seventy and over.[7] As of 1997, 53.1 percent of males and 25.9 percent of females aged between sixty-five and seventy-four who lived in Tokyo participated in the labor force.[8] Within Central Tokyo, the percentages of males (56 percent) and females (25 percent) aged sixty-five and older in Inner Tokyo were higher than in Outer Tokyo (48 and 17 percent, respectively).[9] In Tokyo, the proportion living alone of those aged sixty-five and over was higher in Inner Tokyo than in Outer Tokyo and the growth of older persons between 1997 and 2000 was higher in Inner Tokyo than in Outer Tokyo (Table 21.2).

Compared with older persons in the rest of Japan, fewer of Tokyo's older persons have children—7.2 percent versus 12.3 percent for the country as whole. Among those who have children, compared with parents in the rest of Japan, fewer of Tokyo's older persons were living with their children—39.8 percent versus 54.3 percent for the country as a whole (Table 21.3).

The Long-Term Care Needs of an Aging Population

Yo-Kaigo-Nintei (the official recognition of eligibility for long-term care services), the computer-aided decision-making process, determines not only whether a condition requires long-term care—for example, a bedridden condition or senile dementia—but also the extent to which long-term care is needed. Although eligibility for long-term care services does not take family-caregiver capacity into consideration, preparation of a long-term service plan requires intense assessment of this capacity.

Table 21.2. Persons 65+ Living Alone:
Tokyo and Japan, 1998, 2000 (as percent of age cohort)

	65+		85+	
	1998	**2000**	**1998**	**2000**
Tokyo	17.3	19.8	15.0	20.2
Inner	20.8	24.7	18.1	23.0
Outer	18.1	20.0	16.4	19.2
23 Wards	18.9	21.6	16.9	20.3
Japan	13.2	13.8	——	——

Source: Tokyo Statistical Association (1998, 2003); Statistics and Information Department, Minister's Secretariat, Ministry of Health, Labor, and Welfare 1998, 2003.
Note: % of elderly living alone = # of elderly living alone × 100 / # of elderly given age group.

Table 21.3. Living Arrangements of Persons 65+:
Tokyo and Japan, 1995 (as percent of all persons 65+)

	Living with Children	**Living Separately**	**No Children**	**Unknown**
Tokyo	39.8	36.8	12.3	11.1
23 Wards	39.5	34.5	13.2	12.8
Japan	54.3	32.2	7.2	6.2

Source: Japan Census 1995.

In the context of Central Tokyo, crowded housing, higher rates of living alone, and the increasing employment of women result in limited ability of families to care for older relatives. In addition, that women outlive men by several years means that those at the oldest ages and with the greatest need for care are far more likely to be female.

Care need level. Most older persons in Tokyo are healthy, and the proportion of healthy older persons has steadily increased. A comparison of Yo-Kaigo Do—the official assessment of the degree of nursing care needed under Japanese long-term insurance for care and assistance for older persons—across Tokyo's neighborhoods and Japan provides some insight into this phenomenon (Table 21.4). As of December 2000, 11.3 percent of people aged sixty-five and over nationwide have

Table 21.4. Level of Care Need among Persons 65+: Tokyo and Japan, March 2001

	Inner Tokyo (%)	Outer Tokyo (%)	23 Wards (%)	Tokyo (%)	Japan[a] (%)
65+ population[b]	341,318	854,812	1,196,130	1,685,171	22,137,784
Needing assistance	5,353 (1.6)[i]	11,810 (1.4)	17,163 (1.4)	24,206 (1.4)	320,809 (1.4)
Needing care	39,120 (11.5)	93,521 (10.9)	132,641 (11.1)	188,293 (11.2)	2,176,974 (9.8)
Level 1[d]	11,743	27,263	39,006	55,719	670,271
Level 2[e]	8,348	20,825	29,173	41,568	466,664
Level 3[f]	6,636	15,849	22,485	31,513	352,238
Level 4[g]	6,544	15,168	21,712	30,780	364,870
Level 5[h]	5,849	14,416	20,265	28,413	322,931
Needing assistance and care	44,473 (13.0)	105,331 (12.3)	149,804 (12.5)	212,199 (12.0)	2,497,783 (11.3)

Sources: Personal communication, M. Yoshida, April 5, 2001; Ministry of Health, Labor, and Welfare.

Note: In combination with case management, computer-aided decision making for the degree of care need is based on functional assessment (of mental and physical conditions). As level of need care certification increases, the degree or intensity of nursing care increases in general. The upper limit of the amount of services that elders can receive at home or in an institution differs according to level of care need. With care-plan maker (the care manager), elders and their family are also participating in the decision making with respect to the selection of in-home versus institutional services (Office for Preparing for the Enforcement of the Kaigo-Hoken System, Health and Welfare Bureau, April 2000).

[a] Data are for December 2000

[b] Data are for 1997

[c] Day-care service twice a week

[d] Various types of daily home-helper service

[e] Various daily services including day care three times a week

[f] Services twice a day, including home-helper service at night or in early morning; in case of great need of medical care, visit and nursing 3 times a week; in case of senile dementia, daily service including day care 4 times a week

[g] Services 2–3 times a day, including home-helper services at night or in early morning; in case of great need of medical care, visit and nursing 3 times a week; in case of senile dementia, daily service including day care 5 times a week

[h] Services 3–4 times a day, including home-helper services at night and in early morning; in case of great need of medical care, visit and nursing 3 times a week

[i] Figures in parentheses are for the population 65+ needing assistance and/or care, as a percent of all persons 65+

been officially recognized as eligible to receive long-term care services because of their mental and physical conditions; 1.4 percent of these required day-care service twice a week (need assistance), and 9.8 percent required various forms of nursing care (need care levels 1–5).

Inner Tokyo has a higher concentration of older persons (13 percent) in a condition requiring various long-term care services (expressed as D/A) as compared to Outer Tokyo and the rest of Japan, 12.3 and 11.3 percent, respectively (Table 21.4). Nationwide, the overwhelming majority (76 percent) of beneficiaries of the long-term care system are aged seventy-five and above (Table 21.5). Living alone usually heightens the probability of requiring long-term care.

Indicators of Supply of LTC

The lower capacity of long-term care beds in Inner Tokyo raises several questions: How does it affect the choice of long-term care facilities and services? Do older

Table 21.5. Persons Requiring Long-Term Care, by Age Group and Gender: Japan, 2001

	40–64 %	65–74 %	75–84 %	85+ %	Total %
Male	7.7	28.4	38.5	25.3	100
Female	2.7	15.1	38.8	43.4	100
Total	4.4	19.6	38.6	37.3	100

Source: Ministry of Health, Labor, and Welfare 2001; available at www.mhlw.go.jp/toukei/saikin/hw/kaigo/setai00/kekka-2.html.

Table 21.6. Institutional Long-Term Care Beds: Tokyo and Japan, 2000

	Tokyo Prefecture	Japan	Range	High/Low Ratio
LTC beds per 100,000 older persons	2,018	2,912	2,018–5,188	2.57

Source: Ministry of Health, Labor, and Welfare 2001; available at www.mhlw.go.jp/toukei/saikin/kaigo. For population figures: Japan Census 2000.
Note: Institutional LTC beds include special nursing homes, health-service facilities for the elderly, and long-term care hospitals.

persons in Tokyo choose more home care, as a result? Or do they end up in general hospitals as cases of social hospitalization more frequently because they have no other place to go? Do they out-migrate from Tokyo to benefit from institutional long-term care? If so, what does this mean to their family caregivers? Definitive answers to these questions are beyond the scope of this chapter, but I present some initial analysis that sheds light on them.

Institutional care capacity. The Tokyo Prefecture's long-term care bed capacity was the lowest among all prefectures in Japan as of 2000 (Table 21.6). This may be the reason why approximately one-third of Tokyo's older persons needing institutional long-term care are using facilities outside Tokyo (Table 21.7). Even within Central Tokyo there is a large variation for both Special Nursing Homes and Health Facilities for the Elderly (Table 21.7). Ten (43 percent) of twenty-three wards did not have Health Facilities for the Elderly.

Although the provision of institutional long-term care services is not the primary goal for TMG, Tokyo's less than adequate capacity with respect these services could work against the cost effectiveness of the long-term care system because of the unintended effects, such as substituting general beds for long-term care recuperation and allowing more permissive policies with regard to "social hospitalization."

Home helpers and medical and public health personnel. In 1996, home helpers were more available in Inner Tokyo than in Outer Tokyo (22.1 versus 20.2 per one thousand households with at least one person sixty-five or over).[10] The supply of physicians and public health nurses in Inner Tokyo is, respectively, more than threefold and double that in Outer Tokyo (Table 21.8). As indicators of community-health resources, public health nurses, in particular, play a critical role in the long-term care system, since their primary practice is community-health education, case management, and home visits for optimal community-based disease prevention and health promotion.[11]

Table 21.7. Institutional Long-Term Care Beds: Tokyo, 1998 (per 100,000 older persons)

	Inner Tokyo	Outer Tokyo	23 Wards	Tokyo
Special Nursing Homes for the Aged	827.5	784.1	796.6	1299.6
Health Service Facilities for the Elderly	133.3	193.5	160.9	266.1
Total	960.8	977.9	957.5	2,523.2

Sources: Tokyo Metropolitan Government 1998; for population figures, Japan Census 1995. Tokyo Metropolitan Government, Fukushimap 1998, available at *http://nenrin.or.jp/choju/fukushimap.*

Table 21.8. Medical and Public Health Personnel: Tokyo, 23 Wards, and Japan, 1996

	Inner Tokyo	Outer Tokyo	23 Wards	Japan
Physicians[a]	454.5	134.3	226.7	131.9
Public health nurses[b]	27.2	11.8	16.2	17.3

Sources: Tokyo Metropolitan Government 1998; Tokyo Bureau of Hygiene 2000.
[a] Per 100,000 persons 65+, 1995
[b] Per 100,000 persons 75+, 1995

Indicators of Use of LTC

Decreasing family size and increasing numbers of older persons, as well as other demographic and social factors affecting family structure, have given rise to formal institutions to share or take over some of the family's traditional responsibilities. While these institutions are necessary and respond to a real need, particularly for physical care, the question of whether they have proven to be acceptable substitutes for the family in providing emotional, psychological, and social support will require close examination in future studies. The debate continues as to the proper balance between family and government assistance, and the appropriate means and ways of helping families continue to be responsible for their frail older members.

Home-care use. While the distribution of home versus institutional care recipients for each category is unknown for Tokyo, approximately two-thirds of long-term care recipients throughout Japan selected home services in 2000. Before the enactment of Long-Term Care Insurance, Tokyo's older persons had used more home helpers and day services than the national average. In 1996 and 2000, the use of home helpers was higher in Inner Tokyo than in Outer Tokyo (Table 21.9).

The higher rate of home-care use can be a function of both living arrangements and the nature of the family system. Although approximately 40 percent of older persons in Tokyo are living with their children, one could speculate that urban families may have less rigid familial roles and are more open-minded to extrafamilial sharing, compared to families in rural areas. If this assumption is correct, the importance of family ties for providing care to older relatives is inversely related to the importance of the family's caregiving.

Historically, home care, compared with institutional care, has been provided to a less functionally dependent population, but new long-term care policies have been designed to try to encourage home care in lieu of institutional care. In 2000, nationwide, 56.2 percent of older persons requiring care levels 1 through 5 chose home-care services, and 38.2 percent chose institutional care.

Table 21.9. Home-Helper Visits: Tokyo, 1996 and 1999 (per 100 persons 65+)

	Inner Tokyo	Outer Tokyo	23 Wards	Tokyo Prefecture
1996	220.6	161.1	178.2	164.2
1999	356.1	267.7	292.3	265.1

Source: Tokyo Metropolitan Government 1996, *Annual Report on Social Welfare Statistics, 1996,* Fukushimap home page (2002) available at *http://nenrin.or.jp/choju/fukushimap.*

Home-helper use by level of care need. Overall, 58.7 percent of eligible older persons in Central Tokyo used home-helper services in 2000. As the level of care need increases, home-helper use decreases. In contrast, as the level of care need increases, the use of home-visiting nurses increases, indicating a good division of labor. Overall, 13 percent of eligible older persons used home-visiting nurse services.

Home care use and aging. The proportion of the oldest old (aged eighty-five and above) is strongly and positively correlated to home-helper and home-visiting nurse use, indicating that very old people use more home-care services.

Home-care cost. There is greater variation by ward for home-care cost in Inner Tokyo than in Outer Tokyo, consistent with the greater variation of home-care use in Inner Tokyo.

Institutional care use and issues of social hospitalization. In 2000, approximately half of those nationwide who chose institutional care were persons with a functional level 3 or less, indicating that factors other than physical and mental function, such as family conditions, underlie institutional use. Sicker and more needy older persons (levels 4 and 5) are more likely to be institutionalized in long-term medical facilities than in nursing homes and health facilities.

According to the 1999 Patient Survey, over 20 percent of patients sixty-five years and over and almost 25 percent of patients seventy-five years and over in long-term care beds are categorized as cases of "social hospitalization," that is, hospitalized patients with no medical necessity but with no place else to go.[12] These social issues will worsen in Japan if reliance on family for long-term care is overestimated and no social reform is undertaken to remove some family burden.[13] A study done by Nakai and others found that about 40 percent of institutionalized older persons in Health Facilities for the Elderly said that they do not wish to return home.[14] The longer they stayed in an institution, the less likely their wish to return home; only 30 percent of those who stayed longer than one year wished to return home, compared to 56 percent of those who stayed less than a month. Reasons for not wishing to return to home included not wanting to trouble their family members (38 percent), and no one to take care of them (27 percent). This study underscores the influence of social support systems for older persons on patterns of institutional care use and sheds light on the importance of the expansion of home-care services to reduce social hospitalization.

While social support of Tokyo's older persons is elusive, culturally it means kinship and idealizes women's caregiving in particular. A government survey reveals that more than 80 percent of caregivers were female family members.[15] The rate of longer institutionalization in 1991 among older persons having a daughter or daughter-in-law under the same roof was significantly less than that of older persons without a daughter or daughter-in-law under the same roof (28.8 versus 31.3 percent: p<.001).[16] The rate of longer institutionalization among older persons living alone was highest (34 percent) among other family structural patterns in 1991.[17]

However, within Central Tokyo, inpatient days were not correlated to older persons living alone. They were negatively correlated to physician supply and moderately related to public health nurses, which suggests that the higher the supply of medical personnel, the lower the inpatient days (Table 21.10). Adherence to health screening and inpatient days were inversely related, which indicates that the higher the adherence, the lower the inpatient days. Whether or not shorter inpatient days can be seen as a better health outcome is controversial, yet fewer inpatient days are certainly a better economic outcome. This evidence appears to support the premise that investment in secondary prevention is cost effective.[18]

Inpatient days per capita of persons aged seventy-five and older in 1998 were slightly lower in Inner Tokyo (22.1 days) than in Outer Tokyo (24.7 days).[19] Overall

Table 21.10. Correlations between Inpatient Days of Persons 75+ and Community Medical Resources, 1996 and 1998

	% Living Alone, 1998	Physician Supply, 1996[a]	Public Health Nurse Supply, 1996[b]	% Health Screening Adherence, 1998[c]
Inpatient days per capita, 1998	r = -0.202 p = 0.355	r = -0.573[d] p = 0.004	r = -0.586[d] p = 0.003	r = -0.494[e] p = 0.016

Sources: Tokyo Statistical Association 1998; Tokyo Municipal Government 1998; Tokyo Bureau of Hygiene 2000.

[a] Number of physicians per 10,000 persons 65+
[b] Number of public health nurse per 10,000 persons 65+
[c] Persons received check-up*100 / persons 40+ who are invited
[d] Correlation significant at the 0.01 level
[e] Correlation significant at the 0.05 level

in the Tokyo Prefecture, length of hospital stay (LOS) has always been shorter than the national average: LOS of general hospital beds in 1996 was 28.2 days in Tokyo and 33.5 days in Japan.[20]

Overall, approximately one in two older residents in Central Tokyo underwent health screening, yet the rates by ward range from a low of 14.6 to a high of 73.6 percent, which reveals great variation in the success of screening. The reasons for this are complex and beyond the scope of this chapter. However, empirical studies have explored the relationship to such factors as gender, educational level, and social support.

The Informal Care System in Tokyo

Since long-term care is generally a family decision, Japanese caregiving behavior provides a basis for understanding the dynamics of long-term care demand and supply and helps guide long-term care policies. Rapid modernization in Japan had little impact on traditional help-seeking and help-accepting patterns but has made urban-dwelling older persons more likely to experience alienation and loneliness compared to those in rural areas, where social solidarity remains strong. Ogawa and Retherford also point to the continuing decline in the ability and willingness of family to provide care for older persons throughout Japan.[21]

The sense of loneliness among urban-dwelling older persons was documented in a survey study conducted by Toyokawa and others, who examined the relationship between psychological well-being of older persons and the long-term care infrastructure, including living conditions, in a sample of 1,401 older residents in Edogawa-ku (Outer Tokyo).[22] Most noteworthy are findings that about 30 percent of the study sample had a sense of loneliness related to having no caregivers. Similarly, living in an institution as opposed to living at home, having poor health status, receiving welfare services, and having no caregivers were related to an increased sense of dissatisfaction, while absence of spouse, family structure, and source of finance were not. Availability of caregivers appears to be an important factor affecting older persons' psychological well-being. Preference that caregivers be family members was not studied but would be a critical question in developing a care plan for older persons and LTC policies.

In Tokyo, as in most of the world, the caregiving burden falls heavily on women (76.9 percent), of whom wives (31.8 percent), daughters (23 percent), and daughters-in-law (22.1 percent) are an overwhelming majority. Most caregivers are older persons themselves; about 27 percent are aged sixty to sixty-nine, 22 percent aged seventy to seventy-nine, and 8 percent aged eighty and over.[23] The increasing concern about aging caregivers is documented in a 1999 study by Maeda, who randomly sampled 1,148 primary caregivers caring for older persons who required various care and assistance in one of Tokyo's twenty-three wards. While over 30 percent of the caregivers were aged seventy and older and over 40 percent reported poor health status, age and self-rated health status of caregivers were significantly associated with the ability to seek social support. As caregiver age increased, the ability to seek social support decreased. About 36 percent of the caregivers were participating in the labor force and were more likely to experience impaired well-being as compared to nonworking caregivers.[24] The implication is troubling, since the number of older persons who enter or remain in the job market is increasing in Tokyo.

Conclusion

In summary, this chapter sheds light on two findings: first, a high concentration of the oldest old (eighty-five years and over) and older persons living alone has increased the need for health care and social services in Tokyo, particularly within the urban core; second, use of long-term care services appears to be driven by health and family needs, despite the lack of sufficient services and institutional long-term care beds. While emotional ties and mutual support among family members remain strong in Japan, it is clear that demographic changes will increasingly affect the capacity of families to continue their caregiving roles.

Although the government encourages the concept of "living with independence and choices" as a strategic objective in developing its system of long-term care, there are several research topics about which we will need to improve understanding to ensure a proper balance between family and government assistance. First, the extent to which disparities in service use is attributable to the characteristics of older persons' social and family environments. Second, the extent to which services can be developed to support childless older persons and widows at home in later life. Finally, the extent to which long-term care can alleviate social hospitalization, as well as family-care burdens. As the older population in Tokyo continues to grow, these topics will no doubt continue to preoccupy policy makers in the future.

Notes

1.   Japan has three types of long-term care facilities: long-term care hospitals (LTCH), health facilities for the elderly (HFE), and special nursing homes for the aged (SNHA).
2.   Yoshida M. Personal communication. April, 5, 2001. Tokyo: Ministry of Health and Welfare.
3.   Kato, M., S. Hashimoto, M. Miyashita, M. Hayashi, K. Nakamura, S. Oshima, Y. Matsumura, and K. Fukutomi. 2000. Roujin fukushi taisaku no todoufuken, shichousonn-kan no suii [Trend of differences within prefectures and within municipal local units in long-term care services]. *Kouseino Shihyou*, 47(4): 8–13.
4.   Ministry of Health, Labour, and Welfare. 1996. *Patient Survey*. Tokyo: Health Statistics Office, Vital and Health Statistics Division, Statistics and Information Department, Minister's Secretariat, Ministry of Health, Labour, and Welfare.
5.   TMG. 2000. Annual Report on Health in Tokyo. Tokyo: Bureau of Public Health.
6.   Tokyo Statistical Association. 1997. *Tokyo Statistical Yearbook*. Tokyo: Tokyo Statistical Association.

7.   TMG, Annual Report on Health in Tokyo.

8.   Ibid.

9.   Statistical Bureau of Japan. 1995. Census of Japan. Tokyo: Statistical Bureau of Japan, Ministry of Internal Affairs and Communications.

10. TMG. 1996. Annual Report on Social Welfare Statistics. Tokyo: TMG.

11. The expertise and field of public health nursing in Japan were established pursuant to the 1948 Nurse, Midwife, and Public Health Nurse Law and differ from those of registered nurses.

12. Ministry of Health, Labour, and Welfare, *Patient Survey*.

13. For example, in Japan, the support system for caregivers is relatively inflexible in the sense that the regulatory system limits caregivers to family members living with the elderly (the insured persons). In contrast, the United Kingdom has extended its support system to nonfamily persons caring for the elderly through the Invalid Care Allowance (ICA).

14. Nakai, S., S. Hashimoto, T. Doi, T. Sone, D. Santou, and H. Noda. 1998. Roujinhokenshisetsu no zaaisho kikan to kanren youin [Factors related to the length of stay in health facilities for the elderly]. *Kouseino Shihyou* 45(10): 13–17.

15. TMG. 1995. Survey on home-visit nursing care. Tokyo: Ministry of Health and Welfare.

16. TMG, Annual Report on Social Welfare Statistics.

17. Doi, T., H. Chin, and K. Ohara. 1997. Rouzin hokenshisetsu zittaichousa karamita keizokuzaishosya no kazokuzyoukyou [Family dynamics for older persons living in long-term care facilities]. *Kouseino Shihyou* 44(15): 10–16.

18. Nakanishi, N., K. Tatara, and H. Fujiwara. 1996. Do Preventive Health Services Reduce Eventual Demand for Medical Care? *Social Science and Medicine* 43(6): 999–1005.

19. Okamoto, E. 2002. Inpatient data for Tokyo. Unpublished raw data.

20. Tokyo Statistical Association. 1996. LOS = annual total number of inpatient days / (annual admissions + annual discharges) x 5.5.

21. Ogawa, N., and R. D. Retherford. 1997. Shifting Costs of Caring for the Elderly Back to Families in Japan: Will It Work? *Population and Development Review* 23(1 [March]): 59–94.

22. Toyokawa, H, T. Nakahara, T. Watanabe, S. Takemura, Y. Sasa, N. Yoshida, Y. Satsumabayashi, and K. Higashikawa. 1999. Koureikitou kyozyu idousya no hoken needs to chiikihokeniryoufukushi no kyoukyuu [The relationship between the health needs of mobile older persons and the supply of long-term care and social welfare]. *Kouseikagaku kenkyu/kenkoukagaku sougou kenkyu zigyou.* In 1999 Kouseikagaku kenkyu kenkyuu houkokusho [1999 Research report on health and welfare]. Japanese Ministry of Health, Labour, and Welfare.

23. Bureau of Social Welfare. 1995. *Survey of the Living Conditions of the Elderly.* Tokyo: Bureau of Social Welfare, TMG.

24. Maeda, D. 1999. Koreiki ni okeru syakaiteki shien to well-being no kankei ni tsuite no kenkyu. [The relationship between social support and well-being among the elderly]. In *Chojyu kagaku Sougou Kenkyu Houkoku.* Tokyo: Ministry of Health, Labour, and Welfare.

22. The Continuum of Long-Term Care in World Cities: From Institutionalization to Home Care

Gabriel Montero, Michael K. Gusmano, and Victor G. Rodwin

Discussions of long-term care usually evoke images of "warehousing" frail older persons in nursing homes, hospitals, and other institutional settings. Most long-term care, however, is provided in the community. As the preceding chapters suggest, world cities have a particularly acute need for innovative solutions for the provision of long-term care. Large older populations face a diverse set of chronic conditions that require flexibility and tailored services difficult to provide in institutional settings. Moreover, specific urban characteristics such as limited land and higher population densities make for costly construction of long-term care facilities. As we show, the solution to some of these challenges is to use the existing housing stock and develop more home-care services.

In this chapter, we compare indicators of service provision at each end of the long-term care continuum. Subsequently, we study the organization and development of institutional innovations along the continuum from institutional care to services received directly in the home, as well as the range of intermediary services. A pervasive theme in long-term care concerns the distinction between "social" versus "medical" care. Social care usually refers to assistance with activities of daily living, such as bathing, dressing, and cooking. In the context of long-term care, medical care refers to skilled nursing services, wound treatment, and the administration of medications. This distinction has been taken very seriously by national and local governments, with important consequences for financing and ultimately for the quality of life of dependent older persons.

Institutional Long-Term Care

Institutional long-term care—more commonly known as nursing-home care—is typically defined as the provision of institutional services for frail older persons who require twenty-four-hour nursing services. Rates of institutional long-term care beds (per thousand persons age sixty-five and over) are consistently lower in the urban cores of these cities than in their first rings (Table 22.1). Despite this pattern in the ratio of beds among urban cores and first rings, there are considerable differences in levels of institutional long-term care among both the urban cores and the first rings of New York, London, Paris, and Tokyo. Even after adding a portion of general hospital beds to Tokyo's special homes for the aged, health facilities for the elderly, and long-term care hospital beds, that city's level of institutional services is as low as London's, followed by those of Paris and New York, which has the highest density of nursing-home beds (Table 22.1).

Despite the growing need for publicly provided home care, the United States, the United Kingdom, and France maintain an institutional bias when it comes to funding long-term care. For example, in the United States, Medicare does not reimburse home-care episodes that last more than eight hours a day or twenty-eight hours a week. Indeed, the vast majority of Medicare funding for long-term care continues to be for nursing-home services. For patients with chronic conditions requiring up to twelve hours' or more care a day, the only recourse is Medicaid-funded home care. However, such care is available only for those who meet stringent income requirements. With respect to Medicaid, the overwhelming majority of long-term care patients across the United States receive care in an institution, as opposed to in the home. In France, this bias toward medical services is evident even within institutions, where patients must cover the residential costs of institutional care, while nursing services are reimbursed through national health insurance.[1]

There are important differences among the characteristics of older persons who reside in institutional long-term care facilities and their counterparts who live at home alone. In Manhattan and Paris, the two cities for which data are available, men and women over sixty-five who live alone have much higher levels of educational attainment than those who live in institutions.[2] Although the sample size is small after age eighty-five, this pattern holds for Manhattanites.

In all four cities, the high price of real estate in the urban cores tends to restrict investment in institutional long-term care facilities compared to levels in the first ring and the rest of the country. The shortage of long-term care beds in London has also been exacerbated by reductions in government payments for residential and nursing-home care and policies that make it possible for local governments to divert to other purposes funds originally intended for long-term care beds (Chapter 10). Similarly, there is a shortage of nursing-home beds in Inner Tokyo, in part, because some municipalities are hesitant to expand benefits and services for older persons, raise taxes, and possibly deter younger families from locating there (Chapter 20).

Community-Based Services for Older Persons

Because of unique physical constraints on construction, and in order to lower costs, maintain the autonomy of dependent persons, and provide more targeted social services, each of our cities administers community-based home care. Older persons prefer home care to nursing-home care because it provides greater autonomy. However, the quality of care provided in the home is much more difficult to monitor than that in a regulated facility. Although we do not have adequate information about the quality of care in nursing homes, we know even less about the quality of

Table 22.1. Institutional Long-Term Care Beds: NYC, London, Paris, and Tokyo (per 1,000 persons 65+)

	Urban Core	First Ring
New York, 2000[a]	33.3	48.4
London, 2001[b]	9.9	12.5
Paris, 2001[c, d]	13.3	22.3
Tokyo, 1997[e]	9.7	12.3

Sources: London: I. Struder and T. Warnes (Chapter 10); New York City: New York State Department of Health; Paris: ORSIF; Tokyo: Ministry of Health, Labor and Welfare, Japan.

[a] Includes all nursing-home beds but excludes beds for AIDS patients

[b] Includes all nursing-home beds but excludes residential homes.

[c] Includes long-term care beds in hospitals, "medicalized" beds in retirement homes and in foyers-logement and places within special institutional facilities for older dependent persons (EHPAD).

[d] The city of Paris operates nursing-home beds outside the city, which are excluded from our analysis. Had we included them, the numbers for Paris would be 19 per 1,000 persons 65+ in the core and 18.8 in the first ring.

[e] Includes 30% of general hospitals beds for which lengths of stay are estimated to exceed 30 days

long-term care services provided in the home. Little research has been done on the issue of quality of care with respect to home help and in-home nursing. The data that we present show that the population receiving such services is quite large and, in many cases, growing. Given the significance of this population, it is important that more effort be given to the study of quality of home care.

Home-care services. Home care includes two kinds of service that are typically distinguished from one another: home-help and home-nursing care. Home help refers to nonmedical services such as cleaning, cooking, and personal assistance such as bathing. Within home help, we distinguish further between home-attendant and housekeeping services: the former involves hands-on care for activities of daily living, such as bathing and dressing, whereas the latter does not (e.g., cooking, shopping, and cleaning). Home-nursing care, which is medical in nature, usually involves wound care, the provision of medications, and skilled nursing services. With the exception of London, which relies only on central funding for both these services, the cities provide supplementary locally financed funding for both types of service. London provides local authority funding for home help only.

We present the number of older home-help users for New York and Paris in Tables 22.2 and 22.3. We include detailed tables for these two cities to give a sense of the complexity and specificity of their diversely funded home-help programs. By contrast, Tokyo and London have relatively simple and centralized home-help programs originating from a single funding source: in the former case, the federal Long-Term Care Insurance program; in the latter, local-authority provisions. As we shall see, with the exception of Japan, the provision of long-term care in these cities evinces a similar pattern: a reluctance on the part of national governments to insure nonmedical services for the frail and the dependent. In France and the United Kingdom, in-home nursing services are funded through national health insurance schemes, while the bulk of social services remains means tested and funded through local programs. Similarly, in the United States, the bulk of in-home nursing services is funded through the Medicare program, while the bulk of social services is funded through the federal-state Medicaid program, which is means tested. In contrast to other aspects of the public welfare state, in which the United States tends to lag behind its counterparts in the developed world, many countries with otherwise generous public welfare provide limited, means-tested programs for home help.

Home-care services in New York City. Users of publicly funded home care in New York City face a bewildering and frequently frustrating system of home-care programs, with various and at times conflicting eligibility requirements, points of entry, and service suites. With respect to home help in the city, Medicaid is the single most important source of funds. Because of strict income requirements, Medicaid home-care services are available only for impoverished older persons. Under the aegis of Medicaid, there exists a multitude of service types, depending on one's medical condition, social service needs, and housing situation. These services range from the most intense program, combining in-home nursing care with twenty-four-hour supervision, to the least intense, involving only housekeeping. Older persons who are ineligible to receive Medicaid can receive publicly funded home-care services through the New York City Department for the Aging's (DFTA) home-care program, a local variant of the federal Expanded In-Home Services for the Elderly Program (EISEP). However, services in this program are restricted to housekeeping, as opposed to hands-on care such as bathing and dressing of clients. As noted previously, the situation for older persons of modest incomes who suffer from chronic conditions is perhaps the worst with respect to home care: while they are not eligible to receive home-care services through Medicaid, the services provided by EISEP will not be adequate for those with more debilitating conditions.

With respect to in-home nursing services, national funding through the Medicare program is the most significant source. As noted previously, Medicare reimburses episodes of care that last a maximum of eight hours a day or twenty-eight hours a week. In this sense, we must modify our previous statement and allow a small measure of U.S. exceptionalism: none of the other nationally financed in-home nursing services places such restrictions on the duration of care. In addition, social services of a type found under Medicaid home-care programs are provided only if they "augment skilled medical services in the overall treatment of a beneficiary who needs skilled medical care."[3] Instead, patients primarily receive traditional "medical-ized" nursing services, such as wound care and the administration of medications. The overwhelming majority of in-home nursing services in the city are provided through certified home-health agencies, which are regulated by the New York State Department of Health and certified to receive both Medicare and Medicaid patients. The majority of in-home nursing patients in New York City (around 65 percent) have been referred by a hospital, while 24 percent require short-term rehabilitative care, lasting less than three months.[4] While longer episodes occur, they are much less frequent. Medicare provisions requiring a prior hospital stay as a condition of eligibility for home-nursing services were overturned in 1980. That the majority of patients remain rehabilitative cases may be evidence of a time lag with respect to patients' awareness of their rights under Medicare.

Aside from Medicare, the Medicaid Long-Term Home Health Care program (LTHHCP) provides home-nursing care in addition to home-help services. Unlike Medicare services, however, care episodes often last up to twelve hours or more and are provided only for patients who meet income-eligibility conditions. In addition, a professional assessment of the patient's condition must determine that the cost of care will not exceed 75 percent of comparable care delivered in a nursing home.

Despite the difficulties involved in navigating the long-term care system, older persons in New York City avail themselves of home care in much larger propor-tions than do their counterparts in the rest of the state and country: 7.7 percent of the older population of New York City receives Medicaid home-help services, as opposed to 5.1 for the state and 2.7 for the nation as a whole.[5] In part, these figures reflect the much larger share of older persons in New York who are poor. However, even when we look just within the Medicaid population, New Yorkers receive more home care: 26 percent versus 22 and 19 percent for the state and nation, respectively. Moreover, while in the state as a whole the majority of Medicaid long-term care users receive care in an institution, in New York City the situation is the opposite: 66 percent of Medicaid long-term care users receive services in the home as opposed to an institutional setting.[6]

In order to provide home-help data strictly comparable to the other three cities, we excluded the use of nursing services in the LTHHCP program. Data from the New York State Department of Health (form 519) reveal that 39.0 percent of services received in Manhattan, and 31.3 percent in the first ring, were nursing services. We took this proportion and applied it to the total number of LTHHCP users to arrive at the number who received only personal, home-health, and social care.

Home-care services in Paris. In Paris, we find a variety of funding streams that pay for home-help services. Among them, the national Old Age Insurance Scheme

Table 22.2. Home-Help Users 65+: NYC, 2000

Service	Urban Core	First Ring	Total
Medicaid			
Home attendant, 2002			
n	8,352	36,571	45,103
(%)[a]	(4.5)	(4.9)	(4.8)
Housekeeper, 2002			
n	1,749	5,927	7,676
(%)[a]	(0.9)	(0.8)	(0.81)
Long-term home-health care, 2000[b]			
n	2,478	6 270	8,748
(%)[a]	(1.3)	(0.9)	(0.93)
Total			
n	12,579	48,768	61,527
(%)[a]	(6.8)	(6.5)	(6.6)
EISEP home help, 2000			
n	1,226	3,607	4,833
(%)[a]	(0.6)	(0.5)	(0.52)
Total			
n	13,805	52,375	66,360
(%)[a]	(7.4)	(7.0)	(7.1)

Sources: New York City—Human Resources Administration of New York City, New York State Department of Health, New York City Department for the Aging, US Census 2000, SF3 file.

[a] Figures in parentheses represent home-help users 65+ as a percent of all persons 65 +.

[b] The Long-Term Home Health Care Program (LTHHCP) provides both home-nursing and home-help services. To provide data comparable to the other three cities, we excluded the use of nursing services in this program. Data from the New York State Department of Health (Form 519) reveal that 39.0% of services received in Manhattan and 31.3% in the First Ring were nursing services. We took this proportion and applied it to the total number of LTHHCP users to arrive at the number who received only personal, home-health, and social care.

Social Services Fund, social welfare services, and the needs-based (according to disability levels), means-tested Personal Autonomy Allowance used to finance home-help services (Table 22.3). Services are delivered by communal centers for social action or contracted out to small for-profit and nonprofit organizations. By contrast, and in accordance with what we find in our other cities, the In-Home Nursing Care Services Program is covered under French National Health Insurance for all persons sixty and over or for younger persons with a debilitating condition.

Home-care services in Tokyo. As mentioned previously, Japan's national Long-Term Care Insurance (LTCI) program covers both "social" home-help services and "medicalized" home-nursing services for all older persons, regardless of income. Although everyone forty years old and over contributes to this program, there are two broad categories of beneficiaries for LTCI. Those aged forty to sixty-four must pay insurance premiums but are eligible for services only if their long-term care needs are the result of one of fifteen aging-related diseases. Those sixty-five years and over pay higher premiums deducted from pensions and are eligible for home-care services regardless of the source of their needs. Users are expected to pay 10 percent of the cost of services, the other 90 percent being covered by a mix of municipal, prefectural, and national funds. Premiums in 2000 were around twenty-four dollars per person per month.

Home-care services in London. In London, the Home Care Services Unit of each local authority provides home-attendant services directly or contracts with independent organizations for their provision. Although increasingly rare, house-keeping services are provided as well. It is up to local authorities to decide whether to charge for these services; some have instituted a weekly rate. Older home-care users who must pay generally do so with their attendance allowance, a weekly income supplement for persons sixty-five and over who require personal care assistance. As is the case in New York and Paris, home-care services in London are means tested. By contrast, in-home nursing services are covered for all citizens under the National Health Service and administered by district nurses. District nurses are affiliated with particular general practitioner practices as part of a Primary Health Care Team and are responsible for providing palliative care, rehabilitation, and wound management.

Table 22.4 compares the share of older home-help users in all four cities. Inner London ranks highest among our urban cores (8.1 percent of the older population), followed by Manhattan (7.4 percent), Inner Tokyo (7.3 percent), and Paris (6.0 percent). What is most striking, however, is the extent to which these figures indicate convergence in the use of home help among the urban cores of these cities, and greater divergence among their first rings. Overall, in all four cities, between 6 and 7 percent of the older population makes use of such services. We do not have

Table 22.3. Home-Help Users 65+: Paris, 2002–2003

Service	Urban Core	First Ring	Total
Régime Général			
n	10,554	14,371	24,925
(%)[a]	(3.2)[a]	(2.8)	(2.9)
Departmental Aide			
n	1,849	2,104	3,953
(%)	(0.6)	(0.4)	(0.5)
APA			
n	6,891	9,583	16,474
(%)	(2.2)	(1.9)	(2.0)
PSD			
n	273	814	1,087
(%)	(0.1)	(0.2)	(0.1)
ACTP			
n	614	1,860	2,474
(%)	(0.2)	(0.4)	(0.3)
Total			
n	20,181	28,732	48,918
(%)	(6.4)	(5.7)	(6.0)

Sources: 2002 APA, PSD, and ACTP figures: Department of Research, French Ministry of Health; 2003 Régime Général figures: National Old Age Insurance Fund; 2002 Departmental Aide figures: ORS Ile-de-France; 2002 SSIAD figures: ORSIF.

Note: These figures do not take into account that APA is for persons 60 and over. Given that, in 1999, persons 65 and over made up 78.5% of the 60+ population in Paris, 80.4% of the same population in the first ring, and 79.7% in the region as a whole, and applying these ratios to the respective population of APA users, our figures are an overestimate and could be lowered accordingly: 5.6% in the urban core; 5.1% in the first ring; and 5.3% for the region as a whole. These figures also underestimate the number of home-care users in Paris because they do not include home care received by beneficiaries of the Agricultural Health Insurance Fund (Mutualité Sociale Agricole). Finally, these figures do not include Parisian frail older persons who have opted not to accept APA and who instead receive ACTP (allocation compensatrice pour tierce personne). However, ORSIF estimates that these adjustments would not increase the number of home-care users in Paris by more than 1,600 users, which would increase the Paris figure only from 6.8 to 7.2%.

[a] Figures in parentheses represent home-help users 65+ as a percent of all persons 65+

Table 22.4. Home-Help Users 65+:
NYC, London, Paris, and Tokyo, 2000–2002 (as percent of all persons 65+)

	Urban Core (%)	First Ring (%)	Total (%)
New York, 2000	7.4	7.0	7.1
London, 2001	8.1	4.7	5.8
Paris, 2002	6.4	5.7	6.0
Tokyo, 2002	7.3	6.5	6.8

Sources: New York: Human Resources Administration of New York City, New York State Department of Health, New York City Department for the Aging, US Census 2000, SF3 file; London: Institute of Public Finance; Paris: 2002 APA, PSD, and ACTP figures: Department of Research, French Ministry of Health; 2003 Régime General figures: National Old Age Insurance Fund; 2002 Departmental Aide figures: ORS Ile-de-France; 2002 SSIAD figures: ORSIF. Tokyo: TMG, Bureau of Health and Social Services.

comparable data on the rates of disability or other measures of need across these cities. Based on national estimates of disability, it is possible that older residents of Paris and Tokyo are less frail and require less help with the activities of daily living than do residents of New York City and London. If this is true, then even though a slightly higher percentage of older New Yorkers and Londoners receive home-help services, Paris and Tokyo may be providing home help to a larger percentage of the older persons who need this care.

It is difficult to compare in-home nursing across these cities because the data to which we currently have access are not equivalent. For example, the Medicare home-care figures for New York City include patients receiving short-term rehabilitative care and longer-term in-home nursing. The Medicare home-care data also include the number of people receiving skilled nursing and home-health aides. Nationally, only 41 percent of Medicare home-care patients received skilled nursing care, but we do not have an estimate for New York City. The data on in-home nursing in London present a similar problem. It is impossible, using published data on the extensive in-home nursing program, to separate patients receiving post-acute rehabilitative care from those receiving longer-term home nursing in London.

For Paris and Tokyo, we have comparable data on the number of older persons receiving long-term home-nursing services (Table 22.5). We find, not surprisingly, that a much smaller share of the older population receives in-home nursing services compared with home-help services. However, we would need more information about levels of disability at the city level before evaluating the degree to which the observed levels of in-home nursing meet the needs of older residents. Although

Keiko Honda's analysis of home care in Tokyo (Chapter 21) suggests that the level of in-home nursing increases with the level of need, it is difficult to know whether all those in need are receiving services.

Community-based residential options. Aside from home care and nursing-home care, each of our four cities has developed intermediary forms of care. We call these services "intermediary" because, while still institutional, they do not provide intense nursing care. Such services are usually reserved for older persons who exhibit an intermediary stage of autonomy with respect to state intervention: their medical condition is such that they do not require publicly funded continuous care, yet they have reached a stage where they cannot or do not wish to live alone, either because they lack the support of informal caregivers who can assist them with daily activities, or because, even with such support, they desire the company of others as opposed to individualized home care.

As we document in Table 22.6, intermediary care of this kind takes on two principal guises: congregate housing with common services, or individual apartments with attached and collective services, which we hereafter call "enriched apartments." The former involves the construction of facilities for long-term care use, whereas the latter involves the grafting of services to preexisting housing stock. We find that the latter is much more readily available in the urban cores of these cities, where land is most expensive. Apartments of this kind represent an important innovative use of urban resources. However, because such units are tied in some way to the housing market rather than designated for a particular purpose, they are usually more expensive for patients than are congregate facilities and are rarely fully funded through public means. Instead, various subsidies exist to pay for such housing and presume that the individual has some assets to pay for services. In the case of congregate

Table 22.5. Home-Nursing Users 65+: Paris and Tokyo, 2002

	Urban Core	First Ring	Total
Paris			
n	2,398	3,130	5,528
(%)	(0.7)	(0.6)	(0.6)
Tokyo			
n	5,909	12,392	18,301
(%)	(1.7)	(1.4)	(1.5)

Sources: Paris: ORSIF, SSIAD; Tokyo: TMG, Bureau of Welfare for the Elderly.

Table 22.6. Forms of Intermediary Care:
NYC, Paris and First Ring, and Tokyo (places per 1,000 persons 65+)

	Congregate Housing	Enriched Apartment
New York	13.1	47.7
Paris and First Ring	15.3	19.6
Tokyo	0.6	5.7

Sources: New York: Alternatives in Senior Housing, New York City DFTA, 1999; New York State-Licensed Assisted Living Programs, DFTA, November 2001; Tokyo: Tokyo Metropolitan Government, Bureau of Welfare for the Elderly: Paris: ORSIF.
Note: London is excluded from this table because at the time of this writing, there are no publicly financed programs for enriched apartments

housing, placement is means tested in all four cities and is not readily available for the poor. For example, while Medicaid does fund assisted-living programs in adult homes, only around three thousand such places were available in 2000. This type of subsidized care represents an intermediary form in an economic sense as well, somewhere between publicly funded long-term care and the private care one can procure in any of these cities.

Among the four cities, New York has the greatest variety of such intermediary forms and spans the funding spectrum from private for-profit facilities to government-funded residential programs. For those fortunate enough to forego publicly funded programs, a variety of high- to middle-income apartment complexes exists with attached social and home-health services. To date, twenty-eight of these complexes have become officially recognized NORCs (naturally occurring retirement communities): apartment complexes in which over 50 percent of the population is over fifty years old and which receive public funding to support their services for older persons. At the opposite extreme, there are public housing facilities set aside for older persons, some of which provide common services (see Chapter 5).

Between these extremes, two principal community-based residential options for older persons in New York exist: enriched housing and assisted-living programs. Enriched housing is a means-tested program for persons whose income disqualifies them from Medicaid but who require personal care assistance. Essentially a collective version of the EISEP program described earlier, enriched housing is usually attached to a particular apartment complex with subsidized apartments. Poor older persons who are eligible for Medicaid and who require both personal assistance and noncontinuous nursing services, but whose home environment is not suitable for home-care services, can receive personal assistance in an assisted-living program

(ALP). The essential difference between these programs and enriched housing is that the former have attached medical services.

ALPs are housed in adult homes or enriched housing programs that have been licensed as certified home-health agencies or long-term home health-care programs to provide personal care services and in-home nursing services reimbursable by Medicaid. They serve as a collective form of the LTHHCP program, but differ from nursing homes because they do not provide continuous care. For older persons with monthly incomes less than or equal to US$966 ($1,932 for couples), federal subsidies through Supplemental Security Income (SSI) can help pay for room and board. In essence, ALPs replicate the social/medical split we have seen, with medical services covered under one program (Medicaid), and residential costs covered by another (SSI). Interestingly, here the order is reversed, with national funding paying for social care and state resources contributing to medical services.

For New York, we counted as congregate housing all registered adult homes, which include Medicaid assisted-living programs in adult homes. For individual units, we included enriched housing (including assisted living in enriched housing) and Section 202 housing for the elderly, but exclude public housing for the elderly. Had we included public housing for the elderly, the numbers for individual units would be 46.5 in Manhattan and 32.5 for the outer boroughs. For both Section 202 and public housing, we have taken the original number of units and multiplied it by 1.5. Based on NYC Housing and Vacancy Survey data for 1999, 87 percent of public housing units with householders sixty-five and over had one to two people per unit, whereas 81 percent of Section 202 units with householders sixty-five and over had one to two persons per unit. We therefore used 1.5 as an estimate to determine the average number of older persons that could be accommodated by these units.

Like New York, Tokyo and Paris both provide congregate housing with collective services, or individualized apartments with collective services. In Tokyo, neither type is fully publicly funded, but subsidies do exist. For Paris, as described in Chapter 15, we count residential/retirement homes, which include the *foyers-logements* (individual apartments with collective services) operated by a city agency, as well as the *maisons de retraite* (retirement homes). In both cases, we have excluded medicalized beds, as well as beds for Parisians that are located outside the city. In London, we have considered only congregate care in the form of residential care homes. Unlike New York and Paris, where funding exists from national sources, residential care homes in London, like home-help services there, are financed by each local authority. For these units in London, we have excluded dual-registered beds that include "medicalized" nursing-home services.

In summary (Table 22.7), Paris provides the highest density of such community residential care places, with 73.4 per one thousand over the age of sixty-five, followed by New York City (60.8), Greater London (33.4), and Tokyo (11.9).[7] In addition, in all the cities except Tokyo, there are more community residential places

Table 22.7. Community Residential Options: Four World Cities, 1999 and 2001 (per 1,000 persons 65+)

	Urban Core	First Ring	Total
New York,1999[a]	27.2	33.6	60.8
Greater London, 2001[b]	12.6	20.8	33.4
Paris and First Ring, 2001[c]	34.9	48.5	73.4
Tokyo, 2001[d]	6.3	5.6	11.9

Sources: New York: *Alternatives in Senior Housing,* New York City Department for the Aging, 1999; *New York State-Licensed Assisted Living Programs,* DFTA, November 2001; New York State Department of Aging; 1999 NYC Housing and Vacancy Survey; U.S. Census 2002. London: Struder and Warnes, chapter 10; U.K. Census 2001. Tokyo: Tokyo Metropolitan Government, Bureau of Welfare for the Elderly. Paris: ORSIF.

[a] Includes congregate housing beds and individual apartments with collective services. Congregate housing includes adult homes (including assisted living programs in adult homes). Individual apartments with collective services include enriched housing (including assisted living in enriched housing) and section 202 housing for the elderly, but does not include public housing for the elderly. Had we included public housing for the elderly, the numbers for individual units in Manhattan would be 46.5 and 32.5 for the outer boroughs. For both section 202 and public housing, we have multiplied the original number of units by 1.5. Based on NYC Housing and Vacancy Survey data for 1999, 87% of public housing units with householders 65 and over had 1–2 people per unit; 81% of section 202 units with householders 65 and over had 1–2 persons per unit. We therefore used 1.5 as an estimate to determine the average number of older persons that these units could accommodate.

[b] Includes residential care homes, excluding dual-registered beds

[c] Includes maisons de retraite (congregate housing) and logement-foyers (individual apartments with collective services). In both cases, we have excluded nursing-home as well as residential home beds for Parisian citizens that are situated outside the city.

[d] Total of congregate and individual apartments with collective services. Congregate includes Keihi Rojin Homes (moderately priced homes for the elderly); individual apartments include Koureisha muke Chintai Jutaku (rental housing for the elderly).

for older persons in the first ring than in the urban core. As mentioned previously, in three out of the four cities, there is a much higher density of enriched apartments as opposed to congregate housing, suggesting that existing housing stock is a more readily available resource for long-term care in these cities than constructed facilities for congregate care. Indeed, with the exception of Tokyo, where cohabitation with children is still an important kind of living arrangement, the density of such community-based options is higher than that of institutional care settings (Tables 22.1 and 22.7). Even in London, nonmedicalized residential care places are more readily available than nursing-home beds. Most notably, in Manhattan and Paris, the availability of enriched apartments far surpasses that of nursing-home beds. Whether this is an outcome of deliberate policy or simply a reflection of market forces remains an open question; what is certain is that more care is currently provided in the community than in nursing-home facilities.

Concluding Observations

Each of these cities has the largest older population in its respective nation (see Chapter 1). These are diverse populations, not only in terms of their incomes, but also in terms of their health needs and chronic conditions. Moreover, there are unique urban constraints attached to global city status, in which land and public space become contested sites for a variety of local and global uses—as a result, construction costs for nursing homes are very high, a fact reflected in the smaller number of such facilities in the urban cores of our cities. This circumstance, coupled with the diverse needs of older persons in these cities, compels them to offer relatively high levels of home help, as well as some of their existing housing stock, to provide long-term care for their older population.

For example, New York City differs from the rest of the United States in that more long-term care is provided in the community than in institutions. Similarly, as Honda explains (Chapter 21), the Tokyo Metropolitan Government intends to shift its resources to home-care services, with attendant reductions in funding for nursing-home care. Indeed, in three of the four cities, the community-based residential options outweigh nursing-home bed availability. In particular, the availability of apartments with attached services is more widespread than that of nursing-home beds. This suggests an implicit recognition of the need to diversify services.

We find a striking convergence among these world cities with respect to the number of older persons receiving home help (Table 22.4). In contrast, the greatest difference among them concerns the density of nursing-home beds, particularly among their urban cores (Table 22.1).

These findings raise several questions that merit further study. For example, how do various components of the long-term care spectrum interconnect and affect one another? Is there a trade-off between the density of nursing-home beds and the share of the older population using home-care services? How do intermediary options, for example, community-based residential care facilities, affect the distribution of older persons across the extreme ends of the spectrum? Can these differences be explained by differences in the role of the family, neighbors, and informal caregivers? We are now studying these questions and hope to find some answers in the future.

Notes

1. Doty, Pamela. 1990. U.S. Long-Term Care Financing in Comparative International Perspective: Old Myths, New Ideas. Washington DC: U.S. DHHS, Office of Disability, Aging, and Long-Term Care Policy. April. http://aspe.hhs.gov/daltcp/Reports/mythses. htm.

2. Gossiaux, S., M. Simon, and V. Rodwin. A Paris, plus de six femmes sur dix vivent seules après 80 ans. 2002. *Ile-de-France à la page*. INSEE, no. 210, May–June. www. insee.fr/ile-de-france.

3. *A Profile of Medicare Home Health*. 2001. Washington DC: DHHS, Health Care Financing Administration, Office of Strategic Planning.

4. New York State Department of Health, form 519, FY2000.

5. Ibid., On-Line SURS Information Retrieval System and Demographic Profiles; Center for Medicare and Medicaid Services, Medicaid Program Statistics (MSIS/2082 Report).

6. New York State Department of Health, 2000 Medicaid Profiles.

7. The figures presented here differ from those in Chapter 10, where chapter authors Strüder and Warnes presented the number of residential facilities per thousand persons age *eighty* and over.

23. Growing Older in World Cities: Themes, Interpretations, and Future Research

Michael K. Gusmano and Victor G. Rodwin

New York, London, Paris, and Tokyo confront common challenges resulting from population aging and longevity. But they do so within national health, social, and long-term care policy contexts that are different. While there is a vast literature about these national-level differences, we know less about how these policies are implemented at the local level, the extent of local discretionary policies, and how they affect the availability and use of care by older persons living in world cities.

What can be said, in conclusion, about the health and well-being of older persons in these four cities? Does the hypothesis that world cities are converging hold up against the evidence we have presented on the extent to which the policy responses to population aging are converging in these cities? In this final chapter, we speculate on the key policy implications from the experience of these cities, explore the many gaps in what we know, and propose a research agenda to address the questions raised in this book.

A Portrait of the Older Persons in Four World Cities

As we noted at the outset, population projections for 2015 indicate that Inner Tokyo will have the highest percentage of persons sixty years old and over (35 percent) in comparison to Paris (20 percent), Manhattan (18 percent), and Inner London (14.3 percent). At present, however, Paris has approximately twice the percentage of persons eighty-five years and over (2.8 percent) of that in Manhattan, Inner London, and Inner Tokyo.

Racial and ethnic diversity. Along with the substantial growth in the number of people eight-five and over, these cities have experienced, to varying degrees, an increase in racial and ethnic diversity. The percentage of the older population in New York and Greater London comprised of racial and ethnic minorities increased steadily between 1980 and 2000. By 2000, racial and ethnic minorities made up almost 43 percent of the older population in New York and approximately 20 percent of the older population in Greater London.

We do not have data on race and ethnicity for Paris or Tokyo, but we have information about the percentage of foreign born, foreign born who were naturalized (in Paris), and foreigners (Paris and Tokyo). Roughly one-quarter of the population in Inner London and Manhattan, and about 20 percent of the population in Paris, was born abroad. In Paris, the foreign-born population is higher than in the first ring. Similarly, there is a greater percentage of racial and ethnic minorities in Inner London than in Outer London, but in Manhattan the percentage of racial and ethnic minorities is lower than in the surrounding boroughs. The growth of diversity in these cities creates a challenge for the organization and delivery of services. Cities with diverse populations must develop ways to deliver care that is sensitive to different cultural norms and must recognize the divergent life experiences of their older populations.

Tokyo, which collects data on foreigners rather than on the foreign born, has a far more homogeneous population than do Manhattan and Paris. In Inner Tokyo, 3 percent of the population are foreigners; in the twelve outer wards, only 1.6 percent are foreigners. These data, however, understate the inter-Asian diversity within Tokyo, as they do not account for Japanese of Korean descent or illegal immigrants from Asia. Because of a decreasing birth rate and increasing longevity, Japan's working-age population is shrinking; at the same time, the need for formal long-term care providers is growing. To improve economic growth and to ensure an adequate number of formal care providers for Japan's aging population, policy makers are debating the merits of loosening the country's immigration policy. If this change occurs, Tokyo will undoubtedly be the destination for many immigrants, and the lessons from New York and London will be ever more relevant.

The health status of older persons. In contrast to the urban health-penalty literature, evidence from these world cities suggests that the health status of their older residents is the same or better than the health status of those living in their nations. In London, there are no differences between the health of older persons living in London and in the nation, but older persons in Paris and New York are healthier than their counterparts in the rest of their countries. Life expectancy at sixty-five in the urban cores of New York and Paris is slightly higher than in their first rings, while hospital admissions for acute care among older persons, and age-specific death rates, were lower in the urban cores than in the first rings. One possible explanation for this pattern is that Parisians and Manhattanites who choose to remain in the city after retirement are healthier than those who choose to leave. Some scholars have argued that this is the case in Paris, but this explanation does not seem consistent with the historical evidence on migration in New York City.

The evidence for Tokyo is mixed. A higher percentage of older people living in Inner Tokyo require long-term care services compared to those living in Outer Tokyo and the rest of Japan. Yet, while the average life expectancy for residents of Inner Tokyo is lower than for those of Outer Tokyo, it is higher than for the rest of Japan. Furthermore, life expectancy for women at sixty-five is higher in Tokyo than in Japan as a whole.

London stands apart from the other three because the older population living in the urban core of the city is less healthy than in the first ring. In London, life expectancy at sixty-five is lower in the urban core than in the first ring, and age-adjusted death rates are higher. As we found in the other cities, hospital admissions for acute care among older persons are lower in the urban core than in the first ring, but in London this may reflect inadequate access to service, rather than better health.[1]

Within each city, health status varies considerably. The variance in health is most striking in London and New York where there are greater levels of "deprivation," and greater disparities in mortality and morbidity across neighborhoods than in Paris or Tokyo. It is difficult, however, to interpret these findings because they may reflect immigration effects, differences in socioeconomic status, and access to services, as well as differences in the quality of the environments in which older people live. A deeper understanding of these findings will require additional research.

Housing and living arrangements. The quality of housing is a vital component of quality of life for older persons. Without decent, affordable housing, it is impossible to "age in place." Generally, housing for older persons in London is better than it was in the early 1990s and, according to Tony Warnes and Inge Strüder (Chapter 11), "it is no longer the case that poor housing is associated with older occupants." Yet, there is still tremendous variation within the city of London. Most postwar public housing has high standards with basic amenities, but public housing in the poorer boroughs of London is often deficient, without central heating. Neither the government nor private landlords have invested adequately in home improvement in many London boroughs.

Paris has a very old housing stock dominated by small units, and housing in Paris is much older than that in the city's first ring. Likewise, the share of substandard housing units is also higher in Paris than in its first ring. Within Paris, a slightly higher share of older residents live in housing units without bathrooms than do their younger counterparts, and a slightly lower share live in housing units without toilets. In contrast, the quality of housing in New York City is better for older residents compared with their younger counterparts. Nearly all older New Yorkers live in housing units with complete kitchen and bathroom facilities. In London, Paris, and New York, the percentage of older persons living in substandard housing is significantly higher in poor neighborhoods. We do not currently have systematic data on the quality of housing among older persons in Tokyo, but John and Ruth Campbell (Chapter 19) argue that much of the housing in Tokyo is inadequate to meet the needs of frail older persons.

There are millions of people who live alone in these world cities, and the oldest old living alone are the fastest-growing segments of these populations. In all four cities, rates of living alone among older persons are higher in the urban cores than in the first rings. This is true for the population over eighty-five and more generally for those over sixty-five years. Whether or not it is true that big cities promote solitude, as Marie-Eve Joël and Robert Haas contend in the case of Paris (Chapter 14), the increase in older persons, particularly women living alone, has focused greater attention on the importance of social interaction with friends, neighbors, and local programs to assist the frail older old.

Gender, ethnicity, and race are important factors in distinguishing among older persons who live alone. Older women are much more likely than older men to live alone in all four cities. In New York, rates of living alone are significantly lower among Hispanics and Asians aged sixty-five and older, and slightly lower among African Americans in this cohort than among their white counterparts. Likewise, in Greater London, rates of living alone are higher among the white population than among black Caribbean, Indian, and Bangladeshi populations.

Globalization and Policy Convergence?

Debates about the hypothesis that the social and economic characteristics of world cities converge often rest on assumptions that are insufficiently nuanced to capture the "thick description" and complexities we present in this book.[2] For example, discussion of this hypothesis in the literature suggests either that world cities are converging or that Paris and Tokyo are systematically different from New York and London because they benefit from greater central government protection from the forces of globalization. We find some evidence that supports both extremes, and other evidence that is captured by neither.

Few dispute that the challenges faced by these cities are similar. In addition to those associated with competing in a global economy, all four cities are coping with a growing number of persons eighty-five years and over and a growing number of older women living alone. Similarly, all four cities face growing immigrant populations. Disagreements emerge when scholars discuss the responses to and consequences of these challenges.

The convergence hypothesis is supported by the evidence of significant and growing inequalities of income, housing, health, and health care within all four cities. Yet, the critique of the convergence hypothesis, which suggests that differences in history, politics, institutions, and culture lead to different responses to the challenges posed by globalization, is also supported by some of our evidence. For example, the characterization of Paris and Tokyo as "soft" global cities is consistent with the adoption of Japan's LTCI and France's recent expansion of home-care services for frail older persons. Likewise, the characterization of London as a "hard" global city is consistent with efforts to shift the cost of long-term care to older persons.

Complicating matters, however, we also find evidence that conflicts with both perspectives and suggests that the typical descriptions of these cities—and their nations—border on caricatures. For example, New York, which is always characterized as the "hardest" of the four global cities, provides twice as many nursing-home beds as London, Paris, or Tokyo—and both New York and London provide as much home help as do the two "soft" cities in our analysis (Chapter 22).

Further refinement of the convergence hypothesis is beyond the scope of this book, but our evidence highlights the need to move beyond simple characterizations and to develop a more robust understanding of national and city responses to the forces of globalization. Further examination of how cities, and their nations, respond to specific policy challenges will advance this discussion.

Models for the Future

Perhaps the most important lesson from the experience of New York, London, Paris, and Tokyo in adapting to the growth of their oldest old populations is summarized by the thesis of Thorstein Veblen's study of Imperial Germany, in which he invoked the "advantages of backwardness." Indeed, no other cities in the world have as many of the oldest old residing within them as do these world cities. And there may well be some advantages for smaller cities in OECD nations and megacities of developing nations in reviewing some of the policy issues raised by the unprecedented numbers of the oldest old in these cities. We would summarize these as follows:

1. Can we afford to allow frail older persons, particularly those who require institutional long-term care, to remain in the urban cores of world cities?

In each of these cities, there are significantly fewer nursing-home beds in the urban core than in the first ring. Land prices make it extraordinarily expensive to build institutional care beds in cities that contain "massive chunks of the most lucrative parts of the global economy's sector," as Emanuel Tobier put it.

In Paris, in contrast to the other three cities, we were able to obtain data on the share of older frail Parisians (30 percent) who spend their final years in nursing homes outside Paris (Chapter 15). New York and London do not have the capacity to track older residents in this way. Japan should, in theory, be able to track the movement of older persons from one ward to another as they move into institutional care, but to date has not made these figures available to the public. Despite these data limitations, the relative paucity of nursing-home beds in Manhattan, Inner London, and Inner Tokyo suggests that the situation in these cities is comparable to that of Paris.

As Naoki Ikegami argues (Chapter 16), the problem of dispersing frail older persons from their residence in the urban cores of world cities to their peripheries raises the issue of whether we can afford to support the costs of aging in place for the most vulnerable residents of world cities, or whether this is a luxury that these societies are not willing to support. The answer will depend, in part, on the extent to which we are able to develop alternative models of assisted living, strong home-care programs, and other innovations that provide less costly alternatives to nursing homes and hospitals.

2. How can we implement central government policies, while at the same time developing local policies to fill in the gaps left by higher levels of government?

Even the centralized unitary states of Japan, France, and the United Kingdom have been unable to meet the needs of the oldest old without close collaboration with local government, nonprofit organizations, community and neighborhood organizations, and families. First, none of the public pension schemes in these countries provide adequately for lower-income older persons. Beyond this, the needs of most frail older persons go well beyond what pensions can cover. National health programs address many of these needs, but not all. In particular, national health programs do not cover social services. In all these places, the financing and delivery of social services tends to be more decentralized. Even city governments find it useful to rely on nongovernmental organizations to identify and respond to the needs of the oldest old.

Japan has the most centralized system of long-term care, but since there is an important financial contribution by prefectures and municipalities in funding this program, Tokyo Metropolitan Government and the individual wards within Tokyo share financial risk with central government. They therefore have an incentive to plan the configuration of long-term care services and, to whatever extent possible, reduce the amount of institutional care people receive. This requires them to assess the housing, transportation, health, and social service needs of older persons within their jurisdiction. Some wards can afford to provide more services than others. For example, as Etsuji Okomoto notes, Nakano, Shinagawa, Ota, and Shibuya Wards all provide preventive activities that are not financed by the other wards in Tokyo (Chapter 20).

In France, although the financing of home help for persons with significant disabilities (APA) is more centralized than in Japan, Paris authorities are still required to produce a local master plan for long-term care services, which include social services, some of which are locally financed and provided. Furthermore, Paris provides cash allowances for very poor older persons, who are typically eligible neither for a pension nor for the APA. Paris also offers a range of services for frail older persons living alone, which are more generous than those available in most other parts of France. In the United Kingdom, the boroughs of London have responsibility for participating in the financing of, and deciding on placement for, older persons in social housing. Other examples, across all four cities, include city funding for telephone help lines, meal delivery for homebound older persons, and transportation and rent subsidies.

Although housing and long-term care can be strongly reinforced by such central government policies as preferential mortgage loans and long-term care insurance (as in Japan), there will always be a role for local government in implementing these policies, coordinating services, and making its own policies—as in London and New York for housing and residential care; in Paris for provision of nursing and residential homes; or in New York, London, and Paris to manage contracts for the provision of meals to frail older persons.

Since addressing the needs of older persons requires an in-depth understanding of local conditions (see Chapter 14), future models for enhancing the lives of the oldest old point to increased collaboration at the neighborhood level among an immense number of nonprofit organizations.

3. How can we cope with diverse older persons, taking into account increasing ethnic minorities and inequalities in socioeconomic and health status?

All four world cities, even less diverse Tokyo, have recognized that the oldest old are a heterogeneous group. Differences in culture, educational levels, income, and health status make it impossible to set uniform policies without allowing a good deal of discretion and choice at local levels. New York City's Department for the Aging (DFTA)has responded to the city's growing diversity by arranging for meals that meet the preferences of different ethnic groups, and its Department of Health and Mental Hygiene has established district public health offices in response to the higher risks faced by racial and ethnic minorities. In Paris, the development of the *café sociale* in the nineteenth arrondissement is an effort to meet the needs of the growing older population from North Africa. In London, as in New York, there are severe health disparities by ethnicity, and the National Health Service has made the delivery of culturally appropriate care a priority.

4. How can we best provide information to older persons and give them voice?

In all four world cities, municipal governments have invoked the rising importance of providing older persons with information about the multiplicity of services available to them and involving them in plans for the future. With respect to giving older persons a greater voice, the Paris gerontological master plan called for a "Rights of Older People Charter," which is designed, in part, to provide older Parisians with an opportunity to voice their policy preferences. As Okamoto reports in Chapter 20, Tokyo conducted a consumer survey to evaluate the satisfaction of older persons with the implementation of LTCI. Furthermore, efforts to allow a greater voice for older persons vary within these cities. For example, in Tokyo, Nakano Ward is notable for encouraging the direct participation of residents in policy making. In this same spirit, Age Concern in the United Kingdom has advocated on behalf of "giving voice to all age groups" (see Chapter 8).

As for getting information to older persons, in Paris, the neighborhood coordination centers, or Emerald Paris Points, provide information about existing services, address inquiries, and assist older persons and their families and caregivers with decision making. In New York City, DFTA provides a wealth of information about federal, state, and local programs for older persons, including tools that help people determine their eligibility for different services. There are questions about how many older persons access this information on the Internet, but this is an important innovation that is likely to be used by an even larger portion of future cohorts of older persons.

5. How can we support the oldest old living alone and identify the most isolated and vulnerable among them?

In Manhattan, Inner London, and Paris, over half the oldest old live alone. However, within this group we do not know the relative share of those who are isolated and lonely versus those who have the ability to remain independent. Learning more about the location of a city's most vulnerable oldest old is crucially important. The 2003 August heat wave in France served as a dramatic example of how a city with a high concentration of older persons can be completely unprepared to cope with its aging population. In Paris, the result was thousands of deaths. But many people do not realize that a comparable event took place in Chicago in 1995. Similarly, thousands of older New Yorkers were left stranded and dangerously isolated during the days immediately after 9/11. In both France and the United States, major cities were unprepared to cope with their aging populations.

As Eric Klinenberg reports in his book on Chicago's heat wave, social isolation led to higher mortality rates among older residents living in neighborhoods with abandoned lots and little street life than in equally poor neighborhoods with a more congenial built environment and more social interaction.[3] Furthermore, he found that the built environment influenced the degree of social connectedness—what Lisa Peattie calls conviviality in city neighborhoods.[4]

Fortunately, there is a new awareness about the vulnerability of the oldest old and recognition that municipal governments have a responsibility to identify and reach out to the vulnerable oldest old who live in isolation. The challenge for these cities is to find methods for identifying and tracking vulnerable older persons without violating their civil liberties.

Future Research

One goal of this book was to identify gaps in our knowledge about older persons in these four world cities. We have identified three crucial and related issues about which we know little: the social isolation of older persons, the role of informal care services in supporting them, and the extent to which both formal and informal health and social services vary by neighborhood. We know that many older persons live alone, but living alone is not the same as being alone. For some older persons, living alone facilitates independence. For others, it leads to social isolation. Currently, we have limited information about the health status and quality of life of community-dwelling older people in these cities.

How do formal and informal care services vary across diverse neighborhoods of world cities? What is the interaction among them? To what extent are gaps in publicly financed long-term care met by privately financed formal long-term care or informal care provided by family, friends, and neighbors? Existing publicly available sources of data reveal very little about these questions. In the future, it will be important to extend the examination of formal services for older persons in these cities to include informal services in selected neighborhoods, as well as innovative programs at the neighborhood level.

Urban neighborhoods and the health of older persons. Existing research indicates that a neighborhood's characteristics influence the health of its residents.[5] Although there is vigorous debate about whether the relationship is causal, community socioeconomic status, measured as median household income, is strongly associated with poor health, even controlling for individual income.[6] Similarly, neighborhood-level inequality is associated with health, violence, and "collective efficacy."[7]

Crime rates can also influence the health of neighborhood residents. Aside from the obvious dangers of injury, high-crime areas can increase the stress of neighborhood residents, thereby aggravating medical conditions that are sensitive to stress. Stress may also encourage a variety of unhealthy behaviors, including smoking, drinking, and drug use.[8] There are a number of additional ways in which neighborhoods can affect their residents' health.[9] We review these next, with an emphasis on the connections among neighborhood characteristics, local institutions, social interaction, and health.

The built environment. One of the most important neighborhood determinants of health is housing.[10] The risk of fires, accidental injuries, and lead poisoning are all related to the quality of housing.[11] The prevalence of infectious disease is strongly correlated with housing factors such as waste disposal, presence of vermin, food storage, and overcrowding. Finally, chronic diseases such as asthma and other respiratory conditions are associated with dampness, poor ventilation, dust, and pest infestations.

In addition to housing, the "built environment" more generally has an impact on health and health behaviors.[12] Poor quality streets and sidewalks, for example, can put older persons at greater risk for falls. In contrast, the existence of benches and other places to rest may encourage older persons to walk more frequently. Also, the ways in which physical space structures social behavior and social interaction demonstrate the complex relationships among neighborhood characteristics and health.[13]

Institutions and local organizations. Medical resources in cities are often distributed unequally, reflecting the unequal distribution of wealth, income, and goods and services.[14] For example, there are high concentrations of medical and social services in areas where high-income-yielding jobs are most dense and in those neighborhoods where most residents work in these jobs, with low concentrations elsewhere. Neighborhoods in which higher-income people live also have higher rates of utilization of medical and social services compared with lower-income neighborhoods.[15]

City neighborhoods also vary with regard to local organizations, voluntary associations, and formal programs or institutions designed to improve service delivery and enhance the quality of life for older people. For example, in New York City, about a dozen housing developments with people who have "aged in place" have been designated naturally occurring retirement communities (NORCs) and receive funding from the state and city to provide services to their older residents.

Social interaction. A growing body of literature suggests that social networks and social interaction have a significant effect on mental and physical health.[16] Studies have found that, among older people, social networks are related to rates of suicide,[17] morale and notions of self worth,[18] perceptions of health,[19] and life satisfaction.[20] Social networks also appear to promote recovery following an acute medical condition.[21]

Precisely how social networks and social interaction promote health is less well understood, but there appear to be several mechanisms at work.[22] First, social interaction provides emotional support that promotes self-esteem and helps individuals cope with stressful situations.[23] Furthermore, there is evidence that older people who engage in productive activities, for example, caregiving, enjoy greater physical and psychological well-being.[24] Second, members of a social network provide instrumental support:[25] help with meal preparation, assistance with other household chores, provision of transportation, and many more activities traditionally associated with informal care.[26] Third, social interactions often encourage health-promoting behavior, such as exercise and nutrition counseling. Fourth, social networks lead to better communication of information to older persons, enhancing the effect of formal health-education programs,[27] promoting adherence to treatment protocols, improving the communication between older people and formal care providers, and possibly improving their choice of providers. Fifth, social networks provide informal monitoring that can help ensure the safety and well-being of older people in the community.[28] Finally, strong social networks may also allow political organization of neighborhood residents to address the conditions that influence their health.[29]

Next steps for research on aging in cities. The International City/County Management Association recently recognized that social policy innovations are addressing the needs of an aging society and urged local governments to "begin with an analysis of the distribution of population and amenities as these pertain to older adults and active living."[30] Yet not enough action has been taken by these four cities on this agenda and too little is known about how policies, institutions, and neighborhood characteristics shape the social interactions and health of older city residents.

Imagine if one could adapt the kinds of mapping tools used by the police to fight crime (such as Compstat) for the multiplicity of city departments and nonprofit organizations that promote healthy and productive aging and serve frail older persons in each of these cities. Programs and service delivery might be dramatically improved by effective use of targeting. Such use would not even demand a huge investment. Instead, it would require analysis of existing data sources and collection of some new data to improve understanding, at the neighborhood level, of the relationship between the needs of older people and the availability of services for them.

Conclusions

The unprecedented convergence of population aging and urbanization presents great challenges and opportunities for cities and their older residents. The chapters of this book provide a detailed account of how the four largest cities in some of the wealthiest nations of the world—New York, London, Paris, and Tokyo—are confronting these changes.

One challenge that each of these cities confronts is how to balance the desire of most people to age in place with the tremendous cost of growing older in world cities. One response to this challenge has been to disperse frail older persons out of the urban core of each city. Over the coming decades, these cities, and no doubt many others, will have to decide whether to continue sending large numbers of older persons to facilities outside the city when they become too frail to care for themselves, or whether to invest in alternatives that make aging in place a possibility for more residents.

Many of the institutions, neighborhood characteristics, and other social factors that influence the health of older people may be beyond the reach of city government and must be addressed at the national level. Cities are limited in their ability to redistribute income and address neighborhood-level poverty and inequality.[31] Similarly, many environmental issues must be addressed at a regional level.[32] Nevertheless, we should not underestimate the ability of city governments to address social issues, including the health and well-being of older residents.[33] Nor should we overestimate the capacity of the existing national welfare states to serve those who fall through the cracks of a host of health and social welfare programs. Cities and other local governments address many social problems that are not addressed adequately by the national government.

In the wake of September 11 and the Paris *canicule* of 2003, the need to address the needs of vulnerable older persons living in cities is more apparent than ever. Older persons—particularly isolated older persons—are typically an invisible population that does not receive attention from policy makers, the media, or the general public. Greater appreciation of the needs of this vulnerable population is probably the only positive outcome from these catastrophic events.

Notes

1. Warnes, A. 1997. *The Health and Care of Older People in London: A Report to the King's Fund London Commission*. London: King's Fund.
2. The term "thick description" is from Geertz, C. 1983. *Local Knowledge: Further Essays in Interpretive Anthropology*. New York: Basic.
3. Klinenberg, Eric. 2002. *Heat Wave: A Social Autopsy of Disaster in Chicago*. Chicago: University of Chicago Press.
4. Peattie, L. 1988. Convivial Cities. In M. Douglass and J. Friedmann, eds. *Cities for Citizens*, 247–254. New York: John Wiley.
5. Yen, I. H., and S. L. Syme. 1999. The Social Environment and Health: A Discussion of the Epidemiologic Literature. *Annual Review of Public Health* 20:287.
6. Kawachi, I., and T. A. Blakely. 2001. When Economists and Epidemiologists Disagree. *Journal of Health Care Politics, Policy, and Law* 26(3): 533–541; Milyo, J., and J. M. Mellor. 2003. On the Importance of Age-Adjustment Methods in Ecological Studies of Social Determinants of Mortality. *Health Services Research* 38(6): 1781–1790..
7. Morenoff, J. D., R. J. Sampson, and S. W. Raudenbush. 2001. Neighborhood Inequality, Collective Efficacy, and the Spatial Dynamics of Urban Violence. *Criminology* 39(3): 517–559.
8. Newman, K. S. 2003. *Different Shade of Grey: Midlife and Beyond in the Inner City. New York: New Press,*52.
9. Gould-Ellen, I., T. Mijanovich, and K. N. Dillman. 2001. Neighborhood Effects on Health: Exploring the Links and Assessing the Evidence. *Journal of Urban Affairs* 23(3/4): 391–408.
10. Mayor, S. 2003. Poor Housing Continues to Affect Health Adversely. *British Medical Journal* 326(7397): 1111.
11. Wallace, R., and D. Wallace. 1998. *A Plague on Your Houses: How New York Was Burned Down and National Public Health Crumbled*. New York: Verso.
12. Jackson, R. J. 2001. What Olmsted Knew. *Western City*, March, 1–3; Lantz, P. M., J. S. House, P. J. Lepkowsky, D. R. Williams, R. P. Mero, and J. Chen. 1998. Health Behaviors Don't Explain High Death Rates among Poor. *JAMA* 279:1703–1728; Seelye, K. Q. 2003. Cities Made for Walking May Be Fat Burners. *New York Times*, June 21; Tanaka, A., T. Takano, K. Nakamura and Schiko Takeuchi. 1996. Health Levels Influenced by Urban Residential Conditions in a Megacity. *Urban Studies* 33(6): 879–894.
13. Klinenberg, *Heat Wave*.
14. Andrulis, D. P. 1997. The Urban Health Penalty. American College of Physicians On-Line Position Paper. www.acponline.org/hpp/pospaper/andrulis.htm; Fossett, J., and J. Perloff. 1995. The "New" Health Reform and Access to Care: The Problem

of the Inner City. Washington, DC: Kaiser Commission on the Future of Medicaid. December; Politzer, R., D. Harris, M. H. Gaston, and F. Mullan. 1991. Primary Care Physician Supply and the Medically Underserved. JAMA 266:104–109.

15. Lantz et al., Health Behaviors.

16. Cattell, V. 2001. Poor People, Poor Places, and Poor Health: The Mediating Role of Social Networks and Social Capital. Social Science and Medicine 52(10): 1501–1516; Felton, B. J., and C. A. Berry. 1992. Do the Sources of Urban Elderly's Social Support Determine Its Psychological Consequences? Psychology and Aging 7(1): 89–97; Kawachi, I., B. Kennedy, K. Lochner, and D. Prothcow-Stith. 1997. Social Capital, Income Inequality, and Mortality. American Journal of Public Health 87(9):1492–1498.

17. Conwell, Y., and R. P. Duberstein. 2001. Suicide in Elders. Annals of the New York Academy of Sciences, The Clinical Science of Suicide Prevention 932 (April):132–150.

18. Litwin, Howard. 2001. Social Network Type and Morale in Old Age. Gerontologist 41(4): 516–524.

19. Fees, Bronwyn S., Peter Martin, and Leonard W. Poon. 1999. A Model of Loneliness in Older Adults. Journals of Gerontology 54B(4): 231–239.

20. Gustafsson, T. M., D. G. L. Isacson, and M. Thorslund. 1998. Mortality in Elderly Men and Women in a Swedish Municipality. Age and Ageing 27(5): 584–593.

21. Mutran, E. J., D. C. Reitzes, J. Mossey, and M. E. Fernandez. 1995. Social Support, Depression, and Recovery of Walking Ability Following Hip Fracture Surgery. *Journals of Gerontology* 50: S354-S361; Oxman, T. E., and J. G. Hull. 1997. Social Support, Depression, and Activities of Daily Living in Older Heart Surgery Patients. *Journal of Gerontology* 52:1–14.

22. House, James S., Karl R. Landis, and Debra Umberson. 1988. Social Relationships and Health. *Science* 241:540–545.

23. Felton, Barbara, and Carolyn A. Berry. 1992. Do the Sources of the Urban Elderly's Social Support Determine its Psychological Consequences? *Psychology and Aging* 7(1): 89–97.

24. Morrow-Howell, Nancy. 2000. *Productive Engagement of Older Adults: Effects on Well-Being*. St. Louis: Center for Social Development, Washington University.

25. Mendes de Leon, Carlos F., Deborah T. Gold, Thomas A. Glass, Lori Kaplan, and Linda K. George. 2001. Disability as a Function of Social Networks and Support in Elderly African-Americans and Whites: The Duke EPESE, 1986–1992. *Journal of Gerontology* 56B(3): S179–S190.

26. Ibid., S190.

27. Herman, Mindy. 1999. Using Health Networks to Enhance Education, *Journal of the American Dietetic Association* 99(5): 8–10.

28. Klinenberg, *Heat Wave.*

29. Dreier, Peter, John Mollenkopf, and Todd Swanstrom. 2001. *Place Matters: Metropolitics for the Twenty-first Century*. Lawrence: University Press of Kansas, 72.

30. Active and Living for Older Adults: Management Strategies for Healthy and Livable Communities. *activeliving@icma.org.*

31. Judd, D. R., and T. Swanstrom. 1994. *City Politics.* New York: HarperCollins, 314–315.

32. Sclar, E. 2003. Urban Planning. Conference on Health and the Built Environment, Co-Sponsored by the New York Academy of Medicine and the Centers for Disease Control and Prevention. March 25.

33. Peterson, Paul E. 1981. *City Limits.* Chicago: University of Chicago Press; Stone, Clarence N. 1989. *Regime Politics, Governing Atlanta, 1946–1988.* Lawrence: University Press of Kansas.

Contributors

Robert N. Butler, M.D., is the founder and president of the International Longevity Center-USA. He is also Professor of Geriatrics and Adult Development in the Henry L. Schwartz Department of Geriatrics at the Mount Sinai School of Medicine. From 1975 until 1982, he was the first director of the National Institute on Aging of the National Institutes of Health. In 1982, he founded the nation's first department of geriatrics at the Mount Sinai School of Medicine, where he served as Chairman and Brookdale Professor of Geriatrics until 1995. Dr. Butler, the author or coauthor of numerous articles, book chapters, and books, in 1976 won the Pulitzer Prize for *Why Survive? Being Old in America*. He is the coauthor, with Myrna I. Lewis, of the books *Aging and Mental Health* and *Love and Sex After 60*. An internationally recognized leader in gerontology and geriatrics, Dr. Butler has received numerous honors from various professional and other associations in his fields.

John Creighton Campbell, Ph.D., is Professor and Associate Chair of the Department of Political Science at the University of Michigan. Professor Campbell is interested in how policies change from agenda setting through implementation, and in the relationship between politics and substantive public policy. He works mostly on Japan, often in comparative perspective, these days mainly about social policy, including health care and Japan's new public, mandatory long-term care insurance system. Currently he is following up on an old avocation by directing a project of secondary data analysis called Losing Faith in Politics? Trends in Citizen Attitudes and Behavior in Japan and the United States. Other interests include the auto industry, U.S.-Japan relations, and organization theory. He is the author of numerous books, chapters, and articles, including *How Policies Change: The Japanese Government and the Aging Society* (Princeton, N.J.: Princeton University Press, 1992; Japanese edition, 1995) and, with Naoki Ikegami, *The Art of Balance in Health Policy: Maintaining Japan's Low-Cost Egalitarian System* (Cambridge University Press, 1998) and *Long-Term Care for Frail Older People? Reaching for the Ideal System* (Springer-Verlag Telos, 1999).

Ruth Campbell, M.S.W., is an Adjunct Lecturer and the Associate Director of Social Work and Community Programs at the University of Michigan Geriatic Center. Her research interests include, aging, long-term care, caregivers, and social work practice. Her publications include *The Delicate Balance: Case Studies in Counseling and Care Management for Older Adults* (with Berit Ingersoll-Dayton) (Health Professions Press, 2001) and "An Ideal Long-Term Care System: From the Perspective of the Older Adult" (*Keio Journal of Medicine* 47, Supplement 2 [1998]).

Marjorie Cantor is Professor Emerita and Brookdale Distinguished Scholar of Fordham University Graduate School of Social Service and the Scholar in Residence of Lighthouse International. Professor Cantor is a nationally and internationally recognized leader in the field of aging. Her areas of research expertise include elderly in the urban setting, the effect of ethnicity and culture on elderly lifestyles, and the role of family and other informal supports in providing care for older people. She is the author of more than seventy articles, books, chapters, and papers presented in the United States and abroad.

Florence de Maria is a Research Scientist (Chargée d'études) in public health at the Observatoire Régional de Santé d'Ile-de-France, in Paris. Her research is focused on gerontology, and she serves as a consultant to the Medical School at Creteil on issues of statistics and epidemiology.

Marc Esponda is a demographer in charge of socioeconomic studies for the urban planning agency of Toulon in the south of France. Previous to this position, he worked for the urban-planning agency of Paris, the Atelier Parisien d'Urbanisme (APUR), where he conducted socioeconomic analyses of gentrification in Paris and initiated studies on Paris's older population.

Maria Evandrou is a Reader in Gerontology at Kings College in London. Her research interests include social policy issues concerning older people, in particular the retirement prospects of future cohorts of elders; health, disability, and access to health and social services; health and socioeconomic position of minority ethnic elders; the changing economic and family-care roles of individuals in midlife; tools for policy making: dynamic microsimulation modeling; and the socioeconomic position of informal carers. Her publications include "Demographic Change in Europe: Implications for Family Support for Older People" (with J. Falkingham), in P. Kreager and E. Schroeder-Butterfill, eds., *Elderly without Children* (Oxford: Berhahn Books, 2004), and "Family, Work, and Quality of Life: Changing Economic and Social Roles through the Lifecourse" (with K. Glaser) (*Ageing and Society* 24 [1]: 1–21).

Michael K. Gusmano, Ph.D., is an Assistant Professor of Health Policy and Management and Lauterstein Scholar in the Mailman School of Public Health, Columbia University. He is also the Co-Director of the World Cities Project at the International Longevity Center-USA. His research interests include politics of health-care reform, Medicare, Medicaid, and comparative welfare-state analysis. Before joining the ILC, Professor Gusmano was a senior research associate in the Division of Health and Science Policy at the New York Academy of Medicine. Previously, he was a research associate in the Department of Epidemiology and Public Health and a lecturer in the Department of Political Science at Yale University, where he conducted research on health-care politics and policy. Professor Gusmano holds a doctorate in political science from the University of Maryland at College Park and a master's in public policy from the State University of New York at Albany. He was also postdoctoral fellow in the Robert Wood Johnson Foundation Scholars in Health Policy program at Yale University. His publications include (with G. Fairbrother and H. Park) "Exploring the Limits of the Safety-Net: Community Health Centers and Care for the Uninsured" (*Health Affairs*, 21 [6 (2002)]: 188–194); and (with M. Schlesinger and T. Thomas) "Policy Feedback and Public Opinion: The Role of Employer Responsibility in Social Policy" (*Journal of Health Politics, Policy, and Law*, 27 [5 (2002)]: 731–772).

Robert Haas is an attorney with the Association Notre Dame de Bon Secours who works primarily on assisting older persons in the Paris region.

Keiko Honda, Ph.D., received her Ph.D. in Public Health from New York University in 2002. Currently, she is a National Cancer Institute (NCI)-sponsored Postdoctoral Fellow in Cancer Epidemiology at the Mailman School of Public Health, Columbia University. Dr. Honda is also a Fellow in NCI's Cancer, Culture, and Literacy Institute.

Naoki Ikegami is Professor and Chair of the Department of Health Policy and Management at the Keio University School of Medicine, Japan. His research areas are health policy, long-term care, and pharmacoeconomics. His publications include *The Art of Balance in Health Policy: Maintaining Japan's Low-Cost Egalitarian System* (Cambridge University Press, 1998) and *Long-Care for Frail Older People? Reaching for the Ideal System* (Springer-Verlag Telos, 1999), both with John C. Campbell.

Marie-Eve Joël, Ph.D., is a Professor of Economics at the University of Paris-IX Dauphine and the Director of Laboratoire d'Economie et de Gestion des Organisations de Santé (LEGOS). Her research interests include the social protection of frail and dependent older persons in Europe, the economics of long-term care and chronic disease, and the politics of public health. Her publications include "Health Status and Work Burden of Alzheimer Patients' Informal Caregi-vers: Comparisons of Five Different Care Programs in the European Union" (with A. Colvez, A. Ponton-Sanchez, and A.C. Royer), *Health Policy*, May 2002; and "Penser un modèle d'intervention en réseau pour la prise en charge des personnes âgées dépendantes," *Editions La dispute*, September 2002.

Kenneth A. Knapp, Ph.D., is Research Analyst at the International Longevity Center-USA. Currently, he is involved in the Productive Engagement initiative at the ILC, the main purpose of which is to discover ways to expand opportunities for paid work and to reduce unnecessary obstacles for the continued labor-force participation of older people. Dr. Knapp has presented papers based upon Productive Engagement research at conferences in Belgium, Canada, and the United States. He is also involved in the Arkansas Aging Project, a collaboration between the ILC and the University of Arkansas that will assess the Arkansas approach to aging in the public and private sectors and put that approach in a national context. Dr. Knapp's other main research interest is in the housing of older people. He recently presented "Human Settlements of Older Urban Residents" before the NGO Committee on Aging in New York. A former graduate teaching fellow and adjunct professor at Brooklyn College and assistant professor at St. Francis College in Brooklyn, Dr. Knapp has taught corporate finance, money and banking, statistics, urban economics, and other courses in economics. In 1996, he served as a research consultant to the Citizens Housing and Planning Council, a nonprofit think tank based in New York City. Dr. Knapp earned a Ph.D. in economics from the Graduate School at the City University of New York, and a joint B.A./M.A. degree in economics from the City College of New York.

Yukiko Kudo, Ph.D., is the Research Director at the International Longevity Center-Japan and a Senior Specialist for Textbook Examination, Elementary and Secondary Education Bureau, Japanese Ministry of Education, Science, Sport, and Culture. Her recent publications include "Young People and Pensions in a Fluid Era" (*Pension and Employment* 20[3]) and "Integrated Care or Older Persons and Children: Toward the Development of New Care for Older Persons" (*Social Insurance Bulletin*, Social Insurance Institute, 20[61]).

Véronique Lucas-Gabrielli is Researcher (Maître de recherche) at the Institut de Recherche et de Documentation en Economie de la Santé (IRDES) in Paris.

Gabriel Montero is a doctoral candidate in Sociology at Princeton University. Mr. Montero served as a research scientist for the World Cities Project in the Robert F. Wagner School of Public Service from 2001 until 2005. Previously he was a research assistant in the Division of Health and Science Policy at the New York Academy of Medicine. His publications include (with M. K. Gusmano and V. G. Rodwin) "Neighborhoods and Health: Public Health Interventions in World Cities" (*Journal of Urban Health* 79[1 (2002)]: S119–S120).

Etsuji Okamoto, M.D., M.P.H., is the Chief of the Section of Management Administration, Management Science Division of Japan's National Institute of Public Health. Dr. Okamoto is interested in the application of health insurance claims data to health technology assessment. He is also interested in estimating the disease burden in communities and conducting economic evaluations of preventive health services. He is the author of numerous journal articles, including "Estimation of Disease-specific Costs in Health Insurance Claims: A Comparison of Three Methods" (with E. Hata) (*Japanese Journal of Public Health* 51[11]) and "Reduction of Influenza-related Outpatient Visits among Community-dwelling Elderly who received Influenza Vaccination" (*Japanese Journal of Pharmacoepidemiology.* 8[2]: 55).

Philippe Pépin received his Ph.D. in demography from the University of Paris and works as a Research Scientist (Chargée d'études) at l'Observatoire Régional de Santé d'Ile-de-France, in Paris.

Victor G. Rodwin, Ph.D., M.P.H., is Director of the World Cities Project at the ILC-USA and a Professor of Health Policy and Management at the Robert F. Wagner School of Public Service at New York University. He is a recipient of a 1999 Robert Wood Johnson Investigator Award in Health Policy for his research project "Health and Megacities: New York, London, Paris and Tokyo." Previously, he was Assistant Professor of Health Policy at the University of California, San Francisco's Institute for Health Policy Studies, and postdoctoral research fellow at UCSF's Program in Medical Anthropology. He was also instructor and postdoctoral research fellow at the University of California, Berkeley. A visiting professor at the University of Paris-IX, the University of Rennes, France, and other institutions, he is the recipient of a German Marshall Fund Award, a National Institute of Health Fellowship, and others. He is author and editor of several books, including *Japan's Universal and Affordable Health Care*, *Public Hospital Systems in New York City and Paris* (with D. Jolly, C. Brecher, and R. Baxter), *The Health Planning Predicament: France, Québec, England, and the United States* and *The End of an Illusion: The Future of Health Policy in Western Industrialized Nations* (with J. de Kervasdoué and J. Kimberly). He is also author of more than fifty articles, book chapters, reports, and essays. A frequent lecturer on health policy, comparative analysis of health systems, and related topics, he has had considerable experience in France and Eastern Europe. Professor Rodwin has a B.A. in Economics from the University of Wisconsin and a master's degree in Public Health and a Ph.D. in City and Regional Planning, both from the University of California, Berkeley.

David Barton Smith, Ph.D., is a Professor and Chairman of the Department of Health Services Administration in the School of Business and Management at Temple University. Professor Smith received his Ph.D. at the University of Michigan in Medical Care Organization and has held faculty positions at the Graduate School of Management at Cornell University and the Department of Community Medicine at the University of Rochester. He has also served as an IPA Fellow in the Office of Research and Policy of the Health Care Financing Administration. Recent projects have included assisting in community-health needs assessments for local area communities and Philadelphia neighborhoods, as well as in York County Pennsylvania, Broward County, Florida, Loudoun County, Virginia, Indianapolis, Indiana, and Burlington and Monmouth County, New Jersey; and serving as a program evaluator for Temple's Department of Obstetrics and Gynecology Infant Mortality Reduction project and similar projects in the Philadelphia area. In addition, he has served as a consultant to the Shriners Hospitals, Philadelphia Unit, the Prospective Payment Assessment Commission, the National Institute of Medicine, the Health Care Financing Administration, the Health Resources and Services Administration of the Public Health Service, and the Hospital Research and Educational Trust. He received a 1995 Robert Wood Johnson Health Policy Research Investigator Award for research on the history and legacy of the racial segregation of health care. He is the author or coauthor of four books on the organization of health services and of numerous articles in peer-reviewed journals.

Inge R. Strüder is a Senior Lecturer and has taught in various universities in the United Kingdom and Germany. Her research interests center around women and migrant business and she is an expert on Turkish-speaking businesses. Dr. Strüder is the author and coauthor of four articles on global cities and aging.

Yasuo Takagi, Ph.D., is Professor of Health Policy and Management at Kyushu University in Japan. He formerly worked for the Social Insurance Fund and before that as a journalist on health and social policy. He has written widely on issues of health and aging policy in Japan.

Emanuel Tobier, Ph.D., was Professor Emeritus of Economics and Planning at the Robert F. Wagner School of Public Service at New York University. Previously, Dr. Tobier served four years as chief economist of the Regional Plan Association of New York and was an associate professor of economics at Queens College and the Graduate Center of the City University of New York from 1969 to 1971. He served as the chairman of the Rent Guidelines Board under New York City mayor Abraham D. Beame and was on the economic advisory panel in the Office of Management and Budget during Mayor Edward I. Koch's tenure. He also served as a consultant to New York City's Economic Development Corporation, the National Committee Against Discrimination in Housing, the U.S. Civil Rights Commission, the Mayor's Committee on Criminal Justice, the Housing and Development Administration of New York, and the Port Authority of New York and New Jersey. Dr. Tobier, who wrote extensively about urban and regional economics, was an expert on the historic development and interaction of sectors of the city economy, including Wall Street, the garment district, and tourism. He was also an expert on housing and demography and examined the economic effect of state and local taxes. At the time of his death in April 2003, Dr. Tobier was studying the evolution of Manhattan's central business district.

François Tonnellier, Ph.D., is the former Research Manager at the Institut de Recherche et Documentation en Economie de la Santé (IRDES), Paris, France. Dr. Tonnellier worked in the fields of health geography and medical care geography in Irdes (formerly Credes). He published notably with Emmanuel Vigneron *Geography of Health in France* (P.U.F., Que Sais-Je: Paris, 1999); the articles "Geography of health" and "Demography" in the *Dictionary of the Medical Thought*, (P.U.F.: Paris, 2004), as well as "City Medicine: return to demography" in *Health and Territories, Health records of France 2004*, (Dunod: Paris).

Anthony Warnes, Ph.D., is a Professor of Social Gerontology at the University of Sheffield and Director of the Sheffield Institute for Studies on Ageing. Tony Warnes has pursued research in the social demography of later life and older people's residential choices since the 1970s. His interests in gerontology range from the humanities to the potential of genomic medicine. He has strong international links through his collaborative research on cross-national migration in Europe and the development of European social policies. He has researched the well-being of British retirees in several parts of Mediterranean Europe and is a consultant to Spanish developers of assisted-living retirement communities. Presently he is coordinating a Scientific Network on Changing Retirement in Europe funded by the European Science Foundation. He has a long-term interest in the third world, in Latin America and Thailand particularly, and is a Research Adviser to HelpAge International. Tony Warnes was Chair of the British Society of Gerontology from 1994 to 2000. He is an Academician of the Academy of Learned Societies in the Social Sciences and editor of *Ageing and Society* (Cambridge University Press). His recent publications include (with R. King and A. Williams) *Sunset Lives: British Retirement to the Mediterranean* (Oxford: Berg, 2000); (with M. Crane) *Meeting Homeless People's Needs: Service Development and Practice for the Older Excluded*, (London: King's Fund, 2000); and (with L. Warren and M. Nolan, eds.) *Care Services for Older People: Transformations and Critiques* (London: Jessica Kingsley, 2000).

Daniel Weisz, M.D., M.P.A., is a Research Associate at the ILC-USA. Before joining the ILC-USA in 2001, Dr. Weisz was a Fellow with the Health Subcommittee, Ways and Means Committee of the U.S. House of Representatives. From 1982 through 1999, Dr. Weisz served as an attending surgeon in cardiothoracic surgery at St. Francis Hospital in Roslyn, New York, and an assistant clinical professor of cardiothoracic surgery at the Albert Einstein College of Medicine. Previously, Dr. Weisz served as a staff surgeon in cardiothoracic surgery at Long Island Jewish-Hillside Medical Center in New Hyde Park, New York, and Assistant Professor, Surgery at SUNY Stony Brook. Dr. Weisz received his M.D. from the Johns Hopkins School of Medicine in 1967 and his M.P.A. from the Wagner School of Public Service at NYU in 2002.